Chronic Disease Management

Chronic Disease Management

Jim Nuovo, MD

Professor, Family and Community Medicine
University of California, Davis
Director, Chronic Disease Management Program
University of California, Davis, Health System
Sacramento, CA, USA

Editor

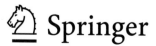 Springer

Jim Nuovo, MD
Professor, Family and Community Medicine
University of California, Davis
Director, Chronic Disease Management Program
University of California, Davis, Health System
Sacramento, CA, USA

Library of Congress Control Number: 2006922571

ISBN-10: 0-387-32927-7   eISBN-10: 0-387-49369-7
ISBN-13: 978-0387-32927-7   eISBN-13: 978-0-0387-49369-5

Printed on acid-free paper.

9 8 7 6 5 4 3 2 1

springer.com

Preface

This book is designed to help you deliver a different kind of care to your patients with chronic disease; hopefully, a more effective kind of care. While the "standard tools" are included in each disease-specific chapter (e.g., medications, consensus guidelines for management, and methods of monitoring), the core of this book is about thinking and doing differently. What does that mean? It means to learn and implement a new set of tools that you can use to provide care; tools that you probably had no exposure to during your training or even with years of practice. This book is divided into two sections. This first introduces these tools, for example, the development of a registry, methods to guide patient's toward more effective self-management, the use of quality improvement interventions, and alternative ways to deliver care (i.e., group visits). The second section focuses on the most common chronic conditions seen in primary care offices. I weighted the amount of discussion to the three most common of these diseases (type 2 diabetes, heart failure, and asthma).

This book is the outcome of a long process that began with concerns in my practice about the quality of care we were giving to our patients. As a residency director of a family practice training program, I felt that too many patients had adverse outcomes related to their chronic diseases. I felt that too many patients were not receiving care consistent with consensus guidelines. I was convinced that we could do better. Fortunately, I had like-minded people in my department. We put together a team to learn about new ways to improve chronic disease management. There were many barriers along the way. I talk about these in the introduction. What never was a barrier was the energy and enthusiasm brought to this effort by all members of the team. To my team (Jane, Sue, Tom, Bridget, Sharon, JoAnn, and Ron), thank you. This project would have ended some years ago were it not for our ability to follow our "lessons learned" and continue to move forward. We have also benefited from leaders at our institution who recognized the importance of this work and gave us their support. To our leaders (Claire Pomeroy, MD, MBA (Vice Chancellor and Dean), Bob Chason, Nabi Mussalam, Phil Raimondi, Deb Gage, and Al Siefkin), thank you. I would also like to thank the many mentors and pioneers who along the way helped guide and inspire us: Ed Wagner, Tom Bodenheimer, Halstead Holman, Kate Lorig, Gordon Moore, Peter Sobel, and Alan Glasseroff.

Jim Nuovo, MD

Contents

Contributors

Thomas A. Balsbaugh, MD
Assistant Clinical Professor, Department of Family and Community Medicine, University of California, Davis, School of Medicine, Sacramento, CA, USA

Bruce Allen Chernof, MD
Adjunct Associate Professor, Department of Medicine, David Geffen School of Medicine, University of California, Los Angeles, Los Angeles, CA, USA

Timothy W. Cutler, PharmD
Assistant Clinical Professor, Department of Clinical Pharmacy, University of California, San Francisco, School of Pharmacy, San Francisco, CA, USA

Bridget R. Levich, MSN, RN, CDE
Clinical Nurse Specialist, Diabetes, Chronic Disease Management Center, University of California, Davis, Medical Center, Sacramento, CA, USA

William Lewis, MD
Associate Professor, Department of Internal Medicine, Division of Cardiovascular Medicine, University of California, Davis, Medical Center, Sacramento, CA, USA

Samuel Louie, MD
Professor, Department of Medicine, University of California, Davis; Director, University of California, Davis, Asthma Network, Sacramento, CA, USA

Edward B. Noffsinger, PhD
Independent Healthcare Consultant on Group Visits, Santa Cruz, CA, USA

Jim Nuovo, MD
Professor, Family and Community Medicine, University of California, Davis, Director, Chronic Disease Management Program, University of California, Davis, Health System, Sacramento, CA, USA

Marilyn Stebbins, PharmD
Clinical Professor, Department of Clinical Pharmacy, University of California, San Francisco, San Francisco, CA, USA

David Stempel, BS
Medical Student, David Geffen School of Medicine, University of California, Los Angeles, Los Angeles, CA, USA

Ernesto Zatarain, MD
Clinical Associate Professor, Division of Immunology and Rheumatology, Stanford University School of Medicine; Chief, Rheumatology Section, Palo Alto VA Medical Center, Palo Alto, CA, USA

Section I
Background

1
Overview of Chronic Disease Management

Jim Nuovo

I want to go into medicine so that I can help large numbers of patients who are suffering from the effects of chronic diseases. I want to be a member of a multidisciplinary disease management team. I want all members of the team to have well-established roles, roles that take advantage of each of our strengths. I want to use information technology in a way that helps provide better care to each of my patients and to the population of patients I care for. I want access to a registry so that I can determine how my patients are doing and so that I can track clinically meaningful outcomes. I want to be able to review the registry data and implement rapid cycle interventions that can be readily monitored and measured, interventions that are linked in cycles and work toward building a safer and more effective health care system. I want to have evidence-based guidelines embedded in the electronic medical record so that I can provide improved point of service care. I want to find ways to be more effective in helping patients learn more about their disease and how to become better at self-management. I want to be comfortable in using motivational interviewing techniques to support the lifestyle changes that are necessary to improve quality of life and outcomes. I want all of my patients to set their own goals and to use an action plan to manage the complications that uniformly occur in chronic disease. I want to be able to recognize the comorbid conditions that occur in patients with chronic diseases and to assist the patients in coping effectively with these challenges.

How many of you went into medicine with these thoughts in mind? Me neither. Few if any of us went into this profession with the mission and vision to deal with chronic disease. No matter what reason we chose for what we do, we are left with a substantial problem in the care of our patients. The burden of chronic disease is enormous. Almost 80% of all health care expenditures are for the care of chronic disease. Our health care system is not up to the challenge of dealing with this problem.

Our health care system is heavily weighted to dealing with the problems of the urgent, problems that are often "best" managed with the patient in a passive role. As interest in building a more effective health care system has increased, more information has become available, indicating the serious nature of this problem. The most consistent information is that few providers or practices deliver care that is consistently high quality as measured by consensus guidelines. Study after study, regardless of the underlying disease, has shown generally poor performance in caring for patients with chronic disease. Our disease management team was highly motivated by this challenge. When we started thinking about setting up a disease management program, we were motivated by an abundance of patients with chronic diseases with an abundance of comorbid complications. Actually, we were highly motivated by the belief that "we stink." Yeah, that was our motto. We were faced with a very large number of patients with chronic problems, mostly diabetes, heart failure, chronic pain, asthma, and depression. We felt overloaded with the number of complex patients with multiple comorbid conditions. It was common to face a patient with diabetes, hypertension, chronic renal failure, hyperlipidemia, and depression in the context of a 15-minute office visit. Many of our patients struggled with substantial barriers of limited English proficiency and with cultural issues that affected "compliance" with our treatment and monitoring recommendations. Sound familiar?

We did the usual things in a practice, using the continuous quality improvement (CQI) model of looking at adverse outcomes in the clinic to address these problems. We did not have a registry, so most of the interventions were actually targeted toward optimizing patient flow or doing random chart audits. It didn't work. Patient flow got better, but the outcomes for patients with chronic diseases didn't. Of course, in the beginning of our program we had no guide to know how we were doing. No way to measure the effect of our interventions. No way to know how we were really doing for a given patient and for the population of patients we care for. Ultimately, we made an important discovery that has had a long-lasting impact on the care we deliver.

We participated in a "learning collaborative" that jump-started everything we have done in disease management. We learned about the chronic care model. We learned how to develop a registry. We learned how to use the registry data to perform rapid cycle PDSA (Plan-Do-Study-Act) activities, all designed to improve the quality of care we provided. We learned how to deliver different models of care, the group visit and the planned visit. We learned how to support self-management, understanding that not all patients and not all providers are ready for this change. We learned that these activities represented a true paradigm shift. That is really what this book is all about: how to go from being frustrated and disheartened with the challenges of dealing with chronic disease to a feeling that you can develop effective interventions using the right guide, the right tools.

My guess is that if you are reading this book you are doing so in part because you are concerned with the quality of care you and your colleagues are providing. Remember, you are in good company. Very few of us are doing a good job when it comes to effectively managing the problems of chronic disease. Many of us have given up. Giving up really seems to have become a problem. To highlight this, let me share a true story from a conference that I went to. I was asked to lead workshops on the management of several chronic diseases. One of the workshops was on the management of type 2 diabetes. I had prepared a case that I thought was really straightforward. The case was that of a patient doing poorly on a two-drug regimen and needing to consider starting insulin. I was also going to use the case to describe the importance of self-management support, a concept presented in some detail in this book. After presenting the case I asked the group if they had any suggestions as to what to do next. The good news with this group was that they were engaged, interested, and uninhibited about expressing their honest and open opinions about how they run their practice. The bad news with this group was that they were engaged, interested, and uninhibited about expressing their honest and open opinions about how they run their practice. So one of the participants raised his hand and said the following: "I'd look the patient right in the eye and say—you can either do what I say or I can give you and your family the number for the local undertaker, cause that's who you're gonna need next." Not only was I impressed with this response but I was equally impressed with the responses of many of the members of the group. "Great idea!" "Yeah, I'm going to give that a try." Certainly an honest answer. Certainly something that has gone through most of our minds as we care for complex patients who do not seem to be motivated to help themselves. From the point of view of the chronic care model, this workshop was not going very well. So I asked the group, "Have any of you ever tried to make a lifestyle change for yourself, like losing weight, eating a more healthy diet, or starting an exercise program?" Most everyone raised their hands. "How would it have felt to you to have had your physician link some outcome like death or disability or disfigurement if you didn't get started on this change? Who would feel that this approach is helpful?" No one raised his hand, thank goodness.

Is this story just an aberrancy? An outlier? An article recently appeared in the journal *Diabetes Care* about how physicians respond to their patients' inadequate glycemic control. In a retrospective cohort of 1,765 patients with diabetes at 30 U.S. academic medical centers, Grant and associates [1] found that the rate at which physicians made appropriate adjustments in medications to properly treat their patients was surprisingly low. For example, fewer than half of patients with elevated HbA1c levels had changes in therapy instituted during the office visit, even when the HbA1c level exceeded 9.0%. Only 10.1% of 208 patients with elevated blood pressure (exceeding 130/80 mm Hg) were started on antihypertensive therapy; among those with blood pressures greater than 150/100 mm Hg, only 13.9% had therapy initiated. Similarly, physicians failed to initiate lipid-lowering therapy for study participants with elevated low-density lipoprotein levels.

Only 5.6% of patients with levels between 101 and 130 mg/dL, 8.7% of those with levels between 130 and 160 mg/dL, and 15.4% of those with levels exceeding 160, received lipid-lowering drugs. Just what is the source of this inertia? What are the barriers to patients receiving evidence-based care?

Even if you are among the group of providers who would never talk to a patient using a "threat" as I've described previously, there are still so many other barriers to improving the care we provide for chronic disease. We are all too busy. Office visits are often rushed. The urgent needs of the patients take precedence over their chronic problems. It is far too common to have the chronic disease addressed as an "oh by the way" at the end of a visit. This is what Ed Wagner, MD has referred to as the "Tyranny of the Urgent." The problem seems to be too overwhelming to address. So who can blame anyone for "giving up"? Some of the lessons we have learned from our disease management program have been "pearls" to remember. One of the most important is: "Working harder doesn't work." Adding yet another burden to the activities of a day is not something that any of us wants to do. To do better disease management is not a matter of starting earlier and staying later. It won't work; it's not sustainable. It is time to consider a system redesign, a paradigm shift. How to do it? The practice components have been described by Hal Holman, MD, who has been involved in assessing the effects of self-management programs for chronic diseases for over 25 years.[2] These practice components include the following:

1. A registry of patients to invite and monitor participation in disease management activities
2. Use of patients' planned visits to prepare individual management plans
3. Use of an action plan, developed with each patient, including responsibilities for different members of the team
4. Access to patient self-management education programs
5. Group visits of patients with the physician and selected staff members, during which the interests and concerns of each are raised and mutual learning occurs
6. Remote management capabilities (telephone, e-mail, home monitors)
7. Case management with remote communication based in the team office
8. An electronic medical record to ensure continuity and integration of care

These are the essential ingredients in setting up an effective care program for patients with chronic diseases. This book is designed to provide you with the details needed to develop such an intervention program. These include the background tools, the use of a registry for quality improvement activities, self-management support, group visits/shared medical appointments/planned visits, and cultural competence. This book also includes a detailed description of interventions for management and monitoring of the most common chronic diseases: diabetes, heart failure, and asthma. Integrated within the content of the disease-specific chapters are themes common to the care of all chronic conditions. They are:

1. Comorbid conditions are common and often affect the ability to achieve optimal care. The most common comorbid condition is depression. Failure to address the effects of depression will usually thwart the impact of any disease management intervention.
2. Self-management skills are the key to maintaining function and improving outcomes.
3. An effective self-management program will provide education and supportive interventions. It should help patients gain skills in problem solving and enhance their confidence in dealing with their condition.
4. When dealing with chronic disease, it is important to assess patients' motivation to deal with their condition. This can be done by asking "How important is it to you to gain better control of your (diabetes, heart failure, asthma, etc.)?" If improved control of the disease is not a high priority, it is critical to determine what the barriers are. Common barriers include psychiatric disease, financial problems, and family stress.
5. In addition to "importance," it is useful to determine how ready the patients are to make the necessary lifestyle changes and how confident they are that they can do something that can benefit their health. You can facilitate this process by helping the patients generate their own short-term goals.
6. Goal setting is an important self-management tool. It is best if the goals are patient generated, short-term, and achievable. We should monitor these goals and recognize our patients' successes, and we should not be judgmental about failures. Use "failures" as an opportunity to explore barriers and to help patients develop a new goal that has a greater chance for success.
7. An action plan can be a means to help patients self-monitor their conditions and determine when an intervention that may prevent a serious adverse event is necessary.
8. Use your registry to develop interventions to address problems with specific patients and the population of patients you care for. When performing rapid cycle PDSA activities, as suggested in *The Improvement Guide*, always ask the following three questions:
   a. What am I trying to accomplish?
   b. How will I know that I achieved this goal?
   c. What are the steps that will help me achieve this goal?
9. Remember that it takes a team. You cannot accomplish, you will not accomplish, sustainable measures of success in dealing with chronic

diseases by acting alone. You must find a way to develop a team, a team in which each member has well-defined roles. Working harder will not work; working smarter will.

From all of us in our disease management program, we hope that you find this book a useful guide for yourself, your team, and your patients, to deal successfully with chronic diseases.

Reference

1. Grant RW, Buse JB, Meigs JB, et al. Quality of diabetes care in U.S. academic medical centers: low rates of medical regimen change. Diabetes Care 2005;28:337–442.
2. Lorig K, Holman H, Sobel D, Laurent D, González V, Minor, M. Living a Healthy Life with Chronic Conditions: Self Management of Heart Disease, Arthritis, Diabetes, Asthma, Bronchitis, Emphysema, and others. Palo Alto: Boll publishing, 2000.

2
Self-Management in Chronic Illness

Bridget R. Levich

Summary

1. Self-management is a core component of all chronic disease. All patients self-manage, some more effectively than others.
2. The most effective strategy for chronic disease management comes from an activated team, a team whose "captain" is in fact the person with the chronic illness.
3. When caring for your patients, you should consider reframing your role to that of a health "coach." A coach:
   a. Helps guide patients to specific, self-generated, achievable goals
   b. Assesses patients for their readiness to change and provides appropriate educational resources that match the patients' needs
   c. Helps patients develop problem-solving skills
   d. Understands the relevance of "importance" and "confidence" from the patients' points of view, particularly when it comes to recommended lifestyle changes
   e. Understands the need to probe for barriers, including common comorbid conditions such as depression and social/financial problems that can easily derail the most effective, evidence-based clinical guidelines
4. One of the goals when working with patients around self-management is to empower patients to manage their health by emphasizing their central role in their own health care.
5. Everything you can do in your practice to support/promote self-management for your patients will likely have a substantial return on your investment.
6. Some of the tools that you can use to support/promote self-management are the following:
   a. Team approach with the patient as "captain"
   b. Assistance with behavior change using the Transtheoretical Model

    c. Motivational interviewing

    d. Agenda-setting/decision wheels

    e. Importance/confidence ruler

    f. Typical day strategy

    g. Hypothetical look over the fence

    h. Exploration of costs and benefits

    i. Appropriate information exchange

    j. Effective use of assessment tools

    k. "Cascade of successes"

    l. Patient-centered care

    m. Shared medical appointments with a team approach

    n. Group support

    o. Goal setting/action planning

    p. Self-management education/training programs

    q. Self-monitoring, data management, and patient registries

7. The goal of self-management education/training is to enable patients to take the information that they learn about their illnesses and then solve problems that are meaningful to them.

8. We need to be aware of our own assumptions when entering into a dialogue with a patient regarding health behavior change. Some of these assumptions may include the following:

    a. "Now is the right time to consider change." In fact, a behavior change may not be the priority of the patient, and perhaps the patient may not have even considered a behavior change.

    b. "If he or she does not decide to change, the interaction has failed." We need to remember that behavior change is a process. Even if the patient does not create a change plan at this appointment, it may be the beginning of a contemplative stage.

    c. "This person wants to change." Perhaps the patient has priorities other than his or her health. Assessment of the patient's stage of change may provide useful information.

    d. "A tough approach is always best." "Scaring" the patient is very rarely a useful approach to effect ongoing behavior change. More effective and successful in the long term is a patient-centered approach in which the person with the illness identifies a behavior he or she wants to modify or change.

9. The stages of change have been described by Prochaska and colleagues. In the process of considering a behavior change (e.g., starting to exercise, eating a healthier diet, losing weight), there are six stages that a person might go through in order to change a behavior. They are the following:

    a. Pre-contemplation: no plan to consider making the change within the next 6 months

    b. Contemplation: intends to make a change within the next 6 months

    c. Preparation: has made some plans to start and intends to begin taking action within the next 30 days

    d. Action: is ready to implement behavior change

    e. Maintenance: has changed behavior for longer than 6 months

    f. Relapse: resumes old behaviors

10. Motivational interviewing is a technique used to support patient empowerment. The spirit of motivational interviewing recognizes that the patients are the experts on their illness experience and that it is the patients who should decide what behavior, if any, should be the focus. The four techniques of motivational interviewing are the following:

    a. Express empathy: Expression of empathy is critical to motivational interviewing. Once we are able to express an understanding of the patients' experience they may feel free to consider a change. When receiving empathetic responses, patients are less likely to feel a need to defend a behavior. Questions such as "What is the hardest thing about diabetes for you?" can be powerful in establishing a dialogue with your patient.

    b. Develop discrepancy: "Motivation for change occurs when people perceive a discrepancy between where they are and where they want to be." Part of our role is to facilitate an understanding of the long-term effects of a behavior. By empowering patients to understand that a behavior may not be leading them to "where they want to go," they may become more likely to consider changing the behavior. This intervention needs to be gentle and gradual and to enable the patients to recognize the long-term effects of the behavior.

    c. Do not oppose resistance: Opposing the patients' resistance to change usually leads them to act defensively. You are free to help patients explore alternative behaviors or actions by using their resistance as energy for possibilities. This technique is described as "rolling with resistance."

    d. Support self-efficacy: When patients feel efficacious with a change, the likelihood that they will continue to attempt more changes is increased. Our role is to help identify patient successes. This can be a very powerful technique in motivating patients to continue behavior change. It is valuable to remember that there is no "right way" to change; when one change is not successful, assist patients to identify alternatives.

11. All patients should be assessed for the importance of changing their behavior and for the confidence that they have that they can accomplish this goal. This can be done with a simple importance and confidence "ruler." For example, a ruler marked 1 to 10 is used to rate the importance of a change to the patient. Number 1 represents no importance at all, and number 10 represents the change as being very

important. The patient is asked to rate the importance of a behavior change. In general, if the patient does not recognize the change as at least a 7 on the scale, it is unlikely that the behavior change will occur.

12. Goal setting is a specific strategy that you can use to support self-management. Although the goal must be patient generated, you should not discount your role in this process. You are the coach. The dialogue between an informed, activated patient and a trusted provider is very powerful. A goal-setting form can be used for any chronic illness. Ideally, you can use this as a talking tool once the patient has verbalized an interest in changing a behavior. The topics for self-care are varied, and the topic of most interest to the activated patient may be different from the topic most important to you. If the patient is electing the change, the patient is more likely to verbalize a higher confidence level in achieving the goal. Setting goals is an exercise that may take some getting used to. Be patient with the process, and know that even if there is not a clearly stated goal after an appointment it may have been your patient's first step toward action.

13. Developing an action plan can be helpful in supporting self-management. The key to an action plan is that the behavior is specific and doable. Included in the action plan is a space to address barriers and possible solutions to these barriers. Once the action plan is designed and documented, encourage the patient to keep a copy in a prominent place (like the refrigerator) and to keep a log of the progress or barriers encountered.

Introduction

It has been said that there are two kinds of patients: those who are compliant and those who are not. Some of us avoid this language in favor of more neutral terms such as *adherent* or *nonadherent*. These labels do little more than to reinforce the stereotypes of an omnipotent and omniscient provider and of a subservient and passive patient. Harsh words? Certainly. An exaggeration of fact? Probably not. I believe that there is a better and healthier way to view this relationship, one that recognizes a basic truth common to all chronic conditions: self-management is a core component of chronic disease. No matter what advise is given, no matter what treatment is prescribed, no matter what education is imparted to our patients, they all self-manage, some more effectively than others. In the recent past the term *self-management* may have conjured up negative stereotypes of self-indulgent behavior in which patients did not follow a prescribed regimen, but in fact took matters into their own hands and elected an action that undermined their medical care: they continued to smoke despite having asthma, they continued to overeat despite having diabetes, they continued to be sedentary despite being overweight.

New terminology has emerged from a method of care specifically designed for patients with chronic medical problems: the Chronic Care Model. This model, developed by Ed Wagner [1], suggests that the most effective strategy for disease management comes from an activated team, a team whose "captain" is in fact the person with the chronic illness. Additional members of the team are proactive medical care providers, educators who offer support for patient self-management, and community resources that empower the patient to take charge of the daily management of the illness. As providers, we need to put aside many of the techniques that we use to treat patients with chronic conditions and, instead, adopt the role of the health "coach." A coach helps guide patients to specific, self-generated, achievable goals. A coach assesses patients' readiness to change and provides appropriate educational resources that match their needs. A coach helps patients develop problem-solving skills to address the many issues that arise. A coach understands the relevance of "importance" and "confidence" from the patients' points of view, particularly when it comes to recommended lifestyle changes. Finally, a coach understands the need to probe for barriers, including common comorbid conditions, such as depression and social problems, that can easily derail the most effective, evidence-based clinical guidelines. It is time for a paradigm shift. All patients self-manage; our role is more effective when we view ourselves as a health coach who works to enhance his or her patients' self-management skills.

Chronic disease presents overwhelming challenges to many patients and their families, many providers, and to the health care system. The passive role that we have set up for most of our patients does not work much of the time. For example, the most effective medications for diabetes, despite proven efficacy in randomized, controlled trials, can be easily made ineffective by patients unable to make changes in their lifestyle. Paraphrasing David Sobel, MD, a leader in self-management support from Kaiser Permanente in Northern California, if there was a drug in the PDR that had the capacity to improve measurable outcomes for all chronic conditions, to improve quality of life indicators, to have incidental side effects of improved mood and confidence, and to have few if any adverse effects, the drug would be an instant hit. Pop-up ads would appear on the Internet promising access to this drug. Canadian pharmacies would be swamped with orders. Pharmaceutical representatives would be standing in the hallways of your offices trying to get a few minutes of your time to detail this drug. That "drug" is self-management. Everything you can do in your practice to support and promote self-management for your patients will likely have a substantial return on your investment. Some of the tools that you can use to support/promote self-management are the following:

1. Team approach with the patient as "captain"
2. Assistance with behavior change using the Transtheoretical Model
3. Motivational interviewing
4. Agenda-setting/decision wheels
5. Importance/confidence ruler
6. Typical day strategy
7. Hypothetical look over the fence
8. Exploration of costs and benefits
9. Appropriate information exchange
10. Effective use of assessment tools
11. "Cascade of successes"
12. Patient-centered care
13. Shared medical appointments with a team approach
14. Group support
15. Goal setting/action planning
16. Self-management education/training programs
17. Self-monitoring, data management, and patient registries

Self-Management/Empowerment Overview

Background

Self-management is the "individual's ability to manage the symptoms, treatment, physical and social consequences, and lifestyle changes inherent in living with a chronic condition" [2]. One of the goals in working with patients toward self-management is to empower them to manage their health by emphasizing their central role in their own health care. "Empowerment is not a technique or strategy, but rather a vision that guides each encounter with our patients and requires that both professionals and patients adopt new roles" [3]. There is a difference between traditional patient education and self-management education. The goal of selfmanagement education and training is to enable patients to take the information that they learn about their illness and then solve problems that are meaningful to them. The goal is for patients to develop a greater sense of confidence and self-efficacy with respect to their chronic condition. Bodenheimer and associates [4] have compared traditional patient education and self-management education, and their results are listed in Table 2.1.

Team Approach with the Patient as Captain

Placing the patient at the center of the care team is definitely a paradigm shift in the way health care is typically delivered. Given that the time we have to see patients in the office setting is very limited, it follows that the patients do the majority of the day-to-day work of their health management and make the majority of decisions in dealing with their illnesses. The

TABLE 2.1. Comparison between traditional patient education and self-management education.

	Traditional patient education	Self-management education
What is taught?	Information and technical skills about the disease	Skills to address problems
How are problems formulated?	Problems are caused by inadequate control of the disease	Patients identify problems they experience that may or may not be related to the disease
Relationship between education and the disease	Education is disease specific. It provides information and teaches technical skills related to the disease	Education teaches problem-solving skills that are relevant to the consequences of chronic conditions in general

Source: Bodenheimer et al. [4].

patients are the ones truly in control. Recognizing the patient as the team captain facilitates the roles of the rest of the team. Using diabetes as an example, Figure 2.1 shows all of the possible members of the team.

Physician, certified diabetes educator, dietitian, behavior medicine specialist, pharmacist, peer coach, and exercise physiologist are all possible supporting members for the patient's team. These resources are not typically available in every clinic, but when the resources do exist in the community, they are options for the patient to pursue.

All patients must be seen as their own self-manager, perhaps not managing in an optimal fashion but, nevertheless, making daily decisions impacting their disease. Therefore, education and training efforts working toward

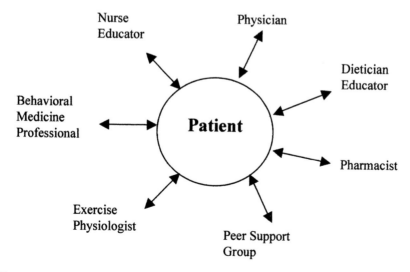

FIGURE 2.1. Example of a patient-centered diabetes team. (Courtesy of UC Davis Medical Group, Sacramento, CA.)

TABLE 2.2. Examples of blaming and empowering comments.

Blaming comments	Empowering comments
1. "I see you haven't lost the whole 10 pounds yet!"	1. "Great job, I see you've lost a few pounds! What made you successful with that?"
2. "I can't help you if you don't stop drinking all the sodas everyday!"	2. "Have you tried to change your soda consumption in the past? (Yes) What got in the way?"
3. "Without more glucose results in your book, I can't possibly come up with a plan to manage your diabetes."	3. "This is a good start at recording your glucose results. Once you have a few more numbers, you may begin to see connections between your actions and your blood sugars. What do you think might help you be able to check more often?"
4. "If your blood sugars don't come down, your kidneys will certainly fail."	4. "Diabetes is a serious illness. We know there is a benefit to controlling glucose numbers. What would have to happen for you to know that this is a problem?"
5. "If you don't start walking, pretty soon you won't be able to walk at all."	5. "Starting an exercise program can be an overwhelming challenge. Do you think you may want to consider receiving some information on beginning a walking program?"

behavior changes chosen by the patients are likely to be most effective. Effective use of assessment tools (to be addressed later) is important in determining action plan ideas for the patients.

Ideally, your role as the primary physician is that of a coach, reinforcing positive actions and working with the patient to identify needed changes. You will spend time exploring possible barriers to self-care efforts but without taking a stance of blaming or shaming the patient. Rather, encourage patients by identifying successes and finding something about which to positively remark, thereby promoting further positive self-management efforts. Examples of these types of comments are listed in Table 2.2.

Shifting to empowering comments is a strategy that emphasizes a positive approach, removes blaming terms such as *noncompliant*, and helps focus all efforts toward a series of achievable goals that can lead to a cascade of successes.

Behavior Change/Transtheoretical Model

We need to be aware of our own assumptions when entering into a dialogue with a patient regarding health behavior change. Some of these assumptions are the following:

1. "Now is the right time to consider change." In fact, a behavior change may not be the priority of the patient, and perhaps the patient may not have yet considered a behavior change.

2. "If he or she does not decide to change, the interaction has failed." We need to remember that behavior change is a process. Even if the patient does not create a change plan during this appointment, it may be the beginning of a contemplative stage.

3. "This person wants to change." Perhaps the patient has priorities other than his or her health. Assessment of the patient's stage of change (discussed later in this chapter) may be useful information.

4. "A tough approach is always best." Scaring the patient is very rarely a useful approach to effect ongoing behavior change. More effective and successful in the long term is a patient-centered approach in which the person with the illness identifies a behavior he or she wants to modify or change.

It is apparent from the large number of no-shows at medical appointments and patient education classes that there is more to behavior change than making these services available. Prochaska and colleagues [5] have done extensive work and identified stages of change. Their process of change is called the Transtheoretical Model. In the process of considering a behavior change (e.g. starting to exercise, eating a healthier diet, losing weight), there are six stages that a person might go through in order to change a behavior. They are the following:

1. Pre-contemplation: Has no plan to consider making the change within the next 6 months
2. Contemplation: intends to make a change within the next 6 months
3. Preparation: has made some plans to start and intends to begin taking action within the next 30 days
4. Action: is ready to implement behavior change
5. Maintenance: has changed behavior for longer than 6 months
6. Relapse: resumes old behaviors

As with many models, the progress through the stages of change can be fluid and dynamic. Many patients can remain at one level for a long period of time just as relapse can occur at any time and out of order.

Motivational Interviewing

To offer appropriate opportunities for behavior change to patients with chronic illness, it is important to first assess where the patient is in terms of readiness to change. Assessing confidence and importance is a helpful tool when working to empower patients. Assessing confidence and importance is one of several strategies employed in a technique called *motivational interviewing*. Motivational interviewing is "a person-centered, directive method of communication used for enhancing intrinsic motivation to change by helping a person resolve her or his ambivalence to change" [6,7]. Motivational interviewing has its roots in addiction medicine and is now used in other settings to achieve many different behavior and lifestyle changes.

Because much of what is involved in chronic illness self-management includes behavior changes, motivational interviewing is one patient-centered strategy to empower patients to engage in self-care. The spirit of motivational interviewing recognizes that the patients are the experts on their illness experience and that it is the patients who should decide what behavior, if any, should be the focus. Achieving a small change may give patients enough confidence to try other changes. By honoring the autonomy of the patients and their choices, there is more likely to be an interaction that can be mutually beneficial. An excellent resource for more information on motivational interviewing is the Web site www.motivationalinterviewing.org

The four techniques of motivational interviewing are the following:

1. Express empathy: Expression of empathy is critical to motivational interviewing. Once we are able to express an understanding of the patients' experiences, they may feel free to consider a change. When receiving an empathetic response, patients are less likely to feel defensive. Questions such as "What is the hardest thing about diabetes for you?" can be powerful in establishing a dialogue with your patient.

2. Develop discrepancy: Motivation for change occurs when people perceive a discrepancy between where they are and where they want to be [8]. Part of our role is to facilitate an understanding of the long-term effects of a behavior. By empowering patients to understand that a behavior may not be leading them "where they want to go," they may become more likely to consider changing the behavior. This intervention needs to be gentle and gradual and to enable the patient to recognize the long-term effects of the behavior.

3. Do not oppose resistance: Opposing a patient's resistance to change usually leads the patient to act defensively. You are free to help the patient explore alternative behaviors or actions by using his or her resistance as energy for possibilities. This technique is described as "rolling with resistance."

4. Support self-efficacy: When patients feel efficacious with a change, there is a greater likelihood that they will continue to attempt more changes. Our role is to help identify patient successes. This has the potential to be a very powerful technique in motivating the patient in continued behavior change. It is valuable to remember that there is no "right way" to change. When one change is not successful, consider assisting the patient to identify an alternative plan.

Agenda Setting

Agenda setting is a tool that can be used to help with motivational interviewing. Negotiating a behavior change is a process, and it can only be used with one behavior at a time. It needs to be very specific; for example, if the long-term goal is to lose weight, the patient needs to narrow it down to specific short-term behaviors, perhaps beginning with walking. One way to set the agenda is to use a decision wheel, as shown in Figure 2.2.

The decision wheel shown in Figure 2.2 was designed for patients with hypertension. All or none of the steps may be of interest to the patient to take control of his or her hypertension, but if the patient can identify one specific area to work on a change, it could promote a collaborative effort. The dialogue could start with something like "There are many things we could talk about regarding your management of your hypertension. These are some of them. Do any of these items interest you?" Following the selection of an area for change, you can work with the patient to design a specific action plan. If a patient responds, "I want to do them all," coach them to targeting one goal first, perhaps the one that they feel the greatest confidence they can achieve.

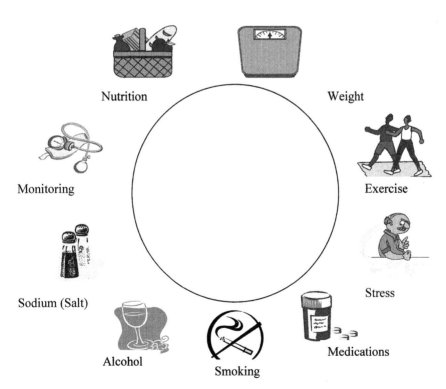

Nutrition   Weight

Monitoring   Exercise

Sodium (Salt)   Stress

Alcohol   Medications

Smoking

FIGURE 2.2. Decision wheel for making lifestyle changes. (Courtesy of UC Davis Medical Group, Sacramento, CA.)

Importance/Confidence Ruler

Another tool to assess readiness is the importance/confidence ruler. Table 2.3 shows an example of such a ruler. To rate the importance of a change to the patient, 1 represents no importance at all, and 10 represents the change as being very important. The patient is asked to rate the importance of a behavior change. In general, if the patient does not recognize the change as at least a 7 on the scale, it is unlikely that the behavior change will occur.

If the change is seen as important (7 or greater), the next ruler asks the patient to rate his or her confidence in achieving the specific behavior change. For example, if a patient rated exercise as important, 8, but could give a confidence level of only 5 for walking 20 minutes 3 times a week, it is appropriate at this point to explore barriers to the change. Perhaps if the patient redesigned the walk to be 10 minutes, the patient would have a confidence level of 8, thereby making it a likely change for the patient. You need to remember that these are the patients' goals, and it is important that they achieve success with their plan. One of the biggest problems physicians have is offering or prescribing only solutions that they develop. Physicians tend to value problem solving as one of their most important clinical skills. However, under these conditions it is best for the physician to refrain from prescribing a solution. Help the patient develop the solution and overcome the barriers.

Typical Day Strategy

The spirit of this strategy is to encourage the patient to verbally paint a picture of a typical day in order for you, as the support person (physician or educator), to appreciate the context of what change may involve. There is no right answer, and it is not an interrogation. The patient describes a typical day for the purposes of establishing rapport and helping you

TABLE 2.3. Rulers to evaluate importance and confidence.

The next 2 questions are about making changes. Please remember there are no right answers . . . and do your best to answer honestly.
How important is it to you to manage your blood sugars?
Not important 1____2____3____4____5____6____7____8____9____10____ Very important

Diabetes self-management often involves changes in behavior, for example, changes in diet or changes in exercise. At this point, TODAY, how ready are you to change one behavior?
Not ready 1____2____3____4____5____6____7____8____9____10____ Very ready

Source: UC Davis Medical Group, Sacramento, CA.

understand the barriers that may exist for the patient. The request may go something like: "I appreciate that change can be tough. Can you take me through your typical day so I can get a picture of what day-to-day life is like for you?" The strategy is most effective if you follow the story but avoid interrogation or forming opinions. This is the patient's experience as the patient sees it. As a partner in the dialogue of a typical day discussion, your responses simply mirror the difficulties or recognize the barriers that the patient is describing.

Hypothetical Look over the Fence

Encourage your patients to "try on" the behavior change before they actually get started. Even a patient who has verbalized a high importance and confidence level for a specific change is still likely to have some misgivings about the change. This exercise gives the patient an opportunity to identify his or her concerns and perhaps find a strategy to deal with them. The exchange could go something like this:

Provider: So, you're thinking you'd like to walk 30 minutes 3 days a week?
Patient: Yes, I know I said a confidence of 8, but I really don't know if I can do it!
Provider: Let's just imagine that you could do it. How would that be for you?
Patient: It would be so awesome! I would feel so proud of myself! But what would I do if it were really cold or raining?
Provider: That may be an important thing to think about. Do you have any thoughts about what you might do?
Patient: Well, there's always the mall, and if I begin walking I will want to make sure I can keep going or I'll likely quit altogether.
Provider: So it sounds to me as if you have a backup plan for weather issues, and you feel pretty confident you'll find a way to walk 30 minutes 3 days a week!
Patient: This actually feels pretty promising! I'm going to try this!

This "look over the fence" allows, and even encourages, the patient to see and feel how the behavior change may work out. It may even identify some unforeseen barriers ahead of time, allowing the patient to think these through.

Exploring Pros and Cons of Changing or Not Changing

This exercise encourages the patient to weigh the "pros and cons" of a behavior change. An alternative exercise is to ask the patient to weigh the "pros and cons" of not making a behavior change. Your role as the provider is to describe a structure in which the pros or the cons can happen and to support the patient in the process. It may be useful to actually write the

TABLE 2.4. Discussing the pros and cons of behavior change: quitting smoking.

Pros	Cons
Improved health	Possible failure
Money saved	Possible weight gain
Better sense of smell	Possible increased nervousness
Possibly making new friends	Possible loss of smoking friends

information down in a chart format. Table 2.4 provides a simple example of exploring pros and cons.

Appropriate Information Exchange

Before giving instructions it is important to determine the patients' knowledge and understanding of their illnesses. Before patients can consider a nutrition change, for example, they may need to receive nutrition information so they can determine the impacts on their typical day. Before giving information, ask patients about their interest in receiving information. This will ensure that the time spent together is useful and productive. If a patient verbalizes a disinterest in a topic of information or a negative opinion about learning more about an issue, clearly it will not be time well spent to do so, and in fact it may undermine the rapport with the patient for future meetings. By simply asking about the patients' interest levels, providers can gain insight into their motivations.

Along the way when delivering information it is a good idea to check in with patients in a nonjudgmental way. Questions such as "Have you heard this information before?" or "Some people find this difficult to do. How does it sound to you?" may help elicit feedback. If there is a lack of information, perhaps offering a class could be an option. Offering a self-management class to a patient is an option, but not necessarily a "magic bullet." Unless the patient elects to participate in the class, it is unlikely that the class will be an effective option. Certainly making the intervention available to the patient is an appropriate step by the provider, but the patient's willingness is important if the training session is to be effective.

Assessment Tools

Throughout this chapter the concept of assessing the patient has come up repeatedly. Motivational interviewing may be a powerful tool to assist patients in designing their action plans. There are many different assessment tools that can be used to determine the most effective strategy to help each patient. Table 2.5 presents a diabetes self-assessment tool. All effective assessment tools must include the previously described concepts of importance and confidence. We use this form in our In Charge and In Control program.

TABLE 2.5. Diabetes self-assessment tool.

This material will become part of your medical record and will remain confidential.
Please bring this completed form with you to the first class.
In Charge and In Control

DATE:_____

Diabetes Self-Assessment

1. General information
   NAME:_____
   ADDRESS:_____
   CITY:_____   STATE:_____
   ZIP:_____
   HOME PHONE:_____ WORK PHONE:_____
   How many people live in your household?_____
   Is there anyone to help with your diabetes care?   Yes   No
   If yes, who helps you?_____
   Your Occupation:_____ Work hours:_____
   Your primary care provider's (doctor's) name:_____

2. What areas of diabetes would you like to learn more about?
   ☐ What is diabetes?   ☐ Diet   ☐ Goal setting
   ☐ Pills for diabetes   ☐ Exercise   ☐ Blood testing
   ☐ High blood sugar   ☐ Stress   ☐ Complications
   ☐ Low blood sugar   ☐ Sick days   ☐ Insulin
   ☐ Other_____

These questions are about caring for your diabetes.

3. How confident are you that you can regularly do all the things that you are supposed to
   do to take care of your diabetes?
   ☐ Hardly confident
   ☐ A little confident
   ☐ Fairly confident
   ☐ Very confident

4. How confident are you that you can keep your diabetes from interfering with the things
   you want to do?
   ☐ Hardly confident
   ☐ A little confident
   ☐ Fairly confident
   ☐ Very confident

5. How much control do you feel you have over your diabetes?
   ☐ None
   ☐ A little
   ☐ Some
   ☐ A lot

The next questions ask about activities during the *past 7 days*.

6. On how many of the last seven days have you followed a healthful eating plan?
                0   1   2   3   4   5   6   7

7. On how many of the last seven days did you do at least 30 minutes of physical exercise?
   (including walking)
                0   1   2   3   4   5   6   7

8. On how many of the last seven days did you test your blood sugar?
                0   1   2   3   4   5   6   7

TABLE 2.5. *Continued*

9. On how many of the last seven days did you check your feet?

    0   1   2   3   4   5   6   7

10. On how many of the last seven days did you take your recommended diabetes medicine?

    0   1   2   3   4   5   6   7

11. How often do you have a dental checkup?_____

12. Do you wear a medical identification bracelet or necklace?_____

13. In general, would you say your health is:
    ☐ Excellent
    ☐ Very Good
    ☐ Good
    ☐ Fair
    ☐ Poor

14. How many times in the last 12 months have you seen your doctor for your diabetes? _____times

15. How many years have you had diabetes? _____ years

16. How many years have you come to this clinic for your diabetes care? _____ years

17. Other than diabetes, do you have an illness that you consider serious?

    ☐ Yes   IF YES, name them

    _____

    ☐ No

18. What is your gender?   ☐ Female   ☐ Male

19. What is your age?   _____ years

20. How would you describe yourself?
    ☐ African American   ☐ Latino/Hispanic
    ☐ Asian/Pacific Islander   ☐ Native American
    ☐ Caucasian   ☐ Other:_____

21. Do you have any ethnic or cultural practices or foods that affect the way you manage your diabetes?

    _____

    _____

22. What is the highest level of education that you finished?
    ☐ Grade school   ☐ Some college
    ☐ Some high school   ☐ Associate's degree
    ☐ High school diploma/GED   ☐ Bachelor's/college degree

The next 2 questions are about making changes. Please remember there are no right answers . . . and do your best to answer honestly.

23. How important is it to you to manage your blood sugars?

    1_____2_____3_____4_____5_____6_____7_____8_____9_____10_____

    Not important   Important

24. Diabetes self-management often involves changes in behavior, for example, changes in diet or changes in exercise. At this point, TODAY, how ready are you to change a behavior?

    1_____2_____3_____4_____5_____6_____7_____8_____9_____10_____

    Not ready   Ready

Thank you for sharing with us. Please bring this with you to class.

Source: UC Davis Medical Group, Sacramento, CA.

Cascade of Successes

Almost all of us have experienced a "cascade of successes" at some point in our lives. It involves the successful achievement of one goal and the subsequent creation and achievement of an additional, and perhaps harder, goal. This is a powerful phenomenon and one that is largely elicited by the patient. All of the strategies described thus far can be utilized to promote this cascade of successes. The important variable, however, is that the plan is made by the patient and that the goal be achievable and specific in detail. Your role as the provider, again, is that of a coach, perhaps commenting on the achievement or initiating a conversation regarding the success of the patient's action plan. The cascade of successes is a significant tool and one that can empower additional behavior changes in your patients.

Patient-Centered Care

It is important to recognize that self-management can be promoted in multiple ways. There are some additional patient-centered strategies that can support self-management. Some of them are shared medical appointments, group support, case management, goal setting and action plans, patient education and training sessions, and documenting self-management goals in the medical record or patient registry.

Shared Medical Appointments

There are many different models for a shared medical appointment. These models are described in detail in Chapter 3. They are based on having multiple patients scheduled for the same appointment. Team members participating in the appointment can include physician(s), a nurse, a behavioral medicine professional, and perhaps an educator. The appointment usually takes place in a space large enough to accommodate 5 to 12 patients and one or two providers. The appointment may use a teaching component in addition to the physician–patient exchange. In general, one of the most powerful impacts of the shared medical appointment is that the patients are able to share their experiences of a chronic illness with other patients in a supportive group setting.

Peer support can be a significant benefit for a patient, and the candid sharing that goes on in a group of patients may pleasantly surprise a provider. We have occasionally called groups of patients with a commonly shared chronic illness together for repeated groups. By utilizing this strategy, the group is able to form a bond and look forward to "checking in" with members of their group to learn of each other's successes or barriers. This can contribute to the positive cascade mentioned previously. Whether the shared medical appointment is a core group of patients returning for quarterly follow-ups or a one-time group formed to see a provider and educator, the built-in support of a group is able to take place.

Goal Setting

Goal setting is a patient-centered strategy that can be useful when working with patients one-on-one or in groups. Although the goals must be patient generated, you should not discount your role in this process. You are the coach. The dialogue between an informed activated patient and a trusted provider is very powerful. There are several tools that may be of help with this.

One is the goal-setting form. Table 2.6 presents a goal-setting form for diabetes. Such a form can be developed for any chronic illness. Ideally, you can use it as a talking tool once the patient has verbalized an interest in changing a behavior. The topics for self-care are varied, and the topic of most interest to the activated patient may be different from the topic most important to you. When patients themselves decide which changes to make, they are more likely to verbalize a higher confidence level in achieving the goal. Setting goals is an exercise that may take some getting used to. Be patient with the process, and know that even if there is not a clearly stated

TABLE 2.6. Goal-setting form.

Diabetes Self-Management: Setting Goals

You, the patient, are the most important person to manage your diabetes.

We will guide you and offer support as you manage your diabetes. Setting self-care goals will help you gain and maintain control of your diabetes to reduce damage to your blood vessels and nerves.

Choose a goal that you are willing to work on to manage your diabetes.

Examples of goals for diabetes care:
I will check my feet daily. If I notice a sore or irritation I will seek medical attention.
I will exercise (walk, run, bike, swim, etc.) _____ days per week.
I will follow my carbohydrate meal plan to lower my blood sugar.
                              Or
I will eat a lower fat diet to reduce my risk for heart disease and stroke.
I will cut back on smoking or quit smoking.
I will check my blood sugar (<u>frequency</u>) and bring my results with me to my medical appointments.

I will take an aspirin or enteric-coated aspirin every day.

Selected Goal: _____
Action Plan: _____
Barriers/Solutions: _____
_____
_____

Source: UC Davis Medical Group, Sacramento, CA.

TABLE 2.7. A diabetes action plan form.

An action plan is one specific activity that you are going to do in the coming week. An action plan must be:
1. Something that is IMPORTANT to you and that you WANT to do.
2. Something that is safe and that you are physically able to do.
3. Be specific—Avoid making global goals such as "I will lose weight." Identify a behavior that will help with this global goal but is clearly and specifically stated, such as "I will only drink one soda each day." What, where, how often, when, with whom? The more specific the better.
4. Design an action plan involving something you are confident of doing. On a scale of 1 to 10, your confidence should be at least 7, preferably 8. If your confidence level is less than 7, rethink the action plan and modify the plan until you can state a confidence level of at least 7.

Example: This week I will walk 3 times for 20 minutes with Susan. We will walk at 7 PM on Monday, Wednesday, and Friday in the mall.

SAMPLE ACTION PLANNING FORM

Date:

This week I will _____ (type of activity) _____.
I will do this _____ times for _____ (time or amount of activity).
I will do this when, where, with whom? The more specific the better.
On a scale of 1–10, my confidence that I will complete the entire plan is _____.
Things that might get in the way of this plan are:

_____

Ways I might overcome these problems are:

_____
_____

Source: UC Davis Medical Group, Sacramento, CA.

goal after an appointment, it may have been the first step toward action by your patient.

Action Plans

Discussions of action plans are frequent in the literature regarding chronic illness care. Table 2.7 presents one example of an action plan. This form can be used for almost any behavior change or chronic condition. As you can see, the important part of the plan is that the behavior be specific and doable. Included in the action plan is a space to address barriers and possible solutions to these barriers. Once the action plan is designed and documented, encourage the patient to keep a copy in a prominent place (such as on the refrigerator) and to keep a log of the progress or barriers that they encounter. It is also a powerful tool for you, as the provider, to check back on at the next appointment; this requires a way for you to include the action plan in the chart or electronic medical record.

There are other models of action plans. The one presented in Table 2.8 is for heart failure and implements the "green, yellow, red" format to which

TABLE 2.8. Action plan: congestive heart failure zones for management.

Green zone: all clear	Green zone means
Your goal weight	Your symptoms are under control
No shortness of breath	Continue taking your medications as
No swelling	ordered
	Continue daily weights
No weight gain	Follow low-salt diet
No chest pain	
No decrease in your ability to maintain your activity level	**Keep all physician appointments**

Yellow zone: caution	Yellow zone means
If you have any of the following signs and symptoms:	Your symptoms may indicate that you need an adjustment in your medication
Weight gain of 2 or more pounds in a day or 3 to 5 in a week	Call your physician, nurse coordinator, or home health nurse
	Name: _____
	Number: _____
	Instructions: _____

Red zone: medical alert	Red zone means
Unrelieved shortness of breath: shortness of breath at rest	This indicates you need to be evaluated by a physician right away
Unrelieved chest pain (even at rest)	Call your physician right away
Wheezing, especially at night	Physician: _____
Need to sit in chair to sleep	Number: _____
Call your physician immediately if you are going into the red zone	

Source: www.improvingchroniccare.org.

patients can refer for an action designed by themselves and their primary provider. This action plan for heart failure is based on signs and symptoms of acute decompensation. It asks the patient to call a designated person when these signs or symptoms occur. There are other plans that will give actual information for adjusting medication(s), based on the signs or symptoms. You will need to discuss the format with your team to determine which is best for your needs.

Self-Management Education and Training Programs

An education and training program implies an active role by the recipient of the program. Self-management is the focus of such programs. For example, in order to have a teaching program recognized by the American Diabetes Association (ADA), 10 clearly mandated areas of education and training must be met. The overall focus of ADA recognition is that the program involves self-management training and action plans by the participant; this philosophy follows the information in Table 2.1. Didactic teaching alone does not meet the ADA criteria for recognition.

When a diabetes (or asthma or heart failure) patient group comes together for training, the initial meeting needs to outline the agenda of the sessions(s) and give the participants a chance to verbalize their own struggles, challenges, and successes with management of the condition. We utilize the self-assessment form for such a purpose. The form is mailed out one week before the initial class meeting, and the participants are asked to bring the form with them to the first class. The facilitator of the training sessions begins the introductions by setting the tone for the training. By making it clear from the outset of the class that the focus will be on action and successes, patients usually feel free to share their own struggles. The facilitator of a diabetes session should state that the instructors are not the "food police" or the "diabetes patrol." This usually helps set the tone for the group and encourages participation and peer support.

The overall goal of the training session is that patients learn how to strategize and make their lives work for them rather than giving each patient a recipe that will prescribe a plan. Even though patients frequently ask for "a diet," most can attest to the fact that it comes back to the patient making daily choices. An ongoing theme of self-management and training classes for chronic illnesses is that it is a daily struggle and most people find it hard to adhere to their action plan every day. Rather than patients giving up when they experience an "indiscretion," the facilitator encourages them to own the action, not to blame themselves, and to continue on with the program. Another important step is for patients to celebrate successes and congratulate themselves for their ongoing efforts.

In the world of obesity, diabetes, sedentary lifestyles, and fast foods, it becomes clear that the self-care lifestyle and behavior changes discussed in this chapter are good for almost everyone! This is another message delivered in the training sessions: the action plans designed by the patients are healthy for everyone, not just those with a chronic illness.

Self-Monitoring, Data Management, and Use of Registries

How often has a patient with diabetes asked you, "Can I eat _____?" The food item could be anything from chocolate ice cream to carrots. Because we understand from a nutritional perspective that the issue is carbohydrates, it may be useful to encourage the patients to "be Dick Tracy" and figure it out for themselves. By performing a fingerstick glucose test 1 to 2 hours after eating the food in question, they can see for themselves what happens with their blood glucose level. Perhaps the food in question is okay but the amount is suspect. In other words, there are no hard and fast rules, but rather we invite the patients again to be the captains of their own team. This example holds true for many behavior changes.

Experiences teach patients more effectively than most providers if the patients are encouraged to use themselves as their own best expert. In like manner, the provider can gather a wealth of information from an activated patient. For example, the patient who comes in with a logbook, in which data are connected to activities or to lack of activities, can be a much stronger coach than the clinic appointment in which a patient asks for a blanket type of food to eat. The first example engages the patient and the provider in a healthy dialogue in which the patient is given an opportunity to go on to the next action plan.

By keeping a log, patients can also gather information on the processes of their daily lives. Realizing the effects of exercise on glucose, blood pressure, or cholesterol levels can be dramatic when patients have made a conscious effort to note the beginning dates of behavior changes.

Summary

It is important to recognize that chronic illness is largely self-managed whether we as providers are involved the in the process or not. There are many different strategies and tools that can support self-management. The patient's perception of importance and confidence are extremely important and often overlooked. If you just started with this strategy for all of your patients with a chronic disease, you will likely see benefits to yourself and your patients. More advanced techniques involving motivational interviewing can help patients who are interested in a behavior change. Personal action plans and goal setting are ways to have the patient commit to a change. Remember to recognize successes and to view "failures" as an opportunity to review barriers. In the final analysis, the most effective and positive changes are those arrived at mutually by the patient and the provider. These create a trust-filled launching pad toward more successful action plans and a cascade of successes.

References

1. Wagner E. The chronic care model. Available at www.improvingchroniccare. org.
2. Barlow JH, Cullen LA, Rowe IF. Educational preferences, psychological well-being and self-efficacy among people with rheumatoid arthritis. Patient Educ Couns 2002;46:11–19.
3. Funnell MM. Patient empowerment. Crit Care Nurs Q 2004;27:201–204.
4. Bodenheimer T, Lorig K, Holman H, Grumbach K. Patient self-management of chronic disease in primary care. JAMA 2002;288:2469–2475.
5. Prochaska JO, DiClemente CC, Norcross JC. In search of how people change: applications to addictive behavior. Am Psychologist 1992;47:1102–1114.
6. Miller WR, Rollnick S. Motivational Interviewing: Preparing People to Change Addictive Behavior. New York: Guilford, 1991:191–202.

7. Resnicow K, et al. Motivational interviewing in health promotion. Health Psychol 2002;21:444–451.
8. Miller WR, et al. Motivational Enhancement Therapy Manual: A Clinical Research Guide for Therapists Treating Individuals with Alcohol Abuse and Dependence. Rockville, MD: National Institute on Alcohol Abuse and Alcoholism. NIAAA Distribution Center, PO Box 10686, Rockville, MD 20849-0686.

3
Use of Group Visits in the Treatment of the Chronically Ill

EDWARD B. NOFFSINGER

Summary

1. Group visits, otherwise known as *shared medical appointments* (SMAs), provide a tool for better meeting the psychological and physical needs of the chronically ill.
2. Shared medical appointments provide an innovative alternative and reverse the trend of putting evermore responsibilities onto the shoulders of the physician—and are particularly helpful when it comes to meeting the complex mind–body needs of chronically ill patients and their families.
3. Shared medical appointments represent the delivery of medical care in a supportive group setting with other patients dealing with similar issues—so that the help, encouragement, and emotional support of other patients is integrated into each patient's experience. This includes the sharing of important information, helpful tips, successful coping strategies, and effective disease self-management skills.
4. Potential benefits of SMAs include the following:
   a. An additional health care choice
   b. Improved access and more time with the patient's own provider
   c. Greater patient education
   d. Reduced repetition of information
   e. Increased attention to mind (psychosocial, emotional, and behavioral health) as well as body needs
   f. "Max-packed" visits and updated health maintenance
   g. The help and support of other patients
   h. The professional skills of a behaviorist
   i. Improved compliance with recommended treatment regimens
   j. Increased patient and physician professional satisfaction
   k. The opportunity for closer follow-up care
5. Three major group visit models of national significance have emerged during the past 15 years:

    a. The Drop-In Group Medical Appointment (DIGMA) model
    b. The Cooperative Health Care Clinics (CHCC) model
    c. The Physicals Shared Medical Appointment (Physicals SMA) model

6. Although DIGMAs are occasionally used for intake visits and new patient appointments, they tend to focus on return appointments and are open to most or all established patients in the provider's practice.

7. The DIGMA is run just like a series of individual office visits but includes other patients as observers. The central focus from start to finish is on the delivery of medical care, with the exact same medical care being delivered as in traditional office visits (history, examination, counseling, medical decision making, documentation), but sequentially to one person at a time in a supportive group setting, while others listen, learn, share experiences, ask questions, and interact.

8. The following are distinguishing characteristics of the DIGMA model:
    a. Different patients typically attend DIGMA sessions.
    b. Sessions are most commonly held weekly for 90 minutes, although they can be held as often as daily and for longer or shorter durations.
    c. Sessions are open to most or all of the provider's patients.
    d. "Drop-in" convenience is offered, although the vast majority of patients are typically prescheduled into DIGMA visits by scheduling staff just as they are for traditional individual office visits.

9. The DIGMAs model is especially well suited for routine follow-up care; relatively stable chronically ill patients; patients who can benefit from peer support and more time with their provider; patients with extensive informational, psychosocial, behavioral health, and emotional needs; patients who are difficult, time consuming, and problematic; patients who are noncompliant or high utilizers of health care services; and patients for whom the physician needs to keep repeating the same information over and over.

10. For DIGMAs to succeed, the physician must take primary responsibility for inviting patients. The invitation from the physician needs to be positively worded and reflect the physician's own belief in the program in order to be fully effective.

11. The DIGMAs are staffed by:
    a. The provider (physician, nurse practitioner, podiatrist, osteopath, physician assistant, or pharmacist), who is in attendance throughout the session
    b. A behaviorist (typically a psychologist or social worker, but occasionally a nurse, diabetic nurse educator, or other midlevel

provider; ideally, this person has group management skills, is able to address psychosocial issues, and is adept at fostering group interaction)

    c. A nurse and/or medical assistant to take vital signs, keep injections and health maintenance current, and perform other "special duties" as needed

12. There are three types of DIGMA models: homogeneous, heterogeneous, and mixed.

    a. In the homogeneous type, each session is open only to patients who have a specific condition or diagnosis—such as diabetes, chronic heart failure, hypertension, asthma, or arthritis.

    b. In the heterogeneous type, each session is open to most or all patients in the physician's practice—regardless of diagnosis, condition, sex, age, utilization behavior, and so forth.

    c. In the mixed type, the physician's practice is divided into four patient groups—one for each week of the month. For example, a Mixed Primary Care DIGMA might be structured as follows: cardiopulmonary patients are the focus the first week of the month; diabetes and weight management, the second week; all gastrointestinal patients, the third; and women's health, the fourth. During the couple of months a year that have five weeks, the fifth session could be open to any group(s) of the provider's choice.

13. The single greatest ongoing challenge to running a successful DIGMA, and by far the greatest weakness of the DIGMA model, is the fact that—because different patients attend each DIGMA session—ongoing attention must consistently be paid to maintaining targeted census levels during each and every session.

14. Although DIGMAs are not for all physicians, some physicians fear that a DIGMA will not work for their particular practice. This concern has been tested and disproved many times over in actual practice. Physicians who initially worried that their DIGMA was at high risk to fail found that it did not fail as long as they were willing to try one for their practice and give it their best effort.

15. Another weakness of the DIGMA model is that, like all group visit models, it has specific facilities, personnel, and promotional requirements that must be met for success to be achieved. The DIGMAs require a relatively large group room capable of seating 20 to 25 people and keeping them comfortable, and a nearby appropriately equipped examination room. This group room needs to have comfortable chairs as well as adequate ventilation for such a large number of people.

16. The CHCC model was originally designed to provide better and more accessible care for high-utilizing, multi-morbid geriatric patients—with

the overall objective of reducing resource utilization and the associated costs of delivering care while increasing the quality of care provided.

17. In the CHCC model, the same group of 15 to 20 high-utilizing medical patients is followed on a monthly basis over time so that outcomes measures can be made with comparative ease.

18. These older patients experiencing multiple chronic health problems are complex patients, and they often bring to their medical visits an extensive "laundry list" of mind–body needs that cannot be fully met during the brief amount of time allocated to a relatively short individual office visit. These wide-ranging patient needs can often be better met during the CHCC because of the greater amount of time available, the extensive patient education provided, and the help and support provided by both the care team and other patients.

19. The CHCC model has been shown through randomized controlled research studies to enhance quality of care; improve patient outcomes; increase patient and physician satisfaction; enhance the patient–physician relationship; reduce the number of referrals to medical specialists; and reduce emergency department, hospitalization, and nursing home costs for this small but expensive group of patients.

20. In the Specialty CHCC subtype of the CHCC model, the patients in attendance are usually experiencing the same diagnosis or health condition (e.g., diabetes, congestive heart failure, or asthma). Also, Specialty CHCCs often meet irregularly, according to best practices rather than monthly.

21. The Physicals SMA model typically consists of a series of privately conducted examinations run concurrently with group interaction among the rotating group of patients not roomed for examinations. This phase is then basically followed by a small DIGMA with all patients in attendance. The group experience provides an opportunity for education, counseling, medical decision making, and so forth, around health issues important to the participants (as the physician sequentially addresses the medical issues of one patient after another in the group setting, while all are able to listen and learn). This format allows the physician the opportunity to present health maintenance topics just once to an entire group, rather than having to repeat the same material to each patient.

22. Key features of the Physicals SMA model include high-quality, team-based care; high levels of patient and physician satisfaction; dramatically increased physician productivity in delivering physical examinations; improved patient access to physical examinations; and one physician–one patient encounters throughout.

23. Physicals SMAs can be widely applied to a multitude of primary care and specialty practices.

Introduction

Group visits (which are more appropriately referred to as *shared medical appointments* [SMAs]) are a tool for "working smarter, not harder" and are ideally suited for better meeting the psychosocial and physical needs of the chronically ill. All three of today's major group visit models were born out of frustration: The DIGMA and Physicals SMA models were born out of my personal and professional frustration (both as a patient and as a provider), and Dr. John Scott's CHCC model was born out of professional frustration with trying to meet the multiple complex medical needs of multi-morbid geriatric patients within the time constraints of a relatively brief individual office visit.

Confronted by today's multiple health care challenges, the exciting potential of group visits, in both redesigning the physician office practice and enhancing care for the chronically ill, is just now beginning to emerge. The economic imperatives of today's managed care environment and the fast-paced treadmill of outpatient care have impacted physicians' practices in many ways. They have increased physicians' roles as gatekeepers, diagnosticians, and technicians fighting disease, and have decreased the amount of time physicians have to comfort, console, educate, emotionally support, and get to know their patients. Shared medical appointments are an innovative alternative to the trend of putting evermore responsibilities onto the shoulders of the physician—and are particularly helpful in meeting the complex mind–body needs of chronically ill patients and their families.

Shared medical appointments represent the delivery of medical care in a supportive group setting with other patients dealing with similar issues so that the help, encouragement, and emotional support of other patients is integrated into each patient's experience (which includes the sharing of important information, helpful tips, successful coping strategies, and effective disease self-management skills). Customized to the specific needs, goals, practice style, and patient panel constituency of the individual provider, SMAs offer most of the same medical services as do traditional individual office visits. They also offer a remarkable combination of benefits to patients, physicians, and health care organizations alike. The benefits they can offer to patients are listed in Table 3.1.

Representing a multidisciplinary team approach to medical care, SMAs are meant to enhance quality and outcomes, improve patient–physician relationships, and increase productivity. Meant to be voluntary to patients and physicians alike, SMAs are designed to provide individual one-on-one time with the physician on an "as needed" basis to all patients. They can also address the critically important economic challenges facing health care delivery systems today.

Shared medical appointments work well in combination with traditional individual office visits (which they are not meant to completely replace), and both group and individual visits can play important roles in the future

TABLE 3.1. Potential patient benefits of group visits.

1. Additional healthcare choice
2. Improved access and more time with the patient's own provider
3. Greater patient education
4. Reduced repetition of information
5. Increased attention to mind (psychosocial, emotional, and behavioral health) as well as body needs
6. "Max-packed" visits and updated health maintenance
7. Help and support of other patients
8. Professional skills of a behaviorist
9. Improved compliance with recommended treatment regimens
10. Increased patient and physician professional satisfaction
11. Opportunity for closer follow-up care

Note: Covers most patients in the provider's practice or chronic illness population management program.

of health care delivery. The challenge now facing us is how to optimize the use of both types of appointments so that we can best match the type of service offered to the actual needs of the patient. In this manner, patients best suited to the highly efficient, cost-effective, supportive, and informative SMAs can be promptly seen in that venue, whereas patients needing or preferring individual office visits will always have that option—in fact, office visits should even be more accessible because the group visit program will off-load many individual office visits.

Today's three major group visit models are complementary rather than mutually exclusive. Shared medical appointments are ideally suited for all types of chronic diseases (e.g., diabetes, hypertension, hyperlipidemia, depression, and congestive heart failure). They can help chronically ill patients gain critical patient education (knowledge that can enable them to stay healthier, live independently longer, and avoid complications), become more compliant with recommended treatment regimens, and be better able to self-manage their illnesses.

By providing accessible, high-quality, and high-value medical care to some of our most challenging and costly patients, group visits offer a creative new approach to the effective management of high-risk, high-cost patients with chronic conditions, and have the potential to reduce medical costs in both fee-for-service and capitated health care delivery systems. Shared medical appointments provide a new technology for the care management of all types of chronically ill patients, one that offers patients numerous quality, access, and service benefits. When carefully designed, adequately supported, and properly run, SMAs have the potential to offer many advantages, including benefits to patients, physicians, health care organizations, insurers, and purchasers of insurance alike. In addition, SMAs can be fun for patients and physicians alike.

Because so many health care dollars go toward the treatment of chronic illnesses, highly productive and efficient group visits can help to contain the rapidly rising costs of providing care to the chronically ill. These high-risk medical patients have the potential for both poor outcomes and high costs to the system, and they often have extensive "mind" as well as "body" needs—complex needs that are difficult or impossible to meet in the brief amount of time available during traditional individual office visits.

In addition to being ideally suited to the treatment of the chronically ill, SMAs can play equally important roles in the following:

1. Improving physician management of busy, backlogged practices.
2. Better meeting the medical needs of all patients (those with routine and acute issues as well as patients with chronic conditions).
3. Providing improved access benefits to both follow-up visits and physical examinations—and therefore in achieving Advanced Access goals.

As can be seen, there are wide-ranging applications for group visits—the actual extent of which is much broader than one might at first envision. In fact, SMAs can play an important role in managing busy and backlogged practices, in outpatient ambulatory care for virtually all medical subspecialties in both primary and specialty care, and in some inpatient settings as well.

Group Visits Address Psychosocial and Medical Needs of the Chronically Ill

There can be a significant emotional and psychosocial overlay to chronic illness, especially serious chronic illness, which can create behavioral health needs that increase both utilization and cost of health care. Chronically ill patients typically have extensive psychosocial as well as physical medical needs—needs that are often better addressed by the biopsychosocial SMA models than by traditional individual office visits.

Because chronically ill patients need extensive medical information and effective disease self-management skills, they appreciate the additional time with their own provider and health care delivery team that group visits offer. They crave more medical information, as well as the reassurance of others who understand and care because they are *in the same boat*. They are comforted by the prompt access to barrier-free, high-quality care and the relaxed pace of care that well-run SMAs can offer, as well as by the encouragement and support of others dealing with similar issues. Chronically ill patients know what it is like to wake up in the middle of the night, feeling alone and isolated—yet not want to burden their friends and family with their health problems. They understand what it is to be stressed, depressed, angry, anxious or worried about their medical limitations and uncertain future. They wonder "Why me?" They can feel beleaguered, unable to cope, and frustrated by their inability to perform normal roles and duties.

The chronically ill can feel overwhelmed by the stress of coping with their illness experience—and by the multiple lifestyle changes now being thrust upon them. They need time to adjust to their condition and to learn the disease self-management skills that can help them to cope with the impact of their illness. Many feel fatigued and face debilitating treatments, while some are told to make significant lifestyle changes (such as diet, exercise, weight loss, or smoking cessation), and others are told to begin taking numerous medications—some of which can have challenging side effects. These multiple, complex issues are not always well-suited to the limitations and time constraints of the traditional office visit; however, they are ideally suited to the benefits that well-run SMAs can offer.

Three Current Major Group Visit Models

Three major group visit models of national significance have emerged during the past decade and a half:

1. Drop-In Group Medical Appointment (DIGMA)
2. Cooperative Health Care Clinics (CHCC)
3. Physicals Shared Medical Appointment (Physicals SMA)

What sets these models apart is that they are shared medical appointments (SMAs)—typically with the patient's own provider. They are not classes, health education programs, support groups, psychiatry groups, or behavioral medicine programs. Also, all three models are team-based approaches to quality care in which as many duties and responsibilities as possible and appropriate are delegated from the physician to less costly members of the care team to increase efficiency and control costs. These models need to be integrated into normal clinic operations to secure ongoing staff and administrative support. By focusing on patients' mind and body medical needs and on the efficient delivery of quality medical care in a supportive group setting, these SMA models can leverage existing resources, contain costs, and play a major role in the efficient, cost-effective delivery of high-quality, high-value care to the chronically ill.

The DIGMA Model

Solving access problems to follow-up appointments with existing resources, improving population management programs for the chronically ill, achieving better management of busy and backlogged practices, and enhancing quality of care and service to patients are all hallmarks of the DIGMA model [1–5]. I developed the DIGMA model in 1996 at Kaiser Permanente Medical Center in San Jose, California. It was born out of personal frustration with health care as it was being delivered while I was seriously ill with a complex cardiopulmonary condition between 1988 and 1992.

Although DIGMAs are occasionally used for intake visits and new patient appointments, they tend to focus on return appointments and are open to most established patients in the provider's practice. During DIGMA sessions, the provider sequentially attends to the unique medical needs of each person individually while fostering some group interaction. In fact, from beginning to end, DIGMAs are run just like a series of individual office visits with other patients as observers. In DIGMAs, the central focus from start to finish is upon the delivery of medical care, with the exact same medical care being delivered as in traditional office visits (history, examination, counseling, medical decision making, documentation, etc.)—but sequentially to one person at a time in the supportive group setting, while others listen, learn, share experiences, ask questions, and interact.

Triple Productivity

Although there are occasional circumstances in which DIGMAs can only double productivity (typically for providers who are already extremely productive, such as primary care physicians who only offer 10-minute appointments), DIGMAs are designed to triple the provider's productivity. Here, we are referring to tripling the provider's actual productivity over individual office visits during the same amount of clinic time as the DIGMA session lasts—that is, not the number of patients scheduled, but rather the number actually seen on average during 90 minutes of clinic time (as there are typically some no-shows and late cancellations, plus some provider down time, that reduce the provider's actual productivity for traditional office visits from the number of patients scheduled).

Although it may not seem like much to triple a provider's productivity during 1½ hours of clinic time each week (e.g., for DIGMAs held on a weekly basis), this actually translates to a substantial net gain in productivity for the entire week. As will be discussed later, for every properly designed DIGMA you run in your practice (i.e., that triples your actual productivity during normal clinic hours), your productivity for the entire work week will typically increase by approximately 8% to 10% if you are full-time, and by 16% to 20% if you are a half-time provider. Therefore, your productivity for the entire week could increase by as much as 40% to 50% if you are full-time and able to run daily DIGMAs and consistently keep your sessions full.

Furthermore, physicians running DIGMAs in their practice often report that they leave the group feeling energized rather than depleted and exhausted. All of this can be accomplished through DIGMAs with high levels of both patient and physician professional satisfaction and without extra hours being spent in the clinic.

DIGMAs Have Unique Features

The distinguishing characteristics of the DIGMA model are presented in Table 3.2. The DIGMAs are run like a series of individual office visits (like

TABLE 3.2. Distinguishing characteristics of the DIGMA model.

1. Different patients typically attend DIGMA sessions because patients attend only when they have an actual need.
2. DIGMAs are typically for follow-up visits, although they are sometimes also used for intake appointments.
3. Sessions are most commonly held weekly for 90 minutes, although they can be held as often as daily and for longer or shorter durations.
4. Sessions are open to much or all of the provider's practice (e.g., high and low utilizers; acute and chronic conditions; different sexes and ages; underserved patient populations) or to all appropriate patients in a chronic illness population management program.
5. "Drop-in" convenience is offered, although the vast majority of patients are typically prescheduled into DIGMA visits by staff they are for traditional individual office visits.
6. All patient education occurs in the context of the physician working with each patient individually in the group setting—there is no structured, class-like educational presentation.
7. Staffing typically involves the provider, a behaviorist, one or two nursing personnel, and a documenter—plus a champion, program coordinator, and dedicated schedulers in larger systems.
8. Sessions focus on delivery of medical care from start to finish, with the same care (plus more) typically being provided as during traditional individual office visits.
9. Best viewed as a series of individual office visits with observers, DIGMAs from beginning to end sequentially provide one patient–one physician encounters to each and every patient in the room.
10. Although the issue of billing is still evolving and not yet completely resolved, DIGMAs are often billed in the fee-for-service environment according to level of care delivered and documented.
11. Team-based care is provided, with high levels of patient and physician professional satisfaction.
12. There are group subtypes, that is, homogeneous, mixed, and heterogeneous.
13. DIGMAs have been used in almost all types of primary and specialty care practices.
14. A group room capable of comfortably seating 20 to 25 persons, and a nearby examination room are needed.

a series of one doctor–one patient encounters addressing each patient's unique medical needs individually) but in a supportive group setting, where some group interaction is fostered. Because most examinations during follow-up visits do not require disrobing, almost all examinations in a DIGMA are performed, with the patient's permission, in the group setting. Although infrequently needed, private time with the physician is always made available for those patients wanting or requiring a brief private discussion or examination (e.g., one that requires disrobing, such as a breast or abdominal examination).

There is no prepackaged "class" type educational presentation to the DIGMA group as a whole, as virtually all patient education occurs in the context of the doctor sequentially working with each patient individually—while others present are able to listen, learn, ask questions, and interact. There are expanded roles played by all members of the DIGMA team, especially the nurse and behaviorist.

A hallmark of the DIGMA model is the presence of a behaviorist—typically a psychologist or social worker (but sometimes a nurse, diabetic nurse educator, etc., who is capable of addressing psychosocial issues and managing a large group). The behaviorist assists the physician, keeps the group running smoothly and on time, addresses group dynamic and psychosocial issues, and temporarily takes over the group (often focusing upon relevant lifestyle or behavioral health issues) while the physician documents the chart note after working with each patient in the group, or leaves the group room for brief private discussions and examinations.

The DIGMA often includes a documenter to assist in the documentation process, especially for systems using electronic medical records. However, when paper charts are still being used, the provider might prefer to dictate the chart note during group, or to use a chart note template that is largely pre-printed and in a "check-off" format.

In addition to the provider, nurse(s), behaviorist, and documenter utilized during actual DIGMA sessions, larger systems will want to have a DIGMA champion (plus a program coordinator, to assist the champion by handling operational and administrative details, and dedicated schedulers) to ensure success and to help move the DIGMA program forward throughout the system.

Efficiency Is Gained in Two Ways

As is the case for all three major SMA models, DIGMAs make highly efficient use of available resources in two distinctly different ways. First, some efficiency is gained from the fact that DIGMAs provide patients with a group experience. Because care is delivered in a supportive group setting, repetition can be avoided, and the provider only needs to say things once to the entire group of patients simultaneously. Rather than inefficiently repeating the same information over and over to multiple patients individually.

Second, the bulk of the efficiency gains that DIGMAs provide result from the team-based approach to care—that is, as many duties as possible and appropriate are off-loaded from the provider's shoulders onto other, less costly members of the care delivery team. Efficiency is thereby gained through the DIGMA because the provider has to do less—but that less is what the provider alone can do.

Whenever possible, all other duties and responsibilities are deferred to the various DIGMA team members. For example, the nursing and behaviorist roles are maximized in DIGMAs (i.e., far beyond their normal, routine duties in the clinic) and, for systems employing electronic medical records, a documenter is often provided to off-load as many of the physician's documentation duties as possible.

For example, the role of the nurse in a DIGMA is expanded to be all that it can be (i.e., within the nurses' skill sets and scope of practice under licensure) rather than simply a repeat of those limited duties currently routinely performed during normal clinic hours. Instead, the physician and nurse sit down together during the initial DIGMA planning sessions to determine what all of the nursing duties are that the nurse could be providing in the DIGMA setting. This is something that many nurses like about DIGMAs, as it is a chance to do something different, develop professionally, and showcase their skill sets.

The end result is that in DIGMAs, nurses still room patients, take vital signs, and perform the normal duties that typically occur in the routine individual office visit setting. However, they also assist in documenting vital signs and other nursing duties into patients' chart notes, updating routine health maintenance for all patients, bringing all immunizations current (tetanus, pneumovax, flu shots, etc.), and conducting any other "special duties" that the provider might want to have performed in the DIGMA. These "special nursing duties" can include such diverse responsibilities as performing preliminary diabetic foot examinations and checking blood glucose levels for diabetic patients, checking blood oxygen and peak flows for asthmatic patients, and reviewing action plans.

The Issue of Billing

Because no billing codes specific to either group visits in general or to the different types of group visit models in particular have yet been developed, the issues of billing and compliance are still evolving for SMAs and are not yet completely resolved. Right now, health care organizations are trying to do the best they can with existing billing codes and regulations; however, they stand ready to adapt to any future billing and compliance changes that might occur for SMAs—hoping that any such future changes are reasonable and appropriate. It is common practice to bill for DIGMAs and Physicals SMAs (because, from start to finish, they are run as a series of one doctor–one patient encounters attending to the unique medical needs of each patient individually) using existing Evaluation and Management codes according to the level of care delivered and documented. However, to the benefit of insurers, patients are not typically billed either for counseling time (as many patients can be simultaneously benefiting from the same counseling) or for the behaviorist's time (which is treated as an overhead expense to the program in order to avoid patients receiving two bills and co-payments for a single medical visit).

Strengths

The DIGMAs have many strengths; their advantages are listed in Table 3.3. Clearly, DIGMAs will not be appropriate for all patients and providers; nonetheless, it is surprising how large the percentage of patients is that can successfully be treated in the DIGMA setting. Even patients who are

TABLE 3.3. Advantages of DIGMAs.

1. Typically designed to triple a physician's productivity, DIGMAs impact most or all patients in the physician's practice or chronic illness program (not just the same 15 to 20 high-utilizing patients).
2. Sessions can be offered weekly or even daily, with each DIGMA increasing productivity by as much as 8% to 10% for a full-time physician (16% to 20% for half-time physicians).
3. Prompt access to care is afforded because patients can attend sessions whenever they have a medical problem (there is no need to wait for the next scheduled monthly session or else be seen individually in between sessions).
4. Access eventually improves for individual office visits as well (i.e., because many traditional office visits are off-loaded onto DIGMA visits).
5. Visits are max-packed, and everything possible (including most examinations) is conducted in the group setting, where all can listen and benefit.
6. Drop-in convenience is offered (although the vast majority of patients will undoubtedly be prescheduled for their DIGMA appointment).
7. A behaviorist (typically a psychologist or social worker, but occasionally a nurse, diabetes nurse educator, etc., capable of addressing psychosocial issues and managing a large group) is present to help address many of the psychosocial and lifestyle issues that confront chronically ill patients.
8. Patients have continuity of care and more time with their own provider and care delivery team.
9. The focus from start to finish is on the delivery of individualized medical care.
10. Patient and physician professional satisfaction is high.
11. Although outcomes studies are, in general, more difficult to conduct for DIGMAs than for CHCCs, the preliminary data emerging are quite exciting.

painfully shy, uncomfortable in groups, or initially reluctant to attend are frequently won over by their initial DIGMA experience. Once they actually attend a session, such patients very often rate their satisfaction with the DIGMA experience very highly (typically around 4.6 on a 5 point Likert scale and often higher than their satisfaction ratings for traditional individual office visits with the same provider) and are willing to return to a future session for their follow-up care.

It is likewise surprising how large the percentage of providers is who can successfully run a DIGMA (even providers seen by their colleagues as "impossible" or "extremely unlikely to succeed") provided that they are willing to try one for their practice and to consistently invite all of their appropriate patients, during regular office visits, to attend the DIGMA for their next follow-up visit.

DIGMAs can play an important role in the care of chronically ill patients in two distinct ways:

1. By helping providers to improve access to, and to better manage, their own busy and backlogged practices
2. By the critically important role they can play in care pathways and population management programs for virtually all types of chronic illnesses

Typically designed for return or follow-up visits with established patients, DIGMAs are open to most or all patients in the physician's practice—that is, whenever they have a medical need and want to be seen. The DIGMA visits, which should ideally be max-packed, are meant to replace individual office visits whenever possible—and not to add extra visits. Most commonly meeting weekly for 90 minutes and with different patients typically attending each session, DIGMAs are meant to off-load many individual office visits onto this highly efficient SMA format. Whenever possible, the goal is to have patients attend a highly efficient and max-packed DIGMA session in lieu of a more costly individual office visit and for this to be a "one-stop" health care experience that comprehensively attends to the patients' various mind–body needs. In this manner, not only are productivity and efficiency increased, but traditional individual appointments are also freed up and made more available to those who truly need them.

DIGMAs Have Widespread Applications

The following three points underscore the breadth of application of the DIGMA model:

1. DIGMAs have widespread applications for improving access and productivity, for enhancing quality and service, as practice management tools, and for the invaluable role that they can play in chronic illness population management programs.

2. DIGMAs have been successfully used in almost every medical subspecialty—and in a wide variety of primary and specialty care applications. To date, they have been successfully launched in the settings of internal medicine, family practice, allergy, cardiology, dermatology, endocrinology, gastroenterology, general surgery, gynecology, hematology, nephrology, obstetrics, oncology, ophthalmology, orthopedic surgery, pediatrics, physiatry, plastic surgery, podiatry, psychiatry, pulmonology, rheumatology, sports medicine, travel medicine, urology, weight management, and women's health.

3. DIGMAs have been successfully used by all types of providers (e.g., physicians, nurse practitioners, physician assistants, PharmDs, osteopaths, and podiatrists) and in a wide variety of health care systems and settings (e.g., fee-for-service, capitated, military, and public hospitals).

Patients

The ideal group size for DIGMAs is between 10 and 16 patients. In addition, two to six support persons (spouses, other family members, friends, or caregivers) generally also attend DIGMA sessions, because patients are invited to bring a support person with them. Be careful to make it clear to patients that they can bring only one support person along to their DIGMA visit if they wish to—I once had a patient bring 13 family members with him, which was an entire group unto itself. However, patients and support persons alike must sign the full disclosure confidentiality waiver at the beginning of each and every session (Table 3.4).

The DIGMAs are especially well suited for routine follow-up care; relatively stable chronically ill patients; patients who can benefit from peer support and more time with their provider; patients with extensive informational, psychosocial, behavioral health, and emotional needs; patients who are difficult, time consuming, and problematic; patients who are noncompliant or high utilizers of health care services; and patients for whom the physician needs to keep repeating the same information over and over. Meant to provide patients with an additional health care choice and to be voluntary to patients and providers alike, DIGMAs are neither intended to completely replace individual office visits nor are appropriate for every patient and provider.

For example, DIGMAs are not intended for most initial evaluations or one-time consultations (although they have been used in this capacity under certain circumstances, such as for podiatry and surgery intakes).

TABLE 3.4. Some, but not all, important points for the corporate attorney or medical risk department to incorporate into the confidentiality release form.

1. Much of the medical care that the patient will receive will be delivered in the group setting.
2. Patients' medical conditions and issues will be discussed in front of others.
3. All attending must agree to keep the setting safe and not to identify others in attendance, either directly or indirectly, or discuss other patients' medical issues once the session is over.
4. Everyone (patients as well as all support persons accompanying them) must sign the release before entering the SMA group setting.
5. The confidentiality release can also spell out that, during SMA sessions, patients are always welcome to request a brief, one-on-one meeting with the physician to discuss a private matter—although the meeting will typically be held toward the end of the group session so as to not interrupt the flow of the group.
6. The choice of whether to attend a DIGMA or Physicals SMA is a completely voluntary one.
7. Patients are free to leave the sessions at any time, without any repercussions for doing so.
8. Subsequent to attending a DIGMA or Physicals SMA session, individual office visits will continue to be made available to patients in the future, as before.
9. The DIGMA or Physicals SMA is meant to provide patients with an additional health care choice.

Note: These points are provided to be helpful to you; however, each medical group must have its own corporate attorney or medical risk department develop its own confidentiality release form to ensure that it is properly updated; in full compliance with all of the local, state, and national regulatory requirements; in compliance with its own corporate standards; and comprehensive, complete, and fully appropriate for the organization's purposes and circumstances.

Similarly, DIGMAs are not for severe acute infectious illnesses (such as severe acute respiratory syndrome or tuberculosis), which are highly contagious and could get other group members ill—although some systems have implemented successful "Cold and Flu DIGMAs" with the rationale that patients are exposed to these conditions in the lobby anyway. In addition, DIGMAs are not for rapidly evolving medical emergencies (such as acute chest pain) or for patients who refuse to attend a group session. Similarly, they are not meant for monolingual patients who do not speak the language in which the DIGMA is being conducted, or for patients who are too severely hearing impaired or demented to benefit. That having been said, there have been DIGMAs specifically designed for the severely hearing impaired and for demented patients and their caregivers; however, special considerations must be addressed in such DIGMAs for patients and caregivers to understand what is transpiring and to fully benefit. Finally, DIGMAs are not generally appropriate for complex medical procedures or lengthy private examinations, for which the Physicals SMA model is often appropriate—although simple tests and medical procedures (such as nitrogen freezes, brief hearing tests, and trigger point injections) can be provided, typically toward the end of the session.

For DIGMAs to Succeed, the Physician Must Take Primary Responsibility for Inviting Patients

It is important that the provider, and staff, take primary responsibility for keeping all DIGMA sessions full by personally inviting all appropriate patients to have their next office visit be a DIGMA visit. This must be something that providers and staff are willing to do—and to do effectively. Because physicians are often not used to inviting patients and paying attention to census requirements, they can become inattentive to this important responsibility. Should the physician stop personally inviting, in a carefully worded and positive manner, all appropriate patients seen during regular office visits to have their follow-up be in the DIGMA, then this program will be at high risk for failure due to pre-established census requirements not being consistently met—and inadequate attendance is by far the most common reason for DIGMAs to fail.

Experience has shown that nothing is as effective in getting a patient to attend a DIGMA as a personal, positively worded invitation from their own doctor. If the physician fails to personally invite patients in a carefully scripted and positive manner, then nothing else can substitute or compensate for this shortcoming in keeping sessions filled. I have attempted to overcome this problem for some physicians who refused, forgot, or otherwise failed to personally invite their patients; however, nothing really worked sufficiently well to overcome this hurdle and salvage the program on a long-term basis—neither invitations and encouragement to attend from the physician's front office and nursing staff nor redoubled efforts on the part of scheduling staff. Even if nursing, scheduling, or front office staff does its best to invite patients and compensate for the physician's failure to personally invite patients, the process is much less efficient and effective (and certainly more time consuming)—because patients are much more likely to try a DIGMA for the first time if the invitation comes from their physician.

How Physicians Should Invite Patients

To be fully effective, the invitation from the physician needs to be positively worded and reflect the physician's own belief in the program. If a physician does not truly believe in the DIGMA program, or if the physician's invitation is so weak as to be meaningless, the invitation will clearly not be very effective. Consider the physician who says something like the following to the patient: "I would like to see you back in 3 months for your diabetes. You can have either a group or individual appointment. Just schedule it as you leave." When this happens, and the physician has not explained the program to patients or encouraged them to attend, the patients will simply go out and schedule an individual appointment—as this is what they are used to—and they will leave knowing nothing about the DIGMA or the multiple patient benefits it offers.

Contrast the above with the types of invitations that successful DIGMA physicians make. When inviting their patients, they will often say something like the following: "I would like to see you back in 3 months for your diabetes. I have a new program that I recently started that could be very helpful to you. It is only for my patients. We will have 90 minutes together so that I can go into more detail than I ordinarily could in the rush of a short office visit. You will likely get answers to important medical questions that you might not have thought to ask, because others will ask them. Also, you will have a chance to meet some of my other patients dealing with similar issues, some of whom will be further along in dealing with their diabetes and could share helpful tips and suggestions with you. We have some fun together and we even serve snacks! Would you like to come to my DIGMA for your next visit?"

The physicians most successful at inviting their patients even go one step further. Should patients demure, equivocate, or show ambivalence toward this invitation, then the physicians most successful at inviting their patients might add something to the effect that "I'm so sure that you will like this program, would you try it once for me?" Few patients will refuse such an invitation from their doctor. Once they attend a session, experience has shown that patients almost always like it because patient satisfaction with DIGMAs is very high—typically as high as (or even higher than) individual office visits—approximately 4.6 on a 5 point Likert scale. Therefore, the key to success is to get patients to attend their first session. Once the patient accepts this invitation—which should not take more than 30 seconds to a minute to make—the patient should be immediately booked into the next appropriate upcoming DIGMA session.

Staffing

The DIGMAs are staffed by:

1. The provider, who is in attendance throughout the session
2. A behaviorist, typically a psychologist or social worker, but occasionally a nurse, diabetic nurse educator, or other midlevel provider (Ideally, this person will have group management skills, be adept at fostering group interaction, have the professional skills to address the psychosocial issues of medical patients and their families, and be able to work closely with the provider.)
3. A nurse and/or medical assistant, who takes vital signs, brings injections and health maintenance records current, and performs other "special duties."

Some medical practices, especially those utilizing electronic medical records, will include a "documenter" to assist the physician in drafting a comprehensive, contemporaneous chart note during the session on each and every patient in attendance (typically after being trained by the provider and through use of the physician's own chart note template for the DIGMA session).

The Behaviorist's Responsibilities

Let us take a closer look at the role of the behaviorist, which is a hallmark of both the DIGMA and the Physicals SMA models. The presence of the behaviorist adds an important dimension to the comprehensive mind–body care of patients, such as the chronically ill, who are often dealing with important disease self-management, lifestyle, psychosocial, and behavioral health issues. The behaviorist can help to diagnose depression, anxiety, substance abuse, stress, and so forth—conditions that are known to be underdiagnosed and undertreated in the primary care setting, yet when treated can substantially increase the patient's utilization of health care services. By the behaviorist helping to tactfully bring these important issues to the physician's attention, it allows these conditions to be better diagnosed and treated during DIGMA sessions—and for psychotropic medications to be initiated (or for referrals to be made to appropriate treatment programs for these conditions).

The behaviorist must be experienced in managing large groups, adept at fostering group interaction, and understand the complex emotional and psychosocial needs of medical patients and their families. In addition, the behaviorist is charged with arriving early and greeting the patients, giving the introduction and starting the group on time (even if the physician is a few minutes late), managing the group dynamics, keeping the group interactive and interesting, ensuring that the group runs smoothly, taking over the group temporarily, whenever the provider is documenting a patient's chart note, assisting the physician in every way possible, and addressing the behavioral health and psychosocial needs of patients—which are known to drive a large percentage of all office visits.

The behaviorist's experience and skill set need to complement (rather than be identical to) that of the physician, which helps to relieve physician anxieties about managing the group—including worries about having it spiral negatively out of control. Because the role of the behaviorist is a much more active one in a DIGMA than in a traditional mental health group, this can lead to problems in how the behaviorists fulfill their role in a DIGMA—especially if they have not had specific training for these new DIGMA responsibilities. For this reason, I caution would-be DIGMA behaviorists to thoroughly read about (and to fully understand) the role of the behaviorist in the DIGMA model before taking on this responsibility—despite what will likely be some initial feelings to the effect that they know how to run groups and that they can probably just "wing it" with their current professional skills and experience.

If the provider frequently runs late for individual visits during normal clinic hours, then it is important to pair that provider off with a behaviorist who is a "taskmaster" with excellent time management skills. On the other hand, if the physician is excellent at time management (and generally runs on time in the clinic during regular individual office visits), then such a provider can be paired with a "warm and fuzzy" behaviorist who is less of a time manager. Even though they might enjoy working with one another, we would definitely not want to have a "warm and fuzzy" provider–behaviorist pairing, because DIGMA sessions would then run late, probably very late.

How Documentation Is Handled

In addition, especially in systems using electronic medical records, it is highly recommended that there be a specially trained documenter sitting at the computer throughout the DIGMA session to assist in the documentation process. The documenter used in DIGMAs has often been a nurse, resident, medical transcriptionist, or motivated member of the physician's staff with good typing and computer skills who is familiar with medical terminology and able to work closely with the physician. Even other providers, such as nurse practitioners and PharmDs, have been used as documenters with great success, as they can add an important extra dimension to the group—plus the additional benefit of acting in a consultation capacity to the DIGMA with their unique skill sets.

However, before selecting another provider as your documenter, make certain that the overhead expense assessed to the program is the provider's hourly wage and not the revenues the provider could have generated for the system by instead spending the group time seeing other patients himself or herself—which could drive the overhead expense up to the point where the program is no longer economically viable. This problem can often be circumvented by using others only when they are clearly providing extra hours to the clinic at their hourly wage (and preferably not at overtime pay).

Experience has demonstrated that having a documenter can not only dramatically increase the provider's productivity and efficiency but also result in a much better chart note being generated—because it is a contemporaneous and comprehensive chart note documenting all that occurred with that patient while it was occurring. It avoids the problem of physicians forgetting much of what they did when they later draft the chart note—immediately after the session, during lunch, at the end of the day, or when coming in on Saturday morning to "catch up." The longer the interval between the delivery of the medical services and the drafting of the chart note, the more details one seems to forget. Also, it avoids the common complaint that "The doctor looked at the computer the whole time and never looked at me."

Immediately after working individually with each patient in turn in the DIGMA setting, the provider typically breaks away temporarily from the group to (1) review the individualized chart note, (2) make any needed additions or changes, and (3) sign off on the chart note that has been drafted for that particular patient. In the meantime, the behaviorist temporarily takes over running the group, typically focusing on a behavioral health issue relevant to the group.

Even when no documenter is used, the behaviorist performs the same function of running the group while the physician takes a couple of minutes to draft or dictate the chart note immediately after working with each patient individually. For systems still using paper charts, the provider will often use a DIGMA chart note template that is preprinted and in a "check off" form in order to efficiently draft a complete, individualized chart note for each patient in the shortest possible amount of time.

If paper charts are being used and the physician chooses to dictate the DIGMA chart notes, then I would recommend that the chart note dictation be made a teaching point in the group. In this case, after completing the work with each patient in turn, the provider can say something like the following to the entire group: "Listen up everybody. I'm going to dictate a chart note summarizing Mary's case. Let me know if I miss anything or leave anything out." I have found that patients are very interested in hearing their cases summarized by their doctor and that the entire group learns from this experience.

Larger Systems Need a DIGMA Champion, a Program Coordinator, and Dedicated Schedulers

In larger systems (say, 20 or more providers), there typically also needs to be a champion charged with the responsibility of moving the DIGMA program forward throughout the organization. In extremely large systems of multiple large facilities, there may even need to be a champion at each facility. The DIGMA champion attends departmental meetings, gives staff presentations, recruits physicians, develops forms and promotional materials, custom designs each provider's DIGMA, and interfaces with high-level administration.

Larger systems also need to have a program coordinator, whose primary responsibility is to assist the champion in every way possible. The program coordinator attends to any operational and administrative details of the DIGMA program; supervises the schedulers, nurses, and behaviorists used in the SMA program; assists with the forms, implementation details, and training necessary for launching each new DIGMA; and takes primary responsibility for producing the periodic productivity, quality, outcomes, and patient–provider satisfaction reports that are necessary for overall evaluation of the program.

In addition, larger systems often hire DIGMA schedulers, perhaps one full-time scheduler for every 15 to 20 DIGMAs that are up and running. These DIGMA schedulers must have good interpersonal, telephone, and telemarketing skills. They are specifically trained to monitor the census of all DIGMA sessions and to take immediate action when an upcoming session is not filled to targeted levels (i.e., by telephoning and inviting additional patients, as requested by the provider). The job of the DIGMA scheduler is not to take primary responsibility for filling sessions (which much remain the responsibility of the provider, the provider's staff, and the health care system's regular scheduling staff) but rather to "top off" and fill to capacity any upcoming DIGMA sessions that might fail to meet target or minimum census requirements.

It is important to note that the primary responsibility for filling DIGMA sessions must rest with the provider, the provider's staff, and the health care system's regular scheduling staff (but most especially with the provider)—as nothing is more likely to succeed in getting patients to attend a future DIGMA session for their next follow-up appointment than a carefully worded, personal invitation from their own doctor. The DIGMA schedulers, for those systems fortunate enough to have them, have the more limited (but extremely important) role of ensuring that all upcoming DIGMA and Physicals SMA sessions meet their target and minimum census requirements, by taking immediate action and inviting more appropriate patients whenever upcoming sessions are insufficiently filled.

Subtypes of the DIGMA Model

There are three subtypes of the DIGMA model: homogeneous, heterogeneous, and mixed.

The Homogeneous Subtype

There is the intuitively appealing homogeneous subtype, in which each session is open only to patients of a specific condition or diagnosis (e.g., diabetes, chronic heart failure, hypertension, asthma, or arthritis). Although the homogeneous subtype is often used in chronic disease care programs, it can also be used to better manage the physician's own practice. In this case, there is usually a series of homogeneous sessions (each of which is dedicated to a specific condition or group of diagnoses), a sequence that is then repeated over and over in the future.

For example, a homogeneous DIGMA in primary care might be designed as follows: the first session in the series might be for diabetes and obesity; the second for hypertension and hyperlipidemia; the third for all gastrointestinal problems (e.g., gastroesophageal reflux disease, inflammatory bowel disease, irritable bowel disease, or ulcers); the next for all cardiopulmonary problems; the next for women's health; the next for headache, fibromyalgia, and chronic pain; and the next for psychosocial issues, such as stress, anxiety, substance abuse, and depression. Once this entire series of sessions is held, the entire sequence could thereafter be repeated over and over in the future.

In this primary care application of the homogeneous model, which is designed to better manage a physician's practice, it is difficult for patients and staff to keep track of the sequence of sessions—especially if the physician has been absent for a session or two because of meetings, vacation, or illness. In actual practice, when the homogeneous model is used in primary care, it poses many additional operational and census challenges. Because only a comparatively small percentage of the physician's practice qualifies for any given session, it is often difficult to keep all sessions full—especially because patients must not only have that particular diagnosis or condition but must also must have a medical need to be seen at that time.

In addition, the physician's scheduling staff might hesitate to schedule patients into homogeneous DIGMAs for fear of being chastised for scheduling the wrong patient in the wrong session—so they sometimes choose to not schedule anybody rather than to take this unnecessary risk. Finally, the fact that patients tend to bring a laundry list of diverse medical concerns to their appointments poses a particular challenge to the homogeneous model—which will become more heterogeneous in nature if such diverse medical issues are in fact addressed during the session. However, addressing all patient concerns is something that, whenever possible, we want to do in DIGMAs in order to make it a "one-stop" health care experience for those patients who attend.

For example, a patient might enter a diabetes DIGMA session with several medical concerns that have nothing to do with diabetes (such as neck or shoulder pain, sinus problems, or a lesion on the sun-exposed parts of his or her skin), issues that could readily be handled in the DIGMA session. When this happens, most physicians will simply address these issues as they arise in the session to prevent an unnecessary follow-up visit by the patient; however, by doing so, the homogeneous DIGMA automatically becomes more heterogeneous in nature.

On the other hand, the homogeneous DIGMA model can work well in relatively large population management programs for specific chronic diseases (e.g., chronic heart failure, diabetes, hypertension, headache, or asthma), where there is typically a large number of patients (often several hundred or even thousands) having the same condition to draw from, so that, with proper promotion, homogeneous DIGMA sessions can be kept full.

The Heterogeneous Subtype

Although counterintuitive, the most common subtype of the DIGMA model for better managing a busy, backlogged practice is the heterogeneous subtype, which is open to most or all patients in the physician's practice—regardless of diagnosis, condition, sex, or age. Interestingly, experience has demonstrated that patients who attend a heterogeneous DIGMA frequently continue to show interest in the group even when patients are discussing conditions other than those that they themselves have.

When asked why they are interested in hearing about other people's health problems that they do not have, patients often respond by saying that they might someday get such health problems or that someone else they know (mother, brother, neighbor, or friend) also has the same conditions. Other patients point out that these wide-ranging discussions on a variety of health topics are not only interesting and stimulating, but also make the DIGMA like "a mini-medical school class" taught by their own doctor—one in which they learn a great deal about medicine and taking better care of themselves and which they feel fortunate to be able to attend. Other patients simply state that they are interested and find that "it's better than watching ER!"

In a heterogeneous DIGMA, all of the patients not only share that particular physician, but they also have many common concerns even though the specifics of their illnesses happen to differ. Especially for the chronically ill, such common concerns include the realization of now being a medical patient; the frustration of facing new limitations and not being able to do what they used to do; the erosion of self-esteem that comes from not being able to fulfill one's normal roles and responsibilities, and the anxiety created by facing an uncertain future. Patients with severe chronic illness know what it is like to wake up with a jolt in the middle of the night worrying about what tomorrow will bring; to feel sick, fatigued, overwhelmed, and unable to cope; to worry about the impact that their illness is having on their job, family, and friends; and to feel isolated, alone, cheated, and ask "Why me?" As can be seen, even though the DIGMA happens to be heterogeneous, there are still many shared issues and feelings among patients.

The Mixed Subtype

The third DIGMA subtype is the mixed subtype. Here, the physician's practice is divided into four large patient groupings—one for each week of the month. For example, a Mixed Primary Care DIGMA might be structured as follows: cardiopulmonary patients are the focus the first week of the month; diabetes and weight management, the second week; all gastrointestinal patients, the third; and women's health, the fourth week. For those couple of months each year that have five sessions, the fifth session could be open to all patients in the physician's practice, regardless of diagnosis, or to any specific condition(s) of the provider's choosing. The caveat with the mixed subtype is that if the most appropriate session for the patient to attend does not happen to fit the patient's schedule, then the patient is invited to attend any other appropriate session that happens to be more convenient for them.

The mixed subtype is also a common and widely used model for better managing a large, busy practice. However, when the mixed model is initially employed, it is often observed to gradually evolve over time into a straight heterogeneous model. This typically happens as the physician gradually becomes more comfortable in dealing with the multiple types of medical issues that arise in any given session, and as the physician is able to see that many different types of medical patients and issues mix well together during group sessions. Over time, there is a general trend with DIGMAs for the physician to deliver more and more medical care in the group setting and for the physician to become evermore comfortable with a heterogeneous mix of patients.

Two different endocrinologists experienced having their DIGMAs gradually evolve into a fully heterogeneous model after initially beginning with a mixed DIGMA model. For both of these endocrinologists, their initial mixed DIGMA model was structured as follows: Type 1 diabetes was the focus for the first week of each month; type 2 diabetes was the focus for the second and fourth weeks of each month; and all other endocrine disorders (such as thyroid, parathyroid, adrenal, pituitary) were the focus for the third week of each month. Both endocrinologists found their Mixed Endocrinology DIGMA gradually evolved into a heterogeneous model within a year because of both the operational simplicity of the heterogeneous model (since any of their patients could then attend any week that they had a medical need and wanted to come in, regardless of diagnosis, which made their scheduling staff more willing to actually schedule patients into their DIGMA sessions) and the finding that it actually worked quite well in practice to see the various types of endocrine patients together during the same session.

The same experience occurred when an entire neurology department started DIGMAs for its practices during the same week in order to solve severe departmental access problems. The two neurologists in the department who originally opted for a mixed subtype found that it gradually evolved into a heterogeneous model during the subsequent year. Because these two neurologists were initially reluctant to start with the heterogeneous model, they started with the "mixed" subtype of the DIGMA model. They designed their Mixed Neurology DIGMAs so that headache was the focus for the first week of each month; multiple sclerosis, seizure disorders, and younger neurology patients were the focus for the second week; stroke, dementia, Parkinson's disease, and older neurology patients were the focus for the fourth week; and the third and fifth weeks—for those couple of months during the year having five sessions—were open to all patients in their practices. This enabled these two heavily backlogged neurologists to schedule almost all of their neurology follow-up visits into their DIGMAs within 1 to 2 week's time. As was the case for the endocrinologists discussed earlier, both of these neurologists found that their Mixed Neurology DIGMAs gradually evolved into straight Heterogeneous Neurology DIGMAs during the subsequent year.

Flow

After rooming the physician's last patient before the DIGMA, the nurse or medical assistant attached to the DIGMA (typically the physician's own nurse) escorts the early arrivers (i.e., those who have already registered for the DIGMA, received their patient packet for the SMA, and signed the confidentiality release; see Table 3.4) from the physician's lobby to the group room. The nurse or medical assistant then begins calling patients one at a time out of the group room and into the nearby examination room—taking vital signs, providing injections, updating health maintenance, and performing other "special duties." Even if the nursing duties are not completed for all patients by the designated start time for the session, the behaviorist starts the DIGMA on time with a brief 3- to 5-minute introduction. In this introduction (which is given during the first couple of minutes of each DIGMA session), the behaviorist welcomes all attendees, explains the program and its benefits to patients, discusses personal comfort issues, covers what to expect and how to make best use of the session, and addresses confidentiality.

Immediately after the introduction, the physician begins to deliver comprehensive mind–body medical care to one patient at a time while fostering some group interaction—typically starting with any patients who need to leave early. The process of having the physician address the medical needs of each patient individually then occupies the remainder of the group time (except for a few minutes toward the end of the session that can be dedicated to brief private one-on-one discussions and examinations in a nearby room for any patients requiring them).

The goal is for the DIGMA to end on time, which requires that the physician leave the group room on time when the group is over to resume normal clinic duties. Otherwise, if the physician lingers, the patients will tend to stay also. Therefore, it is important for the physician to leave on time as soon as the group is finished. It is the behaviorist who lingers in the group room for about 20 minutes or so to answer any last-minute patient questions (e.g., about where to go for their colonoscopy, for the recommended smoking cessation class), and then to quickly straighten up the group room for the next group visit session.

With DIGMAs, Conduct as Much as Possible in the Group Setting

With DIGMAs, almost everything occurs in the group setting—except for infrequent brief private discussions and examinations that require disrobing. These examinations are conducted toward the end of the group in the privacy of a nearby examination room.

Few, if Any, Patients Will Need to Be Seen Outside of the Group

Patients are told by the behaviorist during the introduction that private one-on-one time with the provider will always be made available to anyone requesting or needing it so that the group dynamic and smooth flow of the session are not interrupted. Interestingly, when this matter is handled properly, only a patient or two (and most frequently no patients at all) need to be seen individually.

This observation runs counter to the initial fears that many physicians have when first contemplating a DIGMA for their practice, as they worry that all patients will want to be seen individually by them during every session—which would make for an overwhelming workload (and a boring DIGMA due to the minimal group interaction, sharing, and patient education that would result).

Weaknesses

Although the DIGMA model has numerous strengths, like all group visit models, it also has weaknesses. The single greatest ongoing challenge to running a successful DIGMA, and by far the greatest weakness of the DIGMA model, is the fact that—because different patients attend each DIGMA session—ongoing attention must consistently be paid to maintaining targeted census levels during each and every session. If sessions fail to consistently meet targeted census levels, then the DIGMA will fail for two reasons: (1) it will fail to achieve economic viability and (2) it will fail to achieve ideal group size from a psychodynamic perspective.

Therefore, it is important to promote your DIGMA program to all appropriate patients to ensure that you consistently reach the optimal group size for all of your DIGMA sessions. Otherwise, you will lose your productivity and economic gains. Furthermore, you will find that it is actually more difficult to run a very small group than it is to run a larger group of ideal size (i.e., between 10 and 15 patients). This makes for a more lively, energetic, and interactive group, and one that is actually less work to run than a small group of only three or four patients. Plus, having such a small group would certainly not be economically viable because you could see more patients than that individually during the same amount of time, without the overhead costs of the program.

In addition, because much about the DIGMA model is counterintuitive and very different from traditional individual office visits, it is easy to make common beginner's mistakes that can frustrate providers and undercut the success of the program. For example, despite having many initial concerns, few physicians give much thought to designing their DIGMA so as to ensure that sessions are consistently filled to capacity (i.e., to targeted census levels), and this is the real issue that will determine whether or not the DIGMA will ultimately be successful. Instead, physicians worry about concerns such as the following: "What if I say something stupid in front of 20 of my patients at once?" and "What if I'm asked a question that I don't know the answer to?" Or the physician might worry about: "What if it doesn't work for my practice?" and "What if I lose control of the group and it spirals negatively out of control?" The simple fact is that, should any of these things happen, the physician could simply say something like: "That wasn't quite what I wanted to say. Let me try explaining it another way." The physician might also simply admit that he or she did not know the answer to the question, but would look it up and let the patient know the next time. All that happens in such cases is that patients see their doctors as being more human and often end up feeling even closer to them as a result.

Patients are Often More Open in the Group Setting

It is also counterintuitive to think that patients would be more comfortable discussing many personal issues in the group setting than when alone with their physician during an individual office visit. Surprisingly, some patients actually find the traditional office visit setting more intimidating. Time and again you will hear patients say something like the following in the DIGMA setting: "I didn't feel comfortable bringing this up in my last office visit, doctor; however, I feel safe with these fine people here . . ." and then go on to say something that might be very important from a medical perspective, yet be something that the patient has not previously disclosed to the physician. This is especially true when somebody else in the group has been discussing a personal symptom that the patient might also have but has been too embarrassed to bring up or that the patient had previously minimized, denied, or dismissed out of hand as being unimportant (which all too often happens with important cardiovascular symptoms).

Although Counterintuitive, the Heterogeneous Model Is Often Best

It is also counterintuitive that the heterogeneous DIGMA model (i.e., rather than the homogeneous model) would generally be the best model, especially for better managing a large, busy, and backlogged practice. The idea of having patients with different diagnoses and a wide variety of seemingly unrelated medical conditions attend DIGMA sessions whenever they have a medical need is not at all intuitively obvious. Physicians fear that such a heterogeneous group experience could prove overwhelming to them, that the group discussions could become too diverse and scattered, that patients would be disinterested in afflictions that they do not personally have, and that they could lose control of the group.

Most Physician Fears Quickly Fade, but Ideal Group Size Remains an Ongoing Issue

In actual practice, all of these initial anxieties have been found to gradually fade over a couple of months' time, as experience is gained in running the DIGMA and as confidence grows. Because of such initial, anxiety-based fears as those discussed, many physicians who could most benefit from the heterogeneous model unfortunately end up shying away from it and opt instead for the homogeneous model. This proves to be a common beginner's mistake because, of all three DIGMA subtypes, it is the heterogeneous model that can most dramatically improve productivity and access to a busy, backlogged physician's practice.

There is much that is counterintuitive about all types of SMAs. However, the single greatest ongoing challenge to running a successful DIGMA or Physicals SMA (and by far the greatest weakness of these models) is the fact that ongoing attention must consistently be paid to maintaining targeted census levels during each and every session—which is itself counterintuitive, as few (if any) providers initially show much concern about it.

Experience with Other Types of Groups Does Not Necessarily Make for a Good DIGMA

Although initial provider anxieties can result in many unrealistic fears and concerns, providers can also have a false sense of security—that is, they believe they know more than they in fact do regarding how to run a DIGMA—often because they have been associated with some type of group or class in the past. However, what is required in a DIGMA, if it is to succeed can in fact be quite different from what is required for success in other types of group programs and classes. In turn, this false sense of confidence can lead to poorly designed, inadequately supported, and improperly run SMA programs—and to many beginner's mistakes.

DIGMA Requirements

Facilities

The DIGMA model, like all group visit models, has specific facilities, personnel, and promotional requirements that must be met for success to be achieved. The DIGMAs have significant facilities requirements in that they need a relatively large group room capable of seating 20 to 25 people and keeping them comfortable. This group room needs to have enough chairs as well as adequate ventilation for such a large number of people. In addition, the group room should be appropriately furnished so as to be pleasant and comfortable, and a properly equipped examinations room should be nearby.

If you lack a sufficiently large group room, consider converting any other appropriate space (storage area, staff dining area, or break room) for your DIGMA, or consider using your lobby area during off hours. Although you might be willing to adapt to whatever space is initially available to you for your DIGMA group room, once you have been successfully running DIGMAs for a while (especially after you have demonstrated both feasibility of concept and the multiple quality, efficiency, and productivity benefits that a well-run DIGMA program can offer), you will probably want to ultimately make the necessary changes to the physical plant.

Personnel

In addition to facilities requirements, as with all types of group visit models, there are also specific personnel requirements for a successful DIGMA program. The DIGMAs and Physicals SMAs are team-based care delivery models wherein as much as possible is offloaded from the shoulders of the physician onto less costly members of the DIGMA team. Besides the provider, the DIGMA requires a behaviorist, nurse(s), and often a documenter—plus a champion, program coordinator, and DIGMA schedulers in larger systems.

Promotional Materials

An additional challenge is that you will need to budget for—and then develop—appropriate promotional materials for the program (i.e., to inform patients of the DIGMA and its many patient benefits, and to encourage them to attend). This is because patients have had a lifetime of expecting an individual, one-on-one office visit with their physician. Patients know nothing about group visits or the multiple patient benefits that the groups offer when they are properly designed and run.

It is extremely important to the success of the program for the physician and staff to invite all suitable patients to attend and for the scheduling staff to be appropriately trained to book patients requesting a follow-up appointment into the appropriate DIGMA sessions. However, it is equally important to develop a variety of high-quality promotional materials for the program, materials that are required in order to inform patients of the program and its multiple benefits and to persuade them to attend the next time they need a medical visit.

These promotional materials include nicely framed wall posters for mounting on the physician's lobby and examination room walls, a program description flier containing all necessary details about the physician's DIGMA, an "invitation letter" to be distributed by staff to all appropriate patients on an ongoing basis, an "announcement letter" to be mailed to all patients on the provider's panel at the very start of the DIGMA program, and "patient packets" (containing handouts, a confidentiality release, a name tag, a sheet of paper for taking notes during the session, and any other important DIGMA materials that the physician might select) to be distributed to patients upon registering for each DIGMA session.

It is important that these promotional materials be of high quality and have a professional appearance, one that accurately reflects the high-quality care that patients can expect to receive in this innovative new type of care delivery modality. It is not enough to simply photocopy a poorly drafted poster or flyer for the DIGMA program and then tape it onto the physician's lobby walls. Another disadvantage of group visits is that a confidentiality release must be developed by risk management personnel in the organization—a form that I recommend be signed by all patients and their support persons before each session (see Table 3.4).

Chronic Illness Outcomes Studies Are More Difficult with DIGMAs Than with CHCCs

Another challenge of DIGMAs results from the fact that different patients attend each DIGMA session; therefore, outcomes studies for the DIGMA model typically need to be larger (and take longer) than is required for CHCCs—where the same 15 to 20 patients attend each monthly session and outcomes studies relative to a matched control group are relatively simple and straightforward. This is especially true of the heterogeneous DIGMA model in primary care, where the relatively healthy patient who comes in for a sprained ankle today might not return for a year or more (and could then be seen for an unrelated medical issue such as sinus congestion or earache), which could make outcomes studies more time consuming and challenging than for CHCCs.

Outcomes studies are less of an issue for chronic illness population management programs, because the homogeneous DIGMA model is most often used for such applications. This is because, even though different patients typically attend sessions, they all still have the same chronic disease or condition—which can make outcomes studies easier. For example, because all patients attending a diabetes DIGMA would have diabetes, measuring outcomes such as improvements over time in blood pressure, lipid levels, or blood glucose control—and then comparing these results with a control group receiving traditional care only—would be a relatively simple matter.

Keeping Sessions Filled When No Access Problems Exist

One must also carefully think out how DIGMA sessions will be kept full once backlogs and waiting lists are eliminated—either because of the productivity and efficiency gains from the model itself or because Advanced Clinic Access goals are achieved. There are a number of possible solutions to this challenging situation, all of which would have the same net effect of increasing demand on DIGMA services, including the following: making the DIGMA more heterogeneous (so that more patients qualify to attend each session), enlarging one's practice and panel size, decreasing the number of individual return visits offered on the provider's schedule, reducing hours spent in the clinic, carving out time in the master schedule for desktop medicine or administrative time, and accepting other providers' patients into DIGMA and Physicals SMA sessions.

In addition, one must ask: "If I were a patient and could have either an individual office visit today or a DIGMA tomorrow, why would I choose to go to the DIGMA tomorrow?" The answer lies in (1) how the provider words the invitation for patients to attend the DIGMA for their follow-up visits (e.g., by emphasizing the benefits that a well-run DIGMA offers, such as more time, support from others, greater patient education) and (2) labeling the program in such a way that patients know that this is the proper venue for them (e.g., "Dr. Smith's Medication and Refill Clinic" or "Dr. Smith's Diabetes Clinic").

DIGMAs Can Exacerbate Preexisting Systems Problems

Because they so dramatically increase productivity and efficiency, DIGMAs tend to stress the systems and to exacerbate any preexisting systems problems. This includes stressing the weaker components of the system that might previously have been marginally acceptable when one patient was being seen at a time, but that rapidly become unacceptable when a bolus of 10 to 16 patients is run through the system at once. For example, a slow receptionist might be marginally acceptable when one patient is registering at a time for a traditional office visit; however, when 10 to 15 patients arrive close together to register for a DIGMA, the receptionist can quickly become overwhelmed—the solution to which will likely require additional training, extra help during the registration process, or a shift in personnel.

The good news is that by solving such preexisting systems problems, the remainder of the work week often flows better because the problems most likely had already been surfacing to some degree during normal clinic hours. However, the bad news is that if you fail to take the necessary corrective action, the preexisting systems problems could actually frustrate patients and staff, undercut the efficiency and effectiveness of your group visit program, and possibly cause your DIGMA to fail.

DIGMAs Represent a Major Paradigm Shift

Remember that all SMAs represent a major paradigm shift from the traditional, individual care model by being a team-based approach to health care, by delivering care in a supportive and highly interactive group setting, and by dramatically ratcheting up efficiency and productivity. These changes require proper facilities, personnel, training, promotional materials, attention to myriad operational and administrative details—as well as an adequate budget and high-level administrative support—to be fully successful. As can be seen, group visits represent a major paradigm shift, one that introduces considerable change that can stress the system. Also, these changes often prove to be more difficult to achieve in actual practice than they might at first appear to be.

The CHCC Model

The Cooperative Health Care Clinics (CHCC) model [6–10] was developed in 1991 by John C. Scott (a pioneer in group visits and a personal friend for whom I have the greatest respect) at Kaiser Permanente in Colorado. The CHCC model was born out of Dr. Scott's professional frustration when trying to adequately meet the complex mind–body needs of his high-utilizing, multi-morbid geriatric patients—needs that he felt he was unable to adequately meet within the time constraints of the traditional office visit. Dr. Scott originally developed the CHCC model with the goal of providing efficient, high-quality health care to these high-utilizing, older patients in a group setting.

The CHCC model has been shown to improve quality of care, outcomes, cost effectiveness, and patient and provider satisfaction. Like DIGMAs, it focuses on follow-up visits for established patients and provides a new model for the physician's office visit. However, because CHCCs differ in substantial ways from the DIGMA model, there are major differences between these models in terms of benefits, staffing, structure, flow, strengths, and weaknesses. Interestingly, the differences between the DIGMA and CHCC group visit models are complementary rather than competitive, which enables the two models to coexist and be used together with great success. Each can be used for its own respective strengths, which can build one on the other.

Strengths

The CHCC model was originally designed to provide better and more accessible care over time for the same group of 15 to 20 complex, high-utilizing geriatric patients—with the overall objective of reducing resource utilization and the associated costs of delivering care. As with patients in DIGMAs and Physicals SMAs, seniors in CHCCs have proved to be quite open to sharing experiences and to discussing highly personal issues in the group setting (including disability, loss of independence, feeling like a burden to friends and family, death and dying, and end-of-life decisions), which has actually enhanced the patient–physician relationship.

Older patients experiencing multiple chronic health problems are complex patients, and they often bring to their medical visits an extensive "laundry list" of mind–body needs that cannot be fully met during the brief amount of time allocated to a relatively short individual office visit. These wide-ranging patient needs can often be better met during the CHCC because of the greater amount of time available, the extensive patient education provided, and the help and support provided by both the care team and other patients. The beneficial outcomes of CHCCs demonstrated in research trials are presented in Table 3.5.

TABLE 3.5. Outcomes of CHCCs (for the same 15 to 20 patients in attendance over time).

1. Enhance overall quality of care
2. Improve patient outcomes
3. Reduce costs (when compared with usual care)
4. Increase patient satisfaction
5. Increase physician satisfaction
6. Reduce the number of referrals to medical specialists
7. Reduce emergency department, hospitalization, and nursing home costs

The CHCCs are ongoing groups for older patients that are not time-limited. The CHCC model is the most intuitively appealing of all three group visit models because the same group of 15 to 20 high-utilizing medical patients is followed on a monthly basis over time and therefore outcomes measures can be made with comparative ease. Because the same patients attend regularly (some CHCC groups have already been meeting for more than 10 years), patient bonding can be very intense—bonds that are sometimes described as being stronger than family. Other strengths of the CHCC model are that it brings routine health maintenance current for these patients, and the levels of both patient and physician satisfaction are high.

Patients

In the CHCC model, the same group of patients is followed over time. The CHCC format permits patients to share personal experiences, support one another, learn from each other (as well as from the multidisciplinary team), and receive medical care that addresses existing medical needs and brings routine health maintenance current. Patients are invited to bring a spouse or support person and are taught to be partners in their own disease self-management—such as in measuring their own blood pressures and blood glucose levels.

Because the CHCC typically follows the same patients on a monthly basis, more patients (perhaps up to 25) need to be invited to ensure that 15 to 20 actually attend each session. Additional members need to be added to CHCCs as patients move, die, drop out, or become too frail to attend. Therefore, the physician and nurse are encouraged to monitor census on an ongoing basis and to add additional patients as necessary to maintain desired census levels, thus ensuring the economic viability of the program.

Staffing

The CHCC is usually staffed by a physician, a nurse, and outside speakers as needed—plus a program coordinator in larger systems to oversee the program and handle operational and administrative details. Because physicians and nurses have typically not received specialized training in the skills required to facilitate and manage groups, they need to receive specific training in conducting CHCC sessions, especially in fostering patient participation and group interaction and in not turning sessions into a class. To minimize costs, tasks are delegated to the most appropriate member of the CHCC care team.

Outside speakers (such as pharmacists, nutritionists, physical therapists, and health educators) are also brought in as part of the multidisciplinary team on an as-needed basis. For example, many CHCCs have added a pharmacy intervention component in which the pharmacist can talk about medications and their interactions, review the medications that patients are taking, ensure that patients understand how to take their drugs properly, identify and resolve potential drug-related problems, and discuss how to appropriately take and store their medicines. In addition, the nurse works collaboratively with the physician to monitor the care provided to CHCC patients outside of the monthly sessions. There can also be a physician champion in larger systems charged with the responsibility of moving the program forward throughout the organization.

It is also important to include administrative support staff and clinic managers in the CHCC so that they become champions and ensure that the necessary nursing and physician resources are available to the program. If CHCCs are not fully integrated into clinic operations, and if key administrative leadership is not included in the CHCC decision-making process, then the necessary resources (personnel, supplies, and facilities) might be directed toward other clinic programs and needs.

Structure

The CHCC addresses routine health care needs through an interactive process of education, social relationships, and shared experiences, as well as care from the physician and multidisciplinary care team. Although routine care needs such as injections and vital sign measurements are provided during CHCC sessions, urgent and emergent medical needs are still obtained as before between CHCC sessions. This expectation needs to be occasionally reinforced by the physician and nurse, who must monitor the group's utilization between sessions and offer appropriate coaching as needed to ensure that patients are behaving accordingly.

Before the first CHCC session is held, the physician's practice is searched for high-utilizing, multi-morbid geriatric patients. These patients are contacted and invited to attend the CHCC. Past experience demonstrates that approximately 40% accept the invitation, 20% are indecisive, and 40% refuse. Because these patients must make the commitment to attend sessions regularly on a monthly basis, the focus turns to the 40% who accept the invitation. An initial session is then held to explain the program, and for patients to develop the norms and rules they want for their group—an important tenant in the CHCC is that the patients participate not only in their own health care decision making but also in the development of the program.

Subsequent to this initial session, ongoing CHCC sessions have an initial 90-minute interactive group segment that is followed by an additional 60-minute segment of individual care in which patients needing to be seen are provided with an individual appointment (typically four to seven patients are seen individually each month). The group component of these sessions is structured into the following segments: warm-up and socialization (approximately 10 to 15 minutes); educational presentation on a topic selected by patients during the last session (approximately 30 minutes); working break (approximately 20 to 30 minutes during which vitals signs are taken, prescriptions are refilled, medical charts are updated [patients are also given their own medical chart summary to take with them], medical care is delivered to patients individually by the physician and nurse, and patients needing to be seen individually during the subsequent hour are identified); question and answer time (approximately 10 to 15 minutes); and planning for the next session (approximately 5 to 10 minutes). Once the 1½ hour group is finished, all patients are invited to leave except those who need to be seen individually during the subsequent hour.

Subtypes

The CHCC model has proved to be versatile and adaptable to many disease states and conditions. In the Specialty CHCC subtype of the CHCC model, the patients are usually experiencing the same diagnosis or health condition (e.g., diabetes or congestive heart failure). Sessions in Specialty CHCC groups are structured similar to the original CHCC format (a 90-minute group segment followed by 60 minutes of individual care for those needing it). In addition, like CHCCs, Specialty CHCCs often focus on high-utilizing patients because that is where the economic cost offset maximally occurs.

However, Specialty CHCCs differ as to both the types of patients in attendance (specialty patients versus multi-morbid geriatric patients in primary care) and the frequency with which sessions are held. In the Specialty CHCC, the sessions might be held irregularly (rather than monthly, like CHCCs), and a provider other than the patient's own physician might be used. Such groups can also be time limited rather than ongoing.

For example, hypertension specialty CHCCs might be designed to initially meet monthly for 3 months, then to meet again in 6 months, then 1 year, and finally 2 years. Older patients with multiple medical problems might enjoy ongoing monthly meetings (and benefit from interacting frequently with both other patients and the CHCC health care team), but younger and healthier working patients will likely not need this intense level of contact and support. Although the Specialty CHCC format might vary according to the needs of various diagnostic groups (so that frequency, content, and duration may differ accordingly), the key components of the CHCC program still apply—and can result in improved quality of care, increased patient and physician satisfaction, and contained costs.

Flow

In the CHCC, the physician, nurse, and multidisciplinary team foster group interaction and participate in group discussions. Patients sit in a horseshoe seating arrangement to foster group interaction and to allow the physician and nurse easy access to patients. During all sessions, the same 15 to 20 patients attend the initial 90-minute interactive group segment; of these, approximately four to seven patients will stay on an as-needed basis to be seen individually during the subsequent 60-minute individual visit segment. The typical format and flow of a CHCC session are discussed below; however, it is important to keep in mind that there is ample flexibility as to how to structure the CHCC session.

Warm-Up

At the start of the session, the patients are paired off and given a warm-up exercise to stimulate discussion (such as to describe the first Christmas or birthday that they can remember). During these 10 to 15 minutes, you can hear the intensity of the discussion escalate as patients (and their support persons) get to know each other better.

Educational Presentation

The warm-up is followed by an educational presentation, that is approximately 30 minutes long, on a topic that has been selected by the patients during the previous session (although there are several core topics that are covered during the first year and repeated as needed thereafter). This presentation can be given by the physician, nurse, or a guest speaker.

Working Break and Delivery of Medical Care

During the 20- to 40-minute working break and care delivery segment that follows, patients' vital signs are taken, injections are given, and certain medical issues are addressed individually by the physician and nurse while other patients eat snacks and talk with each other. It is determined at this time which patients will need to be seen individually during the hour following the group session.

As can be seen, CHCCs differ from DIGMAs in many ways. One difference is that medical care is delivered to patients individually during CHCCs (i.e., while other patients are not listening), both during the working break of the group segment and during the individual visit segment). In other words, in CHCCs, the medical care is not delivered during the group setting where all present can listen and learn; this, from start to finish, is a defining characteristic of DIGMAs. Also, delivery of medical care is the focus during only portions of the CHCC visit (the working break and individual visit segments), whereas it remains the central focus throughout the entire DIGMA session—which, as a result, is best conceptualized as a series of individual office visits with observers.

Questions and Answers

A 10- to 15-minute question and answer session follows during which patients' questions are answered in the group setting, where all can listen and learn, while group interaction between patients is fostered.

Planning for the Next Session

Immediately after the question and answer portion, the patients spend approximately 5 to 10 minutes discussing what topic they would like to have addressed during the educational presentation of the next session.

Individual Visits

The 90-minute group visit segment of the CHCC is then followed by up to 60 minutes of individual care for the four to seven patients in attendance needing it. Those patients who only need to attend the group segment leave after the group is over.

Weaknesses

Although the CHCC model is intuitively appealing because the same high-utilizing patients are followed over time, constant attention must be paid to fostering group interaction and—because of the substantial educational format—to keeping patients from viewing the CHCC as a class. The CHCC model is for high-utilizing patients (i.e., not for low- or moderate-utilizing patients) as this is where maximum economic gain is achieved; however, it must be kept in mind that only 40% of high-utilizing patients will make the required degree of commitment to attend the CHCC regularly on a monthly basis. Also, conducting a CHCC group well requires up-front skill building around group processes as well as coaching and monitoring. Unfortunately, the benefits of the CHCC model are often invisible to the staff, which can result in necessary resources being diverted to more visible demands, and can undercut nursing and administrative support for the program despite the long-term favorable results that a properly run CHCC program can provide.

Because basically the same 15 to 20 patients are followed over time on a monthly basis, excellent medical care and close monitoring can be provided to these patients and strong patient bonding can occur; however, unlike DIGMAs, the CHCC does not impact or improve access to the remaining 1,200 to 3,000 patients in the physician's practice. Also, because CHCCs involve 2½ hours of physician time (1½ hours for the group, followed by 1 hour of individual care) rather than the 1½ hours required for most DIGMAs or Physicals SMAs, a correspondingly larger number of patients must be seen to cover the cost of the program.

In short, CHCCs provide excellent care with extraordinary bonding and continuity of care for those patients who are fortunate enough to receive it. As can be seen, the DIGMA and CHCC models have complementary strengths and weaknesses, which is why they work so well in combination for follow-up visits.

Practice Management Limitations

Specialty CHCCs do not improve access to a provider's practice, and they are not a tool for more efficiently handling patient phone call volume or for optimizing the physician's schedule (i.e., for the rest of the physician's practice, other than the 15 to 20 attendees)—all of which are strengths of the DIGMA and Physicals SMA models.

Limits for Chronic Illness Program Applications

Although they can provide great care for the 15 to 20 patients being followed, having all patients start at one time—and then following the same group of high-utilizing patients periodically over time—can also limit the value of this model to chronic illness population management programs. This is especially true:

1. For larger population management programs in which a great number of different chronically ill patients (perhaps thousands, or even tens of thousands) need to be followed over time, whenever they need care
2. When all levels of disease severity and utilization of health care services are being included (such as many low and mid utilizers, along with some high utilizers)
3. When patients have highly variable health care needs so that periodically scheduled CHCC sessions (or even irregularly scheduled sessions for all in attendance, such as those of Specialty CHCCs) may not be ideally helpful

Other Difficulties

Because patients need to make an ongoing commitment to the program, CHCCs are particularly inappropriate for patients who are uncomfortable in a group setting. As is the case with all SMA models, any economic advantage rests on maintaining an adequate group size and on the resultant savings from improved outcomes and reductions in costly utilization. Also, because the care is delivered during the working break of the group segment while other patients are enjoying snacks and socializing with one another, other patients do not get to listen, learn, and benefit from this one-on-one care segment.

Finally, there could be billing issues in a fee-for-service environment due to the highly educational structure of the CHCC group segment (i.e., for those patients who attend the group but are not seen afterwards during the individual care segment), although such concerns might depend to some degree on what care is delivered, how it is provided, and how it is documented during the working break and care delivery segments. Also, unlike the DIGMA model, the group segment of the CHCC does not closely resemble the traditional individual office visit model of care—at least for those patients who attend only the group segment of the CHCC visit (i.e., the 15 to 20 patients attending the group, except for the four to seven patients typically seen one-on-one during the individual care segment).

The Physicals SMA Model

The third major group visit model, the Physicals SMA model [11–13], stands alone because it focuses on physical examinations rather than return appointments. The Physicals SMA model is of benefit to both chronic illness population management programs (i.e., when a private physical examination is needed) and the physician's entire practice (i.e., for improving access to physical examinations). As with all SMAs models, Physicals SMAs increase patient education and the amount of time that patients have with their physician, and integrate the help and support of other patients into each patient's health care experience.

I developed the Physicals SMA model in 1991 at the Palo Alto Medical Foundation in response to a perceived nationwide need to improve access to, and productivity of, physical examinations—and to do so with high levels of patient and physician, professional satisfaction by delivering consistently high-quality care.

The Physicals SMA model represents an important health care innovation because it can deliver quality care while leveraging existing staffing, dramatically increasing physician productivity and efficiency, and solving access problems for physical examinations. In addition, because new patient intakes often involve a physical examination, the Physicals SMA model is often used in both primary and specialty care for bringing new patients either into the system or into the individual provider's practice. It can similarly be used in any chronic illness population program where timely access to private physical examinations is an important consideration. Table 3.6 describes how efficiency is gained with the Physicals SMA.

TABLE 3.6. How efficiency is gained by the Physicals SMA model.

1. By providing a team-based approach to care that off-loads as many responsibilities as possible from the physician and delegates them to various other appropriate (and less costly) team members.
2. By enabling providers to conduct the actual physical examination in a streamlined fashion using several properly equipped examination rooms—without the delays, interruptions, and inefficiencies that so often accompany traditional physical examinations.
3. By deferring most discussions from the inefficient individual examination room setting to the more productive group room setting—where repetition can be avoided and all present can simultaneously listen, learn, interact, and benefit.
4. By overbooking sessions according to the expected number of late cancels and no-shows, thus making Physicals SMAs immune to these problems (by eliminating the expensive physician down time experienced with individual office visits when patients do fail to attend a lengthy physical examination).

Hallmarks of the Physicals SMA Model

As depicted in Table 3.7, key features of the Physicals SMA model include (1) team-based care, (2) high levels of patient and physician satisfaction, (3) dramatically increased physician productivity in delivering physical examinations, (4) improved patient access to physical examinations, and (5) one physician–one patient encounters throughout. Unlike the DIGMA and CHCC models, which focus on follow-up appointments for ambulatory outpatients, the Physicals SMA model instead focuses on private individual physical examinations, with almost all discussion deferred to the subsequent group setting where all can benefit. Like DIGMAs, there are homo-

TABLE 3.7. Key features of the Physicals SMA model.

1. Offers team-based care
2. Focuses on private physical examinations rather than follow-up visits
3. Is used for routine and intake physicals in primary and specialty care
4. Covers most or all patients in the physician's practice or chronic illness treatment program
5. Yields high levels of patient and physician satisfaction
6. Dramatically increases physician productivity in delivering physical examinations
7. Improves patient access to physical examinations
8. Defers almost all discussion from the examination room to the subsequent group setting
9. Like the DIGMA, offers homogeneous, mixed, and heterogeneous subtypes
10. Can be widely applied to any primary care or specialty practice
11. Typically requires a behaviorist, two nurses, and a documenter
12. In larger systems, also requires a champion, program coordinator, and dedicated schedulers
13. Requires four examination rooms and a smaller group room capable of comfortably seating 12 to 16 persons
14. Is conducted as a series of one doctor–one patient encounters in both the examination and group rooms, attending to each patient's unique medical needs individually
15. Delivers medical care, from start to finish, the same as an individual office visit

geneous, mixed, and heterogeneous subtypes of the Physicals SMA model, and the same care is delivered as in traditional individual office visits.

Analogous to our discussion of DIGMAs and CHCCs, although the term *physician* will usually be used in the discussion that follows, other providers of physical examinations (nurse practitioners, osteopaths, podiatrists, etc.) can also run Physicals SMAs for their practices by using the same types of staffing, facilities, and promotional materials.

Physicals SMAs can be widely applied to any primary care or specialty practice. The following are but a few of the medical subspecialties in which the Physicals SMA model is now being applied: prenatal examinations in obstetrics; breast examinations for fibrocystic breast disease in general surgery; foot examinations in podiatry; skin examinations in dermatology; well-baby checks and school, camp, and sports physicals in pediatrics; intakes for breast reduction and carpal tunnel surgeries in plastic surgery; presurgery physical examinations for cataract surgery in ophthalmology; diabetic foot examinations in endocrinology; digital rectal examinations for prostate problems in urology; pacemaker interrogations in cardiology; and post-transplantation visits for bone marrow transplants in hematology.

Subtypes

Like the DIGMA model, there are heterogeneous, homogeneous, and mixed subtypes of the Physicals SMA model. In Primary Care Physicals SMAs, the mixed subtype is frequently used. This allows patients to be divided by sex and age group so that they share some similar medical issues and concerns. For example, for a primary care physician who does mostly male physicals, the mixed Physicals SMA could divide the examinations into those for men over age 50 years during the odd weeks of the month and those for men under age 50 years during the even weeks. On the other hand, for providers doing mostly female physical examinations, the mixed subtype could divide examinations into those for women over age 45 (or 40) years during the even weeks of the month and those for women under age 45 (or 40) years during the odd weeks.

For providers who see mostly women, but of all ages equally, the mixed model could focus on women 18 to 29 years old during the first week of the month, 30 to 44 years old during the second week, women 45 to 59 years old during the third week, and women 60 years and older during the fourth week. The exact ages used for dividing the groups should take into account not only the different medical issues that affect various age groups but also what divisions will yield enough patients for each session to be consistently filled.

Similarly, for Physicals SMAs that are designed for the medical subspecialties, patients are usually separated into homogeneous groups having similar medical conditions or health care issues. Some examples are prostate problems or incontinence in urology; prenatal examinations in obstetrics; well-baby checks or school, camp, and sports physicals in pediatrics; whole-body skin examinations for melanomas in dermatology; breast lumps in general surgery; hips or knees in orthopedic surgery; and candidates for breast reduction or carpal tunnel surgery in plastic surgery.

Respecting Patient Privacy in the Physicals SMA Model

The Physicals SMA model is the least intuitively obvious of all the SMA models as it is difficult to imagine how physical examinations can be efficiently conducted in a group visit format. At first, the consideration of physical examinations in a group visit format might conjure up many fantasies—including those of patients being nude together or being efficiently ushered from one medical station to another. However, unlike the military physical examinations of World War II, patients in Physicals SMAs are neither examined together nor ushered en masse from station to station.

Instead, efficiency is gained in the Physicals SMA model by deferring almost all discussion from the examination room (except for truly private matters and brief discussions that need to take place in order to complete the private examination) to the group room—where all can listen and learn and where repetition can be avoided. Because it is all the talk that takes so much time during most physical examinations (and because most of the talk is deferred from the examination room to the group room), the actual physical examination ends up taking comparatively little time in the Physicals SMA model.

Facilities

During the initial physical examination segment of the Physicals SMA, four patients are roomed at any given time because four examination rooms are most commonly used. Because many physicians have only two examination rooms assigned to them, they will often hold their Physicals SMA at a time when a colleague is consistently absent from the clinic—a colleague willing to let the physician use his or her two examination rooms as well.

While the physician is providing physical examinations to patients during approximately the first half of the Physicals SMA session, the behaviorist remains in the group room interacting with the rotating small group of patients who are not roomed. It is during this time that the behaviorist (1) asks each patient what medical concerns he or she would like to discuss with the physician today; (2) writes these issues down on a whiteboard or flipchart alongside of the patient's name; (3) makes certain that all present have signed the confidentiality release; (4) distributes handouts preselected by the physician and discusses them with patients; and (5) performs whatever other duties the provider and behaviorist want accomplished during this time.

Overbook Sessions to Avoid Costly Down Time

Because of the considerable length of most physical examination and new patient intake appointments (which often represent the greatest "time sink" in a physician's practice), a great deal of down time can result whenever a patient fails to keep an appointment or cancels too late to refill the time slot. One of the great benefits of all group visit models is that this wasted down time can easily be avoided by doing what the airlines do, that is, by making the program immune to having open time slots by simply overbooking all sessions according to the expected number of no shows and late cancels. This number is fairly predictable and can be determined after only a couple of sessions, by determining how many patients have historically failed to attend that provider's previous SMA sessions—a number that can be further refined by taking other variables into account as well, such as the focus of that particular session (in the case of the homogeneous and mixed subtypes) and the types of patients present.

Although this overbooking strategy is an important advantage for all SMA models, it is especially important for Physicals SMAs because physical examination and new intake appointments often represent one of the greatest time commitments in the physician's schedule. When patients do not show or cancel late, a great deal of time can be wasted, especially when there is insufficient time to schedule another patient into that time slot.

Three Basic Components of Physicals SMAs

The Physicals SMA model can best be conceptualized as consisting of three basic components.

The Initial Patient Packet

When patients are scheduled into the Physicals SMA appointment (unlike DIGMAs, patients do not drop in), a designated person in the physician's support staff sends them patient packet, typically 2 to 3 weeks before the session. The patient packet contains (1) a cover letter signed by the provider that welcomes patients and describes the program (including its patient benefits and what to expect); (2) any handouts that the provider wants included; (3) a detailed health history questionnaire, with sections on personal and family health histories, recent health changes, current medical concerns, and so forth, that the patient needs to complete and return to the office at least a couple of business days before the session; and (4) orders for any lab tests (especially blood screening tests) that need to be completed before the appointment.

The Physical Examination

The first part of the actual Physicals SMA session typically consists of a series of private physical examinations conducted individually on all patients in attendance, usually with four patients being roomed at a time. One important difference between the Physicals SMA and traditional physical examinations is that examinations are conducted with the absolute minimum of talking between the doctor and patient in the Physicals SMA. This involves a learning curve for participating physicians (and may take a couple of months of actual experience to become comfortable and efficient with this approach). Typically, only what needs to be discussed in order to conduct the examination (as well as truly private matters) are discussed in this relatively inefficient individual examination room setting. All other discussion and talk is deferred to the group room, where all present can listen, interact, and learn.

Unlike the DIGMA model, in which the preferred behaviorist is often a mental health professional (such as a psychologist or social worker with group experience and expertise in working with medical patients), in the case of the Physicals SMA model, a gregarious nurse who knows the patients is often preferred for the behaviorist role. This is because the group size is much smaller in the Physicals SMA than in the DIGMA so that group dynamic and group management skills requirements are much less for the Physicals SMA model. However, the ability to present basic medical information while alone with patients is often an important consideration, which can make a nurse behaviorist good choice for a Physicals SMA.

The Interactive Group

The next part of the Physicals SMA session is the interactive group segment, which basically consists of a small DIGMA and is when almost all of the discussion between physician and patients occurs. It is here that efficiency can be increased and repetition avoided, as all present can simultaneously listen, learn, interact, and ask questions.

Census Targets for Physicals SMAs

The target census for most 90-minute Primary Care Physicals SMA sessions is typically seven to nine male patients or six to eight female patients. An additional patient (or occasionally even two) would typically be added to compensate for the expected number of no shows and late cancels. For medical subspecialty Physicals SMAs, where the physical examination is often more limited in scope and therefore quicker to perform, the target census is often higher, commonly 12 to 14 patients. Although the target census is typically set to at least triple the physician's productivity in delivering physical examinations, the minimum census is often set so as to at least double the physician's productivity.

Strengths

Physicals SMAs enjoy most of the same quality, service, access, and pro-ductivity benefits as the author's other major group visit model, the DIGMA model, and also has similar staffing requirements. Although not appropri-ate for all patients and providers, Physicals SMAs typically result in high levels of both patient and physician professional satisfaction.

Physicals SMAs Can Be Employed in a Wide Variety of Chronic Illness Programs

Like DIGMAs, Physicals SMAs can play an important role in the care of chronically ill patients by helping providers both improve access to their services and better manage their busy, backlogged practices. Physicals SMAs also have a crucial role in care pathways and population manage-ment programs for the chronically ill. To date, the Physicals SMA model has been successfully employed in a wide variety of primary and specialty care applications. Like DIGMAs, Physicals SMAs have been successfully used by many types of providers (physicians, nurse practitioners, physician assistants, etc.) have a wide variety of personalities and a wide variety of settings (e.g., fee-for-service, capitated, PPO, HMO, IPA, military, and public hospital settings).

The Physicals SMA model is typically used instead of the DIGMA model (i.e., where almost all examinations are conducted in the group setting) whenever a private, individual physical examination is required in primary or specialty care, such as when disrobing is required or truly private information needs to be discussed.

Although patients for the Physicals SMA are typically drawn from the physician's own practice, they can be drawn from other practices. For example, one primary care provider struggled to keep his sessions full once he had caught up with his own backlogged patients through the productiv-ity gains of his Physicals SMA. He therefore asked his physician colleagues who had access problems to physical examinations whether he could also include their wait-listed patients in his Physicals SMA. Although a couple of colleagues refused this generous offer, others were all too happy to accept it—and ultimately found that doing so helped to improve access to their practices as well.

Staffing

With one possible difference, staffing for a Physicals SMA is similar to that of a DIGMA. Like DIGMAs, staff for a Physicals SMA include (1) two nurses or medical assistants for rooming patients, taking vital signs, giving injections, providing other special duties, and staying ahead of the physi-cian at all times; (2) a behaviorist for running the group of non-roomed patients during the first half of the session (while the physician is delivering private physical examinations) and for managing group dynamics, addressing psychosocial issues, assisting the physician, and keeping the group running smoothly and on time during the subsequent interactive group segment (which is basically a small DIGMA); (3) the provider, who is present throughout the session (initially by conducting rapid, but thorough, physical examinations with a minimum of discussion and afterward by running the interactive group segment); and (4) in larger systems, a champion, a program coordinator, and specifically designated schedulers (for moving the program forward throughout the system and for consistently achieving targeted census levels in all sessions).

The one difference between staffing for DIGMAs and Physicals SMAs is that a documenter, which is highly recommended for a DIGMA, especially for systems using electronic medical records, is a necessity throughout the Physicals SMA session, especially for systems using electronic medical records, because the physician will, in most cases, be seeing three or more times as many patients in the same amount of time and because the documentation requirements for physical examinations are considerably more extensive than for follow-up visits. In Physical SMA sessions, a documenter can dramatically increase the physician's productivity and comfort level alike—as it permits more patients to be efficiently seen during the session while providing a supportive, team-based approach to care.

Also, because a documenter generates a comprehensive and contemporaneous chart note during the Physicals SMA, a superior documentation of medical services delivered can be generated. This is because the physician, after traditional office visits, normally forgets some of what transpired simply because the chart note is generated at a later time (immediately after the appointment, during lunch, after work, or when coming in on Saturday morning to wrap up loose ends). In general, the more delayed the writing, the more that is forgotten. However, in return for having a documenter, the provider should be willing to see at least one—or possibly as many as two—additional patients in the Physicals SMA to cover the added overhead cost.

Who can serve as documenter? Clearly, the documenter must have computer skills, be a good typist and speller, understand medical terminology, be able to work closely with the physician, be a good learner and able to multi-task, and be willing and able to generate the precise type of individualized chart note that the physician wants from the chart note template developed for the program. Depending on available resources, the documenter can come from any of a number of possible disciplines—for example, the documenter could be a nurse, medical assistant, or medical transcriptionist specially trained for this duty. However, the ultimate choice probably depends more on who happens to be available—and on the skill sets and personality of that individual—rather than a particular professional discipline.

Clarify the documenter's role when designing your Physicals SMA. As with DIGMAs, Physicals SMAs are customized to the specific needs, goals, practice style, and patient constituency of the individual provider. Clearly, the documenter will be in the group room during the second half of the Physicals SMA (i.e., during the interactive group segment). However, during the initial planning sessions, the physician needs to decide what to have the documenter do during the first half of the session, when the physical examinations are being conducted. The documenter could accompany the physician from one examination room to another while the physical examinations are being performed (in which case the documenter must be a nurse or somebody licensed to be in the room with disrobed patients), or the documenter can stay in the group room during the initial physical examination segment to document what is occurring there.

Some physicians opt for the former, whereas others successfully opt for the latter. As previously stated, the documenter will be in the group room during the interactive group segment (i.e., when the provider, behaviorist, and all attendees are simultaneously present in the group room), which follows the physicals examination segment of the Physicals SMA. In addition, when custom designing their Physicals SMA program, physicians need to develop the chart note template that the documenter will use for drafting the contemporaneous, comprehensive, and individualized chart note for each patient.

Conduct Physical Examinations First, Before the Group

Although the physical examinations could occur before, during, or after the interactive group segment, in most cases they should occur first, before the interactive group segment. In this way, almost all questions, answers, and discussions that would otherwise occur in the examination room can easily be deferred to the group room in the interactive segment that follows—and the time-consuming need for the physician to repeat the same information over and over to different patients individually can thereby be avoided. To accomplish this, the provider simply needs to tell patients in the examination room: "Good point! Why don't you bring that up in the group that follows so that all can listen and benefit?"

Otherwise, if the examinations are done last (i.e., after the interactive group segment), then the provider will have no choice but to answer any questions that patients might later ask in the inefficient individual setting of the examination room rather than in the efficient interactive group setting because the group would then be over. For this reason, the provider would have great difficulty finishing the session on time as patients seem to always have "a few more questions" when they get the provider alone in the examination room—this tends to occur no matter how many times the behaviorist and provider (as well as promotional materials for the program) might tell the patients during the group that all questions and discussion are to occur in the group setting.

Conduct Your Group Visit Program by Sticking Closely to the Established Models

I recommend that those starting a group visit program begin by closely adhering to the original models as they have been designed and described, because they have been demonstrated to work successfully and are the result of much trial and error. Using this approach keeps physicians from having to "recreate the wheel" and making many of the same beginner's mistakes that the designers made when developing the models, because so much about group visits is counterintuitive.

The models were developed gradually and through numerous iterations over time into their final forms. For example, when developing the Physicals SMA model, I made the beginner's mistake of choosing the more intuitively appealing option of doing the interactive group segment first and the physical examinations last—after which patients could leave. However, this turned out to be a major mistake for the reasons discussed earlier, and I ended up frustrating three physicians because I gave them a flawed model that did not allow them to finish on time. As a result, development of the Physicals SMA model was delayed by at least 8 months.

Therefore, when starting your SMA program, resist the impulse to strike out on your own at the start. If you do not, you could find yourself frustrated, and come to the conclusion that group visits will not work for you—even though they most likely can. Instead, start with whichever established group visit model is best designed to meet the most pressing needs that you have in your practice, and then design and run it as recommended by its originator.

Only later, once you gain comfort and experience in running your own group visit, would I recommend that you consider deviating from the established models—perhaps by changing one parameter at a time so that you can quickly recognize, react to, and correct any mistake that you might make along the way. In the long run, this will likely prove to be a better, more satisfying, and less frustrating long-term approach for you to take in implementing as SMA program.

Subtypes

As is the case for DIGMAs, there are heterogeneous, homogeneous, and mixed subtypes of the Physicals SMA model, with the mixed subtype being most common in primary care, the mixed and homogeneous subtypes being most common in specialty care, and the homogeneous model (with its disease- and condition-specific focus) most common in population management programs for chronic illnesses.

For example, a heterogeneous Primary Care Physicals SMA design for a provider who performs mostly male physicals could include all of the male patients for physical examinations, regardless of age, health status, or utilization behavior. Although the heterogeneous model has been successfully employed in some primary and specialty care applications, it must be used with caution because of the small group sizes of Physicals SMAs. Small group sizes with the heterogeneous model can result in patient groupings that are too diverse to achieve maximum benefit and efficiency, to avoid repetition and redundancy, and to attain high levels of patient bonding and sharing.

Examples of homogeneous Physicals SMAs in specialty care include the following: intakes for breast reduction or carpal tunnel surgery in plastic surgery, follow-up visits for benign fibrocystic breast disease in general surgery, pre- or postoperative bone marrow transplant patient evaluations in hematology, presurgical physical examinations for cataract surgeries in ophthalmology, and prenatal examinations in obstetrics.

Billing

Like DIGMAs, Physicals SMAs are run as a series of one doctor–one patient encounters attending to each patient's unique medical needs individually (i.e., in both the group and the examination room). The individual physical examination segment of the Physicals SMA is clearly a series of one doctor–one patient encounters, but without observers. In addition, the interactive group segment of the Physicals SMA is basically a small DIGMA and is very much like a series of individual office visits with observers. In combination, the physical examination and interactive group segments of the Physicals SMA model provide essentially the same medical care as traditional individual physical examinations—but do so with greater efficiency, patient education, and attention to psychosocial needs (and with high levels of patient and physician professional satisfaction).

It is apparently for this reason that many (but not all) health care systems in the fee-for-service world bill for Physicals SMA (as well as DIGMA) visits very much as they do for traditional individual office visits, that is, according to the level of care delivered and documented using existing Evaluation and Management codes, but without charging for either counseling time or the behaviorist's time (for the same reasons as discussed earlier for the DIGMA model). Although billing issues are still evolving and have not been completely resolved, many health care organizations in the fee-for-service world are currently offering the DIGMA and Physicals SMA visits and are using existing Evaluation and Management codes, although they stand ready to adapt to any future changes in billing (which they can only hope will be carefully thought out and reasonable).

Weaknesses

The Physicals SMA model is unique among today's major group visit models because it focuses on physical examinations and not on follow-up appointments. Although Physicals SMAs work well in both primary and specialty care, many providers do not find this model to be at all intuitively obvious and therefore fail to consider implementing it in their practices. This is especially unfortunate because many physicians actually running them for their practices find their Physicals SMAs to be professionally satisfying and a "no brainer." They say this because of (1) the high levels of patient satisfaction engendered, (2) the dramatic increases in relative value units (RVUs) and productivity that this model can provide in the delivery of physical examinations, and (3) the improved access to physical examinations so often experienced once the model has been started.

Physicals SMAs suffer from many of the same weaknesses as the DIGMA model. For example, they require additional personnel, including a behaviorist, typically two nurses or medical assistants, and a documenter (plus a champion, program coordinator, and often dedicated schedulers in larger systems). These personnel resources might not be readily available within the system, and there will likely be competing demands for them. Because of the extensive documentation requirements that physical examinations entail, having a documenter is even more important for Physicals SMAs than for DIGMAs—yet, it is sometimes challenging to find an appropriate person within the system to act as documenter.

There are also facilities requirements, some of which might not be readily available to the provider. Although the group room can be substantially smaller than that required for a DIGMA, a group room is nonetheless required. A group room only half as large as that often required for a DIGMA can typically be used because only 7 to 10 patients typically attend a Primary Care Physicals SMA (rather than the 10 to 16 common for a DIGMA) and because (unlike DIGMAs) spouses and support persons are often not invited to attend.

Although there are facilities requirements, a benefit of the Physicals SMA model is that, unlike DIGMAs, a nearby examination room is not required. On the other hand, a disadvantage of the model is that two to five examination rooms are typically required for physical examinations (four are most common), although they can be in the physician's own office area rather than near to the group room (as is the case for DIGMAs). For example, in Primary Care Physicals SMAs dedicated to male patients, only two to four rooms might be required; however, in the case of female patients in primary care, four or five rooms are normally needed in order for the nurses to always stay ahead of the physician in rooming patients and performing all nursing duties so that the physician is never left in the hallway waiting for a patient to be roomed.

Another weakness is that the great efficiency and productivity gains provided by Physicals SMAs can create a different type of challenge, that is, from where to draw the patients in order to keep sessions filled once the physician's own backlog of patients has been eliminated. It is surprising how efficient this model is at providing physical examinations and at quickly working down backlogs and waiting lists. Once their own waiting list for physical examinations has been eliminated, the physician will need to create additional demand for the Physicals SMA to keep sessions filled to targeted census levels.

Finally, the behaviorist's job is more difficult. In a Physicals SMA, the provider is typically absent from the group room for approximately half the session when providing the individual, private physical examinations (one patient at a time, but with minimal discussion). As a result, another weakness of the Physicals SMA model is that it typically places greater pressure on the behaviorist than does the DIGMA model. This is especially true when the physician is absent from the group room providing individual physical examinations for all patients in attendance (which usually takes approximately the first half of the session), because the behaviorist is then essentially alone with the revolving small group of non-roomed patients for all of this time. It can be challenging for the behaviorist to keep the group moving and to make the best use of this time spent alone with patients (i.e., to keep the group productive, interactive, interesting, and helpful to all patients in the group room at all times).

The Logistics of Handling the Patient Packet Must Be Addressed

There are logistical and operational issues posed by the Patient Packet that is initially sent to patients when they register for a Physicals SMA, including who (this is typically a receptionist or motivated clerical person on the physician's staff) will (1) assemble and mail the packets to all patients when they initially schedule the Physicals SMA appointment; (2) take primary responsibility for receiving the completed health history forms from all patients (ensuring that they are returned to the office in a timely manner); and (3) follow up with patients who have not returned their health history form or completed their routine blood screening lab tests a few days before the session—explaining that patients must return their completed health history form and get their lab tests done prior to attending the Physicals SMA session (otherwise they will be postponed until the next appropriate session after these two items have been completed).

Final Comments on DIGMAs, CHCCs, and Physicals SMAs

Although improved access to physical examinations can also be important, follow-up visits for established patients are often of primary importance to chronic illness population management programs. Because DIGMAs and CHCCs focus on return appointments, it is these SMA models that are most often used in chronic illness treatment programs. Therefore, it is helpful to consider the differences between these two models to help readers clarify which model they might want to start with when first implementing a chronic illness group visit program. Many consider group visits to be ideally suited formats for better meeting the psychosocial and medical needs of the chronically ill, but one must never lose sight of the fact that SMAs can play an equally important role in improving physician management of busy, backlogged practices. Furthermore, to be fully successful, group visits must be carefully designed, adequately supported, well promoted to patients, and properly run.

DIGMAs Are Particularly Well Suited to Chronic Illness Treatment Programs

The DIGMA model is often considered ideal for chronic illness programs because of the many advantages it offers (see Table 3.3), including the facts that productivity and access are improved, that almost all patients in the chronic illness program can attend any time that they have a medical need, and that DIGMAs are widely used in fee-for-service systems. On the other hand, CHCCs offer the benefits of intense personal bonding for the same 15 to 20 high-utilizing patients in attendance (especially for those groups that have been meeting together for years) and of demonstrated reductions in emergency room, hospitalization, and nursing home costs for those patients who attend.

Which SMA Model Should You Start With?

Because the three major group visit models are very different both theoretically and operationally, it is likely that most health care providers will start with just one SMA model at a time. This is true even though it might evolve that all will be integrated into a chronic illness population management program, which can happen because they are mutually enhancing (not mutually exclusive) models, with benefits that can build upon one another.

In terms of which model to start with, it makes sense to select the model that best addresses your most pressing existing need. If your greatest need is improved access to follow-up visits, better practice management for a large and busy practice, or the development of a large chronic illness treatment program in a fee-for-service environment, then consider starting with the DIGMA model because these are some of its greatest strengths. On the other hand, if you are in a capitated system and have a small group of high-utilizing patients who are driving health care costs up, then consider starting with the CHCC. Finally, if increasing productivity, efficiency, and access to high-quality physical examinations is your primary issue, then start with the Physicals SMA model.

Summary

By developing chronic illness population management programs (particularly those that involve group visits), your patients will be better served not only with the benefits of an additional and effective health care choice but also with accessible, high-quality care that can result in both high levels of patient satisfaction and better outcomes. Patients also enjoy a multitude of additional benefits from properly run chronic illness population management programs involving group visits, including improved access to care; a multidisciplinary program specifically tailored to their needs; more time with their doctors; a more relaxed pace of care; greater patient education; closer attention to their mind as well as their body needs; the help and support of other patients integrated into their healing experience; and closer follow-up care.

Physicians benefit by being able to do something new and different that gets them off the fast-paced treadmill of individual office visit care—a treadmill that somebody always seems to be tweaking to go faster and faster so that evermore patients need to be seen with less and less time per patient. Physicians gain from the productivity and efficiency benefits that group visits offer, as well as their quality and patient education benefits. Physicians also benefit from their enhanced ability to better manage busy and backlogged practices and by having some fun during their work week—as group visits are meant to be voluntary, energizing, and fun for patients and providers alike.

In addition, physicians benefit by having a specifically trained multidisciplinary care delivery team available to them, onto whom they can offload many of their evergrowing responsibilities and duties. By so doing, what physicians are left with is what they most love to do—deliver high-quality, high-value medical care to each and every patient in attendance (and to more fully educate their patients about their illnesses, available treatment options, important lifestyle changes to make, and optimizing their own disease self-management skills).

Similarly, the organization benefits in numerous ways by fully utilizing group visits in chronic illness population management programs by having effective care pathways in place for efficiently treating various chronic illnesses and for achieving better outcomes; by the cost containment that comes from leveraging existing resources, improving access, and increasing productivity; through the competitive advantages that new chronic illness treatment programs can offer in the marketplace; and from the increased levels of patient and physician professional satisfaction that can be achieved (as happy physicians and patients translate into retained physicians and patients).

However, it must be cautioned that to fully capture the multiple quality, efficiency, economic, access, and patient–provider satisfaction benefits that such chronic illness population management programs involving group visits can offer (to patients, physicians, and organizations alike), these programs must be carefully designed, adequately supported, fully promoted to patients, and properly run.

References

1. Noffsinger EB. Increasing quality of care and access while reducing costs through Drop-In Group Medical Appointments (DIGMAs). Group Pract J 1999;48(1):2–18.
2. Noffsinger EB. Benefits of Drop-In Group Medical Appointments (DIGMAs) to physicians and patients. Group Pract J 1999;48(3):21–28.
3. Noffsinger EB. Will Drop-In Group Medical Appointments (DIGMAs) work in practice? Permanente J 1999;3(3):58–67.
4. Noffsinger EB. Enhance satisfaction with drop-in group visits. Hippocrates 2001;15(2):30–36.
5. Noffsinger EB. Solving departmental access problems with DIGMAs. Group Pract J 2001;50(10):26–36.
6. Beck A, Scott JC, Williams P, Robertson BJ, Jackson D, Gade G, Cowan P. A Randomized trial of group outpatient visits for chronically ill older HMO members: the cooperative health care clinic. J Am Geriatr Soc 1997; 45(5):543–549.
7. Scott JC, Conner DA, Venohr I, Gade G, McKenzie M, Kramer AM, Bryant L, Beck A. Effectiveness of a group outpatient visit model for chronically ill older health maintenance organization members: a 2-year randomized trial of the cooperative health care clinic. J Am Geriatr Soc 2004;52(9):1463–1470.
8. Scott JC, Gade G, McKenzie M, Venohr I. Cooperative health care clinics: a group approach to individual care. Geriatrics 1998;53:68–81.
9. Scott JC, Robertson BJ. Kaiser Colorado's cooperative health care clinic: a group approach to patient care. Managed Care Q 1996;4(3):41–45.
10. Noffsinger EB, Scott JC. Understanding today's group visit models. Group Pract J 2000;49(2):48–58.
11. Noffsinger EB. Physicals Shared Medical Appointments: a revolutionary access solution. Group Pract J 2002;51(1):16–26.
12. Noffsinger EB. Operational challenges to implementing a successful Physicals Shared Medical Appointment program. Part 1: choosing the right type of shared medical appointment. Group Pract J 2002;51(2):24–34.
13. Noffsinger EB. Working smarter. Physicians Pract 2002;12(3):18–22.

4
Chronic Disease Care: Creating Practice Change

Thomas A. Balsbaugh

Change is Difficult: Summary

1. Most of our practices are driven by the "tyranny of the urgent": the need to provide services for acute problems.
2. Most of us feel that we are working at maximum capacity, that adding anything more will simply result in working longer hours.
3. It is hard to implement change; very few of us have had any training in other models of care.
4. The Chronic Care Model developed by Ed Wagner offers a structure for developing a disease management program.
5. Start by building a team; improvements in chronic disease care are not likely to occur without the help of a team.
6. Start with a champion. Team building for chronic disease care must start with a champion.
7. To start the improvement project, the team must observe the processes and problems that occur in the office environment.
8. Start with a patient story. Patient stories about what went right and what went wrong can be powerful tools for sorting out process improvement.
9. Designate time to talk about process improvement. Consider using a "huddle" at the beginning of the clinic day.
10. Work to develop team cohesiveness; declare "success" whenever you can.
11. Assessing importance is the most critical task for any team trying to accomplish improvements in chronic illness care. You should always check to ensure that the entire team believes in the importance of any change project. If there is not agreement about the importance of an intervention, it is not likely to be successfully implemented.
12. Assessing the confidence of the team in achieving the goal is equally important. If the members are not confident that they can make a particular intervention work, it is not likely to succeed. Remember the motto: "Pick low-hanging fruit."

13. Ask the three questions recommended by Langley, Nolan, and Nolan in *The Improvement Guide:*
    a. What are you trying to accomplish?
    b. How will you know that a change is an improvement?
    c. What changes can you make that will result in improvement?
14. A study of the *Improving Chronic Care Collaborative* found that teams pursuing change projects were most effective when they chose initiatives directly linked to patient satisfaction.
15. A tool for taking a proposed change and building one successful change upon the next is the Plan-Do-Study-Act (PDSA) cycle.

Background

"Your numbers don't look so good. I know you've been trying hard. How do you want to improve things?"

You might think this is part of a typical conversation between a patient and a doctor, but it could be something else. You might have this conversation with your medical director, or the CEO of your hospital, or the medical director from a health plan. Just as patients need to change for better health, health organizations need to change. Change is difficult. People resist change.

Why is it difficult to make changes in the system for chronic disease? This question has been addressed by a number of experts [1,2]. For the most part, our practices are driven by the "tyranny of the urgent": the need to provide services for acute problems. This drives many of us to apply an acute care model to chronic conditions; care is only given when care is demanded. Another common concern is that "working harder is not an option." Most of us already feel that we are functioning at maximum capacity. "Clinical inertia" is another reason that practices fail to change. Phillips and associates [3] used this term to describe recognition of a problem but failure to act. The Chronic Care Model, developed by Ed Wagner [2], offers a structure for building a disease management program. In addition to the macrostructure of disease management, teams must develop a microstructure to help create practice change. This chapter is dedicated to understanding how to make changes in your clinical system.

Build a Team

Improvements in chronic disease care cannot be accomplished without a team. As the physician, you can perform some, but not all, roles in chronic disease management. For example, you cannot call all the patients in your practice who have diabetes and remind them of the need for a flu shot. You are not going to be able to provide detailed dietary counseling to every patient who needs it. You will not be able to monitor the office flow each day and identify the patients with chronic illness who are not being booked for a planned follow-up visit. We already work in teams with well-delineated roles. The office staff provides many of the activities involved in chronic illness care. Some of these care teams exist explicitly, and some are more difficult to recognize. To successfully implement disease management, you must build a clearly recognizable team focused on improving the care of patients who have chronic medical problems.

Start with a Champion

Team building for chronic disease care must start with a champion. If you are reading this book, you may be the champion. The champion provides initial motivation, guidance, and vision. Some teams will have more than one champion. As teams mature, the champion may change or the role may change. Shortell and associates [4] found that successful teams for chronic disease management were more likely to have a physician champion. Although their study found a critical need for physician leadership, there are other team members who may be effective champions for chronic disease management. The champion needs to be able to get other people interested in improving chronic disease care. Coercion rarely works. A "top down" approach rarely works. The champion has to make the case that chronic disease management is fun and important and will make life easier for patients and providers.

Starting the Process

To start the improvement project, the team must observe the processes and problems that occur in the office environment. The office environment is often referred to as a "microsystem" [5]. Every care team operates in a clinical microsystem. The team members and the activities they perform define the microsystem. As the champion builds a team, team members will help determine the boundaries of the microsystem. If team members stray beyond the boundaries of the microsystem, they face outside influences that they may have little or no control over. Early in the process of developing a team and getting started, this can lead to substantial frustration. For this reason, one of the most important tasks of the team is to ensure that the right team members are included to understand and influence the microsystem.

Effective teams understand each team member's role in the microsystem. One approach used to understand roles is to "follow a patient." This approach is a widely used quality improvement technique and is part of an evaluation by the Joint Commission on Accreditation of Healthcare Organizations. In this approach, your team will follow the care of a patient or a group of patients and observe the processes of care. For example, when our team was working on ways to improve access to care for patients with diabetes, we started with drawing a flow diagram on a chalkboard. The diagram started with the patient trying to set up a visit with his or her provider; went through all of the processes needed to be seen, including checking in to the clinic, having vital signs done, and being placed in an examination room; and ended with the provider ordering laboratory tests and asking the patient to set up a follow-up visit. Everyone on the team had the chance to analyze what could or should happen at each step. The team should learn about the processes involved in a particular aspect of chronic illness care, but they will also learn about the people and their roles.

Start with a Patient Story

During the weekly staff meeting, Dr. Goodman told everyone about Mrs. Johnson and her struggle during a recent visit to the emergency room with asthma. "Because it was a weekend, Mrs. Johnson didn't think anyone from the office could help her. Her albuterol inhaler was expired, and she had been feeling worse since she caught a cold the previous week. She had meant to get it filled during her last visit for a pap smear, but she forgot to mention her asthma. On Friday night, Mrs. Johnson was so desperate that she bought some over-the-counter asthma medicine. After taking it she felt strange, 'like my chest would explode.' She called the doctor on call, but it was someone who was cross-covering and didn't know her. He told her that she ought to go to the ER. The patient knew there would be a long wait in the ER, and she tried to see if her cold would get better on its own. Finally, on Sunday, she was feeling more short of breath and tired. She waited in the ER waiting room for 2 hours, and then was seen by the ER attending. She was found to be significantly hypoxemic, and she appeared to be deteriorating clinically. The ER physician elected to intubate Mrs. Johnson. She received intravenous steroids and improved enough to be extubated the next morning. I got up early this morning to see her in the hospital. As I drove back to the office for our meeting, I just couldn't help wondering if we could have done things differently to avoid this hospitalization."

Personal stories help keep your team grounded. Encourage all team members to share their perspective on a patient's story. Respecting the differing roles of team members is important for effective teamwork. The champion should not dominate this process. Good facilitation is important for clarifying each team member's role. Consider using a rotating facilitator. Each team member is an important part of every microsystem for chronic disease care.

Designate Time: Consider Using a "Huddle"

The pager beeped for the fourth time in 10 minutes. The only physician who was able to attend walked out of the lunch meeting; the two medical assistants and the office manager sighed. The meeting came to an abrupt halt, and the remaining team members ate lunch. A few minutes later, a receptionist walked into the room and announced that the pharmaceutical sales representative wanted to speak with a physician. A nurse walked in saying that she wouldn't be able to make the team meeting because a sick patient had arrived just as lunch started. The two remaining medical assistants decided that they needed to get ready for a busy afternoon. Finally, the office manager gathered the packets labeled "Chronic Disease Management Kick-Off Project," and she returned to her office to work on a pile of insurance company denials.

This may sound familiar to you. As you start your journey toward improved chronic disease management, you will always be reminded about the "tyranny of the urgent." Things that need immediate attention always seem to crowd out long-term projects. Every team needs to designate regular, brief times to meet. If the team can only "add on" time to usual meetings, the approach is rarely effective. As you get started, practice leadership must donate this time in good faith, hoping for a "return on investment." Carving out time demonstrates the value of the activity. It can also create an appropriate sense of expectation. If the pressure of routine operations prevents carving out regular meeting time, a practice could consider the brief team huddle before beginning patient care each day. The huddle can be used after an initial planning meeting. This technique requires the team to gather for 10 to 15 minutes before the beginning of a typical day. It can take place at the point of care. It usually requires a strong facilitator who will guide a brief agenda with careful attention to time.

Every effective meeting will need ground rules. The team in the example given earlier would benefit from ground rules. Your team should choose these together. A simple rule could be something like "Leave your pagers with the person covering the phones" or "Before you oppose an idea, you must propose an alternative." They usually include a few fundamental concepts: respect the opinions of others, use time judiciously, and support teamwork. Your ground rules should help you minimize interruptions, reduce tension between team members, and enable you to enjoy being part of the team.

Meetings for chronic disease management should be fun. If you ask your team to attend a meeting that is not part of the usual day, the members better believe that this meeting will make life better for the patients and the team. Making the meetings enjoyable will encourage attendance and sustain your group when the work is difficult. There are many examples of strategies for effective team building during meetings. One team-building strategy is actually an entire workplace philosophy known as the "Fish! Philosophy" [6]. This program was developed out of a successful management approach at Seattle's World Famous Pike Place Fish. If you ever have been to the Pike Place Market, you probably remember the unique energy and enthusiasm of the team that sells fish. The Fish Philosophy encourages team members to have fun while working to create team energy. It emphasizes the team members' choice of attitude that allows them to be fully present at work for assisting other team members and customers. It uses a cartoon-like fish motif to promote shared principles and goals. There is an instructional video describing the "Fish! Philosophy." You should considering acquiring this brief video and having your team watch it together early in the process of your development.

For effective team building, you should work to encourage participation from all team members in your meetings. Consider starting a "team ritual" used at the end of every meeting. No matter how things go with our team meetings, we've developed the habit of saying "success" in unison at the end of every meeting. Sometimes it is said with great enthusiasm, sometimes with a hint of sarcasm. It tends to make us laugh and put things in the right perspective. Meetings should help you accomplish your goal, but they also play the important role of reaffirming team cohesiveness.

Tools for Helping Clinical Systems Change

There are many parallels between how an organization changes and how people with chronic illness change. For patients, health behavior change theory suggests that importance and confidence are key concepts to explore. Specifically, when you are working with a patient on making a health behavior change, you ask your patient the following two questions: How important is this to you? How confident are you that you can make this change? [7] (see Chapter 2 for more details). These themes can be useful when working with health professionals to change the clinical systems for chronic disease care. This approach builds parallel processes; as clinicians use tools to understand their own organizational change efforts, they become more skilled at talking about behavior change with patients.

> The medical director of the large multispecialty group had recently attended a number of disease management conferences. He decided that one office needed to initiate an asthma improvement project. He decided that it would provide asthma action plans to all patients who were treated for an acute exacerbation. Two months after initiating the project, he found that most of the physicians did not know about the program. The medical assistants reported that they did not have time to review the action plans with patients. A few patients reported that the action plan was confusing to read. The office manager said that she had not been able to plan for the resources necessary to staff the intervention.

Assessing importance is the most critical task for any team trying to accomplish improvements in chronic illness care. To assess importance, your team members need to understand *why* they will address a particular problem. What problems are most important to your organization? Do all the team members view the problem as important? Overestimating the importance of a particular task is a common problem in quality improvement efforts. The example depicted above shows the usual outcome when you overestimate importance and lack buy-in. In behavior change theory, this problem is often referred to as "jumping ahead" [7]. In disease management, a team leader can also jump ahead, particularly if he or she chooses the problem and an intervention without gaining a greater understanding from the entire team. In addition to weakening team dynamics, this approach may lower the likelihood of a successful intervention. To find out the importance of a problem, ask about the perspective of each team member when discussing an overall problem. Hearing these stories will allow the entire team to learn where different people get satisfaction in their work. It also allows the group to build a common goal. Our team used the phrase "pick low-hanging fruit" as a means to reinforce taking on tasks that we felt were doable.

Assessing confidence is another crucial task when trying to make changes. Confidence reflects the team members' belief that the team can be successful. To assess team confidence, your members need to understand *how* they will accomplish a particular goal. To achieve improved chronic illness care, all members must have the appropriate confidence to fulfill their role in the microsystem. Confidence can also be increased by expanding your team to include every role in the processes of care. Langley, Langley, and Nolan's Model for Improvement [8] provides tools for your team to find out what is important, and to build the confidence of its members. The process they emphasize for improvement is based on the following three questions:

1. What are you trying to accomplish?
2. How will you know that a change is an improvement?
3. What changes can you make that will result in improvement?

What Are You Trying to Accomplish?

The first step in the Model for Improvement is to determine what you are trying to accomplish [8]. This would be the overall goal for your chronic disease intervention. Your team may choose to start with a broad problem, such as improved care for patients with heart failure, and then begin to narrow the goal. Alternatively, you could start with a specific problem that has "naturally" presented itself to the team. This overall goal will serve as a guiding principle or "aim statement." Choosing a more specific aim statement may be more helpful in directing your team during their journey toward improvement. One example of a specific aim statement might be "Our goal is to prevent any hospital readmission for patients with heart failure, within one month of discharge." The Institute for Healthcare Improvement [9] suggests five important tasks related to making effective aim statements:

1. State the aim clearly. Clarity will help achieve agreement, provide guidance, and maintain progress.
2. Include numeric goals that require fundamental change to the system. Numeric goals help to create urgency for change and will direct measurement.
3. Set stretch goals. Setting "out of the box" goals can help members to look for novel solutions that will overcome the usual barriers.
4. Avoid aim drift. Try to avoid reducing the stretch goal.
5. Be prepared to refocus the aim. Making the focus more targeted can be helpful.

The aim statement should be crafted by the team and posted for everyone to see. This can serve as a constant reminder for a collective goal. Once you have established your goal, the team can move on to measurements.

How Will You Know That a Change Is an Improvement?

This is the second fundamental question in the Model for Improvement [8]. Your team members will require measurements to determine if they are on the right course toward the overall goal. With measurements, your team can make predictions, learn, draw conclusions, and modify processes.

> The chronic pain management team made an aim statement: "Reduce the number of visits for chronic pain exacerbations by 50%." To measure the progress, the team sought visit data from the computerized scheduling system. The team found that it was unable to determine the reason for a visit from the computer system. Members elected to gather data by hand using a simple survey. They considered giving a survey to the providers each time they saw a patient for an exacerbation of chronic pain, but the providers said that there would not be time to complete it during their busy day. The team decided to survey the patients directly when they arrived for a pain exacerbation visit. They used this data to plan their first change project.

In the earlier example, the team agreed that it did not understand the microsystem well enough to make a prediction. In this example, measurements are used to help the team form a hypothesis. In other situations, the team may already have a working hypothesis about a potential change project. In such cases, measurements are used to test the hypothesis. Finally, when the team agrees that a particular change is helpful for achieving a goal, measurements are used to monitor progress implementing the change.

There are different types of measurements used in improvement projects. *Global outcome measures* are important for determining your progress toward your overall goal. An example of a common outcome measure for a population of patients with hyperlipidemia might be "the annual number of myocardial infarctions." In some cases, the overall goal is very broad or involves many complex processes. For these situations, an intermediate goal might be more helpful in determining your progress toward the ultimate goal. These are known as *proxy outcome measures* or intermediate outcomes. A well-known example for diabetes mellitus is the HbA1c level. When a group of patients has HbA1c levels less than 7%, research has shown that these patients will have fewer microvascular complications. The last type is the *process measure*. Processes describe the workings of the microsystem. These measures determine if the parts or steps of care are working as planned. An example of this is "the percentage of newly diagnosed asthma patients given a peak flow meter by the medical assistant." To facilitate more team learning, it is often helpful to use a combination of these measures.

Teams will usually choose measures as they simultaneously plan changes. Occasionally, the team may choose to avoid an intervention because they believe the measurements will be too burdensome. Measurements are only a tool. Teams could spend a great deal of time picking the perfect measurements or designing elaborate data collection. It may be more productive for the team to choose simple measures and simple methods for data collection. The process of collecting data should be built into the process of care whenever possible. Brief surveys or forms can be used to gather information. Only a sample is needed to test a hypothesis. Improvement projects are not the same as medical research. Learning and changing your microsystem is the goal, not discovering new medical knowledge. Consider simple chart audits to gather information; you do not need a certain sample size with power calculations. You only need enough data to help your team make decisions. Measurements are used to change the degree of belief that an intervention will result in improvement.

What Changes Can You Make That Will Result in Improvement?

The Model for Improvement's third question is the root of every care improvement project and can be alternatively stated as "What changes will help us move to our overall goal?" [8]. Brainstorming is a key activity that will help every team address this question. As discussed above, team members can describe a story to improve the understanding of the processes and decisions involved in care. This type of brainstorming can be visually supported using a flow diagram, as mentioned earlier in this chapter, following a patient through a process.

A whiteboard or poster and pens can be used to illustrate what happens in your microsystem. The team should label steps of a particular problem, including the processes, the decisions, and the various roles of different team members. Advanced technology may aid the team. Programs like Microsoft Visio can be used to map out the problem using symbols and pathways. This will allow the flow diagram to be shared as an electronic document.

Brainstorming possible change projects should be a creative but systematic process. After producing a flow diagram for the current microsystem, the team can write possible changes directly onto the existing workflow. Create new thought patterns by rearranging the steps in a process or challenging the usual boundaries. List all of the "unavoidable" barriers, and write all of the possible ways these would be eliminated no matter how outlandish. This will stimulate a variety of possible change projects. Display the flow diagram near the actual place where your team is working. This will help stimulate ideas that are related to observations. The list of possible changes should be maintained and can be systematically tested, either sequentially by your entire team, or simultaneously by subgroups within your team.

As each idea is discussed, members should ask themselves a number of questions: How is this different? Does this avoid spending more time, money, resources? Are you sure this increases value for patients or customers? Dedicate enough time for creative thinking. A study of the Improving

Chronic Care Collaborative found that teams pursuing change projects were most effective when they chose initiatives directly linked to patient satisfaction [4]. This focus on the customer is usually well received by managers and financial leaders.

> The Anytown Family Practice diabetes improvement team chose to do group visits as part of its change project. At first the members discussed a year-long project in which each provider would try a group visit. They decided that it would be too difficult to have all of their providers doing this trial for all of the patients. Instead, they decided to have three interested providers offer a group visit and a follow-up group for 10 of their interested patients. They agreed that this would help them learn about the value and cost of group visits without dramatically changing the usual business of the office.

The change project that your team chooses should not be too large. The change project is only a step in the journey to your overall goal. Choosing too big of a project can make a team feel overwhelmed or helpless. Small projects may allow more rapid assessment of effectiveness and create more opportunities to try the next logical change. Small projects will also help a team feel successful and encourage participation and enthusiasm.

It is the sequential and iterative nature of changes that helps teams create long-lasting significant change. The tool for taking a proposed change and building one successful change upon the next is the Plan-Do-Study-Act (PDSA) cycle.

A Tool for Testing Changes: The PDSA Cycle

> The public health center staff were trying to lower the rates of smoking for their patients with chronic obstructive pulmonary disease (COPD). A chart audit done the previous year showed that nearly half of their patients with COPD smoked. Their goal was to reduce this rate to 25% in the upcoming year. After a team meeting they decided to try organizing a smoking cessation support group. They believed that most of the patients with COPD had tried quitting, but many restarted smoking after a few months. They hypothesized that a support group would help those who had already quit maintain tobacco abstinence. To measure the effectiveness of their change, the staff surveyed the patients when they first joined the group, to determine who had already quit smoking. They surveyed the group at one month and at

two months to see how many of the patients were still abstinent from tobacco. After two months the team determined that there were very few patients in the group who had actually quit smoking. They also learned that many of the patients who had quit did not attend the two-month meeting, but there were many attendees who were thinking of quitting. The group decided to change the focus of the support group to assist those people who were considering quitting.

Without the concept of a PDSA cycle, this group might have continued to believe that the support group helped maintain patients who had already quit smoking. Without using an iterative approach, the team could have concluded that the support group was a failure. Instead, the team used the PDSA cycle to test a hypothesis. Not only did they disprove their hypothesis but they also learned that many of the patients who wanted to quit continued to attend meetings.

The PDSA process is a familiar idea for health care providers (Figure 4.1). The origin of the PDSA is traced to Edward Deming, who helped

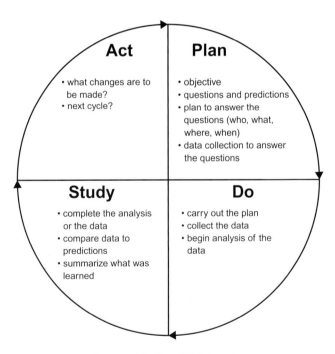

FIGURE 4.1. The PDSA cycle.

rebuild industry in Japan after World War II. The process uses basic principles of scientific thought:

1. Use the available information to form a hypothesis and determine how you could test the hypothesis (Plan).
2. Carry out the test (Do).
3. Gather your observations and analyze. Compare this to your hypothesis (Study).
4. Change your hypothesis and incorporate this change into your next cycle (Act).

Measures play a role in each aspect of the cycle. During Plan, the team will determine what measures they will use. During Do, the team will document the expected and unexpected observations. During Study, the team will analyze the data and compare them with the predictions. During Act, the team will use the conclusions to drive a change in the hypothesis.

Plan

The Plan phase is started with one of the three fundamental improvement questions mentioned earlier: "What changes can you make that will result in improvement?" After the team has chosen the change project, a few other specific tasks must be accomplished as part of the Plan phase. Members should try and make a prediction as part of their plan. For example, "We believe that giving patients peak flow meters will result in earlier presentations of asthma flares." Hopefully, the proposed change project will test their hypothesis. As part of the Plan phase, members should also develop a written plan to determine how they will carry out the change project. This plan should address the following questions: Who will do each part of the task? What are the tools needed? Where will it happen? When will it be done? A well-made Plan should balance completeness with time efficiency. Much of the learning that happens in the PDSA cycle will actually happen in the next phase (Do).

Do

The Do phase is the critical part to completing PDSA cycles. In this part of the cycle team members will execute the actual change. This is often challenging because it occurs in the everyday world outside of meeting time. The Do phase will be what is most visible to many outsiders and has a great effect on the morale of team members. Documenting problems and unexpected observations is critical for the next phases of the cycle.

Study

The Study phase is the integration of the observations and the analysis of measurements. It is often helpful to graphically present data to promote a better understanding of the observations. Members should test observations against their predicted results. This comparison will increase or decrease the belief that a particular change will result in improvement.

Act

The next phase (Act) incorporates the team's learning into a change in the plan. The Act phase is always a prelude to the next Plan. Team members have learned from their prediction and observation, and now they must incorporate this learning into the objectives of the next cycle. The Act phase cannot exist without the next cycle being initiated.

The Diabetes Self-Management Education Team was trying to decrease the number of patients who developed foot ulcers. They predicted that patients who watched a video on foot care were more likely to engage in daily self-foot examinations. They planned an intervention to mail a DVD about diabetic foot care to a group of high-risk patients. Before mailing the video, nursing staff called 20 patients and asked them to report when they had last examined their own feet. They were also asked four simple questions about how they checked their own feet. The reception staff mailed the foot self-examination video to 10 of these patients. Two months later the nurse called the same 20 patients and asked the same questions about foot self-examination. The patients who had seen the video reported higher rates of foot self-examination and had a better understanding of what was done during the examination. The patients who received the video asked the nurse if any other video education material were available. The patients who did not receive the video were surprised and happy to have received a call from a nurse. The Education team met to discuss the results. In this small test, their hypothesis was confirmed; patients who saw the self-examination video were more likely to perform self-examinations. The team learned that patients enjoyed being called and enjoyed viewing video education materials. The team changed their hypothesis for the next cycle. In the next plan, the team predicted that patients who received video education materials and a phone call from an office nurse were more likely to engage in self-care activities.

Linking Your Cycles

To successfully create long-lasting change, your team must link a series of small changes. The learning and energy created by a series of cycles is what will drive continuous improvement. Each individual small change may not appear to be a large step toward the overall goal, but it is the repetition of cycles that allows you to make the greater gains. When the goal of your PDSA cycle is learning, it leaves the door open for an unexpected benefit. These "hidden gems" can propel you toward your overall goal faster than anticipated. For a change to become a fundamental part of the care you give to your patients, there must be a high degree of belief that it will result in an improvement. Your team will test many changes in the journey to these improvements. Each of the PDSA cycles will increase or decrease your belief that the change is an improvement. After each cycle you will compare your actual results to the predicted results and plan the next cycle. This will occur as you develop a change, when you test a change, and when you try implementing a change.

Summary: Lessons Learned

Making improvements for chronic disease care should be an unending process. This journey begins with setting an overall goal, the aim statement. The journey is supported by measurement to serve as a guide for improvement: "How will we know the change is an improvement?" Choose a combination of measures that will allow you to understand the outcomes of your change and the process measures for each step. Brainstorm to find out how you could achieve your goal: "What changes can we make that would result in improvement?" Your team will need to choose the change projects wisely. Understand the different roles of each team member. Make sure that your project is important to the entire team. Assess the confidence for the project to succeed. If confidence is low and the risk of the project is high, consider a smaller project. Use the iterative approach of a PDSA cycle. Form a hypothesis, test it, make conclusions, form a new hypothesis, and start a new cycle to retest. By linking one cycle to the next your team will create a momentum for change. Your team should always be learning. As part of a learning collaborative that our team participated in, one of the most important elements of the process was to take the time to reflect back on "lessons learned." Table 4.1 lists some of the lessons we learned.

This may sound idealized, but working harder is not an option. To support better care we must work together. We must work smarter. Your organization will be more successful if you promote customer service, build teamwork, and promote learning. Go forward team. Declare Success.

TABLE 4.1. Lessons learned.

Lesson	Implication
"Pick low-hanging fruit."	Do not take on too big a project at first. Take on things that are doable, things that your team believes can be done.
"Go for the 80% solution."	When you are coming up with a solution/intervention, don't go for the perfect solution. It is okay to go for an almost perfect solution. You are more likely to be successful.
"When you find an obstacle, go around it."	There are plenty of barriers in getting change projects started and completed. Some of these barriers are processes; some of these barriers are people. Do not waste time, if possible, going up against these barriers. Find creative ways around them.
"Declare success!"	Do this as often and freely as you can.

The office party wasn't for a holiday. It was a team success party. The staff received recognition awards. A large poster told the story of their success, including a graphic showing how the office had reached its overall goal. Staff had prevented every admission for diabetic foot ulcers for six months. The series of changes they accomplished began with gathering information using provider, staff, and patient surveys. Based on this information, the administrative staff started a program to increase overall awareness about foot health and diabetes, including posters and patient handouts. The front desk personnel made sure that patients had received an appointment to a group visit for education and a screening foot examination. High-risk patients received video education materials and a call from a nurse every six months. The team had abandoned a plan for sending all patients an e-mail reminder about foot examinations. A brief PDSA cycle had taught the team that the office did not have the technologic support to track the constant changes in patient e-mail addresses. However, the team did learn from the cycle that patients want some type of reminder. This unexpected finding led the team to send a note by mail to patients to remind them to schedule their screening foot examination. Everyone in the office had a successful role in this project. The team celebrated. As part of the festivities, they planned their next improvement target.

References

1. Bodenheimer T, Wagner EH, Grumbach K. Improving primary care for patients with chronic illness. JAMA 2002;288:1775–1779.
2. www.improvingchroniccare.org.
3. Phillips LS, et al. Clinical inertia. Ann Intern Med 2001;135:825–834.
4. Shortell SM, et al. The role of perceived team effectiveness in improving chronic illness care. Med Care 2004;42:1040–1048.
5. Nelson EC, et al. Microsystems in health care: Part 1. Learning from high-performing front-line clinical units. Joint Comm J Qual Improv 2002;28: 472–493.
6. www.Charthouse.com.
7. Rollnick S, Mason P, Butler C. Health Behavior Change. A Guide For Practitioners. Toronto: Churchill Livingstone, 1999.
8. Langley GJ, Nolan KM, Nolan TW, Norman CL, Provost LP. The Improvement Guide. A Practical Approach to Enhancing Organizational Performance. San Francisco: Jossey-Bass, 1996.
9. www.ihi.org.

5
Medication Management in Chronic Diseases

TIMOTHY W. CUTLER AND MARILYN STEBBINS

Summary

Over the past two decades a significant portion of the biotechnological advances in health care has involved pharmaceuticals. With the combination of the use of novel medications for new and existing indications, and the increasing number of new indications for older medications, prescription drug use and costs continue to be among the fastest growing segments of health care. In fact, over the past decade the Food and Drug Administration (FDA) has increased substantially the number of new drug approvals and has created a fast-track system for pharmaceutical manufacturers to expedite the approval process. This, however, has not come without a price tag from both the financial and utilization perspectives. Financially, there have been double-digit increases in pharmaceutical expenditures, while at the same time prescription drug coverage for individuals appears to be shrinking, thus increasing out-of-pocket expenditures. From the utilization perspective, with more drugs available and more indications for drugs, there has been an increase in polypharmacy, which can place the patient at risk for adverse drug reactions, drug interactions, and medication errors. With the passage of the Medicare Prescription Drug, Improvement, and Modernization Act of 2003 (MMA 2003), Medicare will be offering an outpatient prescription drug benefit for the first time in its 40-year history beginning in 2006. Although older Americans comprise 15 percent of the population, they account for about 40 percent of the drug expenditures [1]. Because of such statistics the new Medicare drug benefit is intended not only to improve access to medication therapy but also to ensure that medications are used safely and effectively [2]. This chapter includes information on polypharmacy, medication errors, and cost containment, as well as strategies for primary care providers to incorporate into their management of chronic diseases.

Polypharmacy

Summary

- Polypharmacy may be present when prescription or over-the-counter (OTC) medications are duplicating the therapeutics of other prescription medications.
- Polypharmacy and nonadherence to medications increase morbidity and mortality.
- Polypharmacy has a negative financial impact on the cost of health care and increases patient out-of-pocket spending.
- Nonadherence is closely linked to the number of medications a patient takes.
- Patients taking five or more medications are at twice the risk for developing medication-related adverse events than those who take fewer medications.
- Complete medication histories are crucial to identifying polypharmacy.
- The elderly are at particular risk for polypharmacy.

Background

The term *polypharmacy* is used to describe the use of multiple, and sometimes inappropriate, medications to treat disease. Polypharmacy can include the following:

- The use of duplicate medications to treat the same condition
- Medications that interact and cause adverse events
- Medications that interact with diseases and cause adverse events
- Medications used to treat unknown, undiagnosed, or poorly described conditions
- Dosing medications too high or too low

Polypharmacy may describe a situation in which the medication therapy treating a condition is not optimized, and multiple medications are used to treat disease when fewer agents could be used.

The overuse of medications to treat chronic conditions has been well documented [3]. Because of the breadth of evidence supporting medication use in chronic conditions, polypharmacy is common in patients with chronic disease. Patients with no chronic diseases fill an average of 1.5 prescriptions per year, while those with one chronic disease fill an average of 7.3 prescriptions per year, and those individuals with five or more chronic diseases fill an average of 52.7 prescriptions per year [4]. The treatment of a chronic condition with a single agent is nearly impossible, as national guidelines increasingly recommend more aggressive treatment and stricter goals [5–7]. For example, the American College of Cardiology recommends at least a four-drug combination for the routine treatment of congestive heart failure [5]. The Third Report of the National Cholesterol Education Program (NCEP) Expert Panel on Detection, Evaluation, and Treatment of High Blood Cholesterol in Adults (Adult Treatment Panel III, or ATP III) guidelines now have an optional low-density lipoprotein cholesterol (LDL-C) level goal of 70 mg/dL for very high-risk patients [6].

Given that chronic conditions are often associated with comorbidities, patients with chronic diseases may be treated for multiple conditions concurrently. The patient with diabetes may not be treated for diabetes alone, but also for the hyperlipidemia and hypertension that often accompany the disease. If long-term complications of diabetes (such as neuropathy, nephropathy, and gastroparesis) are present, then the use of multiple medications increases dramatically. Polypharmacy itself may become a chronic condition that needs management and oversight if left unnoticed. Considering that patients who take more than five medications are at twice the risk of developing adverse drug events from their medication regimen, the treatment of disease with multiple medications poses unforeseen risks to patients [8].

In addition to the risk of adverse events, the greater the number of medications taken, the less likely the patient is to adhere to the regimen [9]. Clinical practice guidelines for the treatment of chronic disease are based on clinical trials. These trials are performed in a highly controlled environment in which the patient may be more adherent to the medication regimen. In the typical "noncontrolled" outpatient setting, adherence to medication regimens may be reduced significantly, and, therefore, the outcomes are less predictable. Improving the adherence of patients with chronic disease may be the most important way to improve their health [9].

Costs

The costs associated with drug-related morbidity and mortality were estimated to exceed $177 billion in 2000 [10].

Epidemiology

Multiple studies have evaluated the issue of polypharmacy in the elderly, but data regarding nonelderly patients are not as well documented [11–13]. The elderly, however, tend to have multiple comorbidities and may be a better predictor of polypharmacy in chronic disease. In the United States it has been estimated that patients over the age of 65 years take an average of five or more medications [13]. A European survey evaluating community dwelling patients over the age of 75 years found that this population takes an average of 4.2 prescription medications and 2.5 OTC medications [12]. These studies indicate that older patients with multiple diseases are more likely to take more medications. Younger patients with multiple chronic diseases are also at risk for polypharmacy.

Management

The first step in evaluating a patient's drug therapy is to obtain complete information. It is critical to ask about all of the medications that a patient is prescribed (and/or taking), including OTC and herbal products. If the patient is a poor historian, have a family member attend the visit or have the patient bring in all of his or her medication bottles. It may become necessary to call the pharmacy (or pharmacies) to find out what the patient has received from the pharmacy, including the prescription fill dates. Patients who have multiple providers may have difficulty remembering all of their medications and who prescribed them. Patients may also receive conflicting information from different providers, and they may only report prescriptions from their primary provider and not other specialists. It has also been shown that medication documentation errors can be common in outpatient clinics [14].

A study performed in the internal medicine clinic at an academic medical center evaluated 39 patient charts containing at least three medications documented by the physician. Of the charts evaluated, 400 medications were evaluated for accuracy. Twenty-two percent of the medications reviewed had some type of error (defined as omitted dosing, incorrect strength, missing OTC medication information, or incorrect assumption of how the patient was taking the medication). Medication documentation errors may also be present at the time of hospital admission. Another study performed at an academic teaching hospital evaluated the errors on medication profiles of patients who reported taking four or more medications at the time of admission [15]. Fifty-three percent of patients evaluated had at least one unintended medication discrepancy. Most of these errors were not considered harmful to the patient, but 38.6 percent of the medical record discrepancies had potential to cause moderate to severe discomfort or clinical deterioration. Complete and accurate medical records are critical to the appropriate management of patients taking multiple medications.

Once complete prescription information is obtained, it is much easier to make informed decisions regarding appropriate medical care. Simple measures such as reviewing the purpose of each medication with patients will enable the provider to find anomalies in patient understanding of medication use. This process may also empower patients to improve adherence to their medication schedules. If patients are empowered, their care will improve [9]. In 2003, the World Health Organization reported on the importance of adherence and patient-centered programs focused on improving the care of the chronically ill. This report detailed that

Table 5.1. Factors that can impair adherence to medication therapy.

1. High-cost medications
2. Difficulty understanding medication directions
   a. Health literacy
   b. Language barriers
   c. Visual impairment
3. Taking multiple medications (pill burden)
4. Medications dosed at awkward or difficult intervals (multiple medications taken BID, TID, QID, and with meals)
5. Adverse events
6. Misinformation from the media or other caregivers
7. Unclear expectations of the effect of the medication (patients skipping doses when they "feel better," discontinuing medications when their condition does not improve, etc.)

empowered patients have better clinical outcomes than unmotivated patients. Empowered patients are more likely to adhere to their medication regimen and are more likely to adhere to lifestyle modifications. The more adherent to medications and lifestyle changes, the better the clinical and economic outcomes. This is evident in patients with metabolic syndrome, where education, diet, and exercise were found to be more effective in preventing the onset of diabetes than metformin alone [16]. Factors that may contribute to medication nonadherence are listed in Table 5.1.

Although there is evidence to indicate that a comprehensive approach is successful in improving medication adherence of the chronically ill, there are other modes to consider for patients with polypharmacy. For example, optimizing therapy to treat several conditions with one medication may reduce the number of unneeded medications and improve adherence. The use of a combination agent to treat several conditions at once or the use of a long-acting medication may simplify the medication regimen and decrease pill burden.

Before utilizing a combination product, the risks and benefits of this technique should be critically evaluated. The patient should be at the appropriate and individualized target dose for all the medications in the combination product. This will minimize the confusion and errors that may occur if one component of the combination needs the dose increased while the other agent stays constant. The costs of the combination agent should also be reviewed. Many combination products are not available on prescription drug formularies, and switching to these agents may increase the out-of-pocket costs to the patient. It is also important to maximize a medication's potential. This may include using its side effects to treat concomitant conditions. For example, a patient with weight loss, depression, and insomnia may be treated with the antidepressant mirtazepine, which has side effects of weight gain and sedation. Table 5.2 provides examples that may reduce polypharmacy and pill burden.

When evaluating a medication regimen, it is important to assess the patient's ability to adhere to the medications prescribed. There is no benefit in prescribing four medications to treat diabetes if the patient is only willing to take two. The key is to recognize that a problem may exist with the drug regimen. Often, in a 15-minute visit, the provider is unable to ask, "How do you take your medications?" or "What types of problems do you have with your medications?" If these questions are not asked, the provider may erroneously assume that the patient is adherent to the prescribed medications. Yet, if the patient is not at goal therapy, the provider may institute medication changes (i.e., increase the dose or add another medication) without realizing that the patient is not adhering to the current regimen. Such misinformation often leads to polypharmacy, poor adherence, and a frustrated provider.

The Elderly Population

The elderly are at particular risk for polypharmacy. Eighty percent of patients over the age of 65 years have one or more chronic conditions, and

TABLE 5.2. Techniques to reduce polypharmacy and pill burden.

1. Combine two medications into a single tablet*
   a. Ezetemide and simvastatin (Vytorin®)
   b. Glyburuide and metformin (Glucovance®)†
   c. Atenolol and chlorthalidone (Tenoretic®)†
   d. Lisinopril and hydrochlorothiazide (Prinivil HCT®, Zestoretic®)†
2. Use one medication to treat several conditions
   a. Mirtazepine for the treatment of insomnia and depression
   b. Hydrochlorothiazide for hypertension and osteoporosis
   c. Venlafaxine for depression and menopausal hot flashes
   d. Beta-blockers for hypertension after a myocardial infarction
   e. Pioglitazone for diabetes, high blood pressure, and high triglyceride level
3. Use extended-release products*
   a. Extended-release diltiazem QD in place of diltiazem immediate-release TID
4. Ensure no duplicate medications exist
   a. Include over-the-counter products, herbal products, dietary supplements, and vitamins
   b. Obtain a complete medication history from the pharmacy, other providers, and the patient's family, if necessary
   c. Do not assume a medication is prescribed for the indication you would expect without documentation listed in the chart (sometimes chart error may also occur, and an inappropriate medication may have been continued unnecessarily)

*This switch may increase the cost of the medication, which may impair the patient's ability to take the medication.
†Indicates that a generic product available.

50 percent have two chronic conditions [17]. The Council of Scientific Affairs for the American Medical Association reported that 66 percent of men and 88 percent of women over the age of 65 years consume at least one prescription medication per week [3]. In fact, patients over the age of 65 years consume over one-third of prescription drugs yet only comprise 15 percent of the population [1]. As the nation's largest health insurer, Medicare was not keeping pace, as it had never included an outpatient prescription drug benefit. With the passage of MMA 2003, Congress sought to create a drug benefit that not only improved access to drugs but also improved the use of medications to result in better patient outcomes and lower overall health care costs. The mechanism identified in MMA 2003 to address improved use of medications is Medication Therapy Management Services (MTMS) [2].

Essentially, health care providers will be reimbursed for their ability to manage polypharmacy as a chronic disease. Those providers (pharmacists, nurses, physicians, and physician extenders) who participate in MTMS are required to improve adherence, assess the health status of the patient, decrease out-of-pocket medication costs, and improve the patient's quality of life. It is clearly stated in MMA 2003 that those people performing MTMS must use an individualized approach and that population-based models (utilizing form letters, formularies, therapeutic substitution, etc.) will not meet the intent of MTMS. Although MTMS is the term used in MMA 2003 to describe medication management of the elderly, the same approach may be used for any patient with chronic disease. Specifically, a comprehensive program that identifies solutions to medication-related problems in chronic disease management is the best way to improve the care of individuals with long-term medical problems.

Another consideration regarding the elderly is their sensitivity and altered response to medications. Therefore, it is important to recognize that there are medications that are potentially inappropriate for the elderly. This list of medications is known as the Beers Criteria for Potentially Inappropriate Medications. First published in 1997, the Beers criteria were quickly adopted by Medicare and incorporated into long-term care regulations. The Beers criteria were updated in 2003 [18]. Although not an all-inclusive list, the Beers criteria help providers recognize potential issues with drug therapy for the elderly. The Beers criteria are separated into those medications that are inappropriate, independent of concomitant conditions, and those medications that are inappropriate based on specific conditions.

Although the Beers criteria have been recently distributed and taught in medical, pharmacy, and nursing schools, it is a relatively new approach to appropriate prescribing for the elderly. Thus, up to 25 percent of outpatient seniors are still prescribed potentially inappropriate and harmful medications (Table 5.3) [19,20].

TABLE 5.3. Medications considered inappropriate for the elderly.*

Drug class	Drugs	Concern
Nonsteroidal anti-inflammatory drugs (NSAIDs)	Indomethacin Ketorolac Naproxen	Indomethacin has the most central nervous system adverse events of the NSAIDs; NSAIDs may cause gastric ulceration
Tricyclic antidepressants	Amitriptyline Nortriptyline Doxepin	Highly anticholinergic and sedating medication and not generally considered the antidepressant of choice for this population
Long-acting benzodiazepines	Flurazepam Diazepam	Long half-life: drug may accumulate and cause excessive sedation, increase risk of falls
Anticholinergic drugs	Diphenhydramine Dicyclomine	Increase fall risk, heat intolerance; may cause constipation, and other adverse events; and may worsen Alzheimer's type dementia
Long-acting sulfonylurea (first generation)	Chlorpropamide	Long-acting antidiabetic medication, which may cause prolonged hypoglycemia and syndrome of inappropriate antidiuretic hormone
Opioids	Propoxyphene Pentazocine Meperidine	May not be an effective oral opioid agent; may cause confusion with chronic use. Meperidine has an active metabolite that may cause central nervous system irritation, confusion, or seizures
Muscle relaxants	Cyclobenzaprine Carisoprodol Chlorzoxazone	May cause sedation, weakness, and confusion; have high anticholinergic activities
Barbiturates (except when treating seizure disorders)	Phenobarbital Butalbital Pentobarbital	Highly addictive and cause sedation in the elderly; When used in combination with other agents to treat headaches, may cause rebound headache
Phenothiazines	Thioridazine Promethazine	High incidence of extrapyramidal effects, sedation; safer alternatives exist
Antiarrhythmics	Amiodarone Disopyramide	Amiodarone may cause QT prolongation and sedation; disopyramide has the most negative ionotropic effects of the antiarrhythmics and is highly anticholinergic. Other safer antiarrhythmics exist

*This list is independent of diagnosis or conditions. The agents listed in this table are considered highest risk. This is not a complete list of all the agents on the Beer's Criteria for Potentially Inappropriate Medications.
Source: Data from Fick, et al. [18].

Medication Errors

Summary

- Safe medication practices are the responsibility of all health care providers.
- Some abbreviations are not safe to use when prescribing drugs.
- Some medications are considered deadly if mistakes occur with their use; these are known as *high-alert medications.*
- The five "rights" of safe medication use are: right patient, drug, time, dose, and route, but this system relies on several individuals for effectiveness, including the prescriber, the pharmacist, and the nurse.
- Manual redundancies and independent double checks may detect 95% of errors [21].
- Errors should be reported and resolved in a nonpunitive environment. The evaluation of errors should focus on the root causes of the error, and organizations should focus on ways to reduce future errors.
- Fifty percent of those individuals with a chronic disease report that they or a family member have experienced a medical error. Only 30% of patients without a chronic disease report that they or a family member have experienced a medical error [22].

Background

The Institute of Medicine (IOM) Report "To Err is Human" highlights the consequences of errors in health care [23]. This report estimates that 44,000 to 98,000 people die each year in the hospital as a result of a medical error. Although the IOM report focuses on the errors related to inpatient hospital stays, the principles highlighted are also applicable to the outpatient setting (Table 5.4).

TABLE 5.4. The four-tiered approach toward improving patient safety in the IOM report *To Err is Human.*

1. Establish a national focus to create leadership, research tools, and protocols to enhance the knowledge base about safety.
2. Identify and learn from errors by developing a nationwide public mandatory reporting system and by encouraging health care organizations and practitioners to develop and participate in voluntary reporting systems.
3. Raise performance standards and expectations for improvements in safety through the actions of oversight organizations, professional groups, and group purchasers of health care.
4. Implement safety systems in health care organizations to ensure safe practices at the delivery level.

Source: Data are from the Institute of Medicine (http://www.IOM.edu).

TABLE 5.5. Patient information: Quick tips for patients receiving a new prescription.

1. Ask questions of your pharmacist or physician.
   a. What is the name of the medicine?
   b. What does the medicine do?
   c. What is the dose of the medicine?
   d. What are the side effects of the medicine?
   e. What other medicines, foods, or activities may interfere with the activity of this new medication?
   f. What do I do if I miss a dose or accidentally take more than I should?
2. When you pick up the medication at the pharmacy be sure it is the same medication prescribed by your doctor.
3. Make sure that your doctor and pharmacist know all of the medications you are taking before staring a new medicine.
4. Make sure you follow up with your physician after starting a new medication.

Source: U.S. Agency for Healthcare Research and Quality (AHRQ) (http://www.ahrq. gov/consumer/quicktips/tipprescrip.htm).

Discussion

The IOM report recommends establishing mandatory reporting systems that would store and receive serious adverse events. The IOM further recommends that providers understand the reason for an error and recognize the process and procedures that need to be changed to prevent further errors from occurring. The Institute of Safe Medication Practices (ISMP) supports this process and further recommends that systems be established that make error prevention cost effective and necessary for health systems [21]. When an error does occur, the IOM and ISMP recommend that a nonpunitive systematic approach that evaluates the root cause of the error be performed.

Medication-related errors are often preventable and cause significant morbidity and mortality [24]. There are several recommendations that providers can give patients to help minimize medication-related errors. These are listed in Table 5.5.

The Joint Commission Accreditation of Hospital Organizations (JCAHO) is also working to reduce medical errors. All JCAHO-accredited organizations are now required to have medication safety programs in place. The JCAHO has also established a list of "do not use" abbreviations that will help to reduce medication-related errors [25]. These are listed in Table 5.6. Although a comprehensive, nonpunitive, systematic approach is recommended to reduce medical errors, each provider of care should take responsibility to ensure that safe practices are utilized when prescribing medications to individuals with chronic disease.

TABLE 5.6. JCAHO official "Do Not USE" list.*

Do not use	Potential problem	What to write instead
U (unit)	Mistaken for "0" (zero) the number "4" (four) or "cc"	Unit
IU (International Unit)	Mistaken for IV (intravenous) or the number "10" (ten)	International Unit
Q.D., QD, q.d., qd (daily); Q.O.D., QOD, q.o.d, qod (every other day)	Mistaken for each other Period after the Q mistaken for "I" and the "O" mistaken for "I"	Daily; every other day
Trailing zero (X.0 mg); lack of leading zero (.X mg)	Decimal point is missed	X mg; 0.X mg[†]
MS; MSO$_4$ and MgSO$_4$	Can mean morphine sulfate or magnesium sulfate Confused for one another	Morphine sulfate; magnesium sulfate

*Applies to all orders and all medication-related documentation that is handwritten (including free-text computer entry) or on preprinted forms.
†Exception: A "trailing zero" may be used where required to demonstrate the level of precision of the value being reported, such as for laboratory results, imaging studies that report size of lesions, or catheter/tube sizes. It may not be used in medication orders or other medication-related documentation.
Source: © Joint Commission on Accreditation of Healthcare Organizations, 2005. Reprinted with permission.

Cost Containment

Summary

- Most providers do not know their patients' prescription drug coverage when prescribing medications during an office visit.
- Generic drugs are regulated and rated by the FDA. If a generic drug has an "AB" rating, it is therapeutically equivalent to the brand name medication and can be safely interchanged.
- Most pharmaceutical manufacturers have "free-drug programs" or patient-assistance programs to help low-income patients.
- Mail-order prescription drug programs can provide significant savings for patients with and without prescription drug coverage.

Background

Access to affordable prescription drugs is arguably the most critical health care issue facing Americans today. Expenditures in the United States for prescription drugs more than tripled during the 1993–2003 period and reached 179.2 billion in 2003, representing more than 11 percent of total health care expenditures [26,27]. This section will address cost-saving strategies for prescription medications that may assist providers in minimizing out-of-pocket expenses for patients.

It is estimated that more than 160 million Americans (64 percent) have prescription coverage from employer-sponsored health plans and that 69 percent of Medicare beneficiaries have some form of prescription drug coverage from sources other than Medicare [28,29]. Because of the increased demand for prescription drugs and rising prescription drug prices, health insurers have had to adopt cost-saving strategies such as formularies, quantity limits, prior authorization, copayments, generic drug programs, tiered formularies, and mail order. In addition to many of these strategies, employers and health plans are shifting a greater portion of prescription drug costs onto the patient and are steering them toward lower cost alternatives.

Unfortunately, many patients do not understand their prescription drug coverage and thus are not maximizing their cost-savings potential. Providers are also faced with a multitude of insurers in their daily practices and may not know how to help patients understand cost-saving opportunities. When prescribing medications, providers need to specifically ask patients about their prescription drug coverage. For example, does the insurance offer lower copayments for generic drugs? Do they have a tiered copay structure in which preferred generic drugs may have the lowest copayment, preferred brand name medications may have a higher copayment, and nonpreferred brand name medications have the highest copayment? Is there an incentive for patients to use mail order through their insurance, and does their local pharmacy allow more than a 30-day supply of medication to be dispensed? Table 5.7 describes how providers can help patients obtain information about their health plans.

Although most Americans have access to health insurance, the number of uninsured Americans is growing. In 2003, the federal government estimated that 45 million Americans (15.6 percent of the population) lacked coverage of any kind for an entire year. Other sources estimate that millions more go without health insurance for shorter periods of time [30].

TABLE 5.7. Patient information: Understanding prescription drug coverage.

1. Call the member services number on your insurance card.
2. Inquire about the pharmacy benefit:
   a. Does the insurance company have a formulary list?
   b. Is there is a difference in copay for different drugs?
   c. What is the copay for generic drugs? Brand name drugs? Nonformulary drugs?
   d. Does it offer mail order services?
   e. Is there a financial benefit to using mail order? What is the benefit?
   f. Can you get a copy of the formulary?
3. Does the insurance company have this information on a Web site that is accessible to patients and providers?
4. Contact your local pharmacy and ask for information specific to your insurance.

TABLE 5.8. Cost-saving strategies.

1. Have an honest and open discussion with patients regarding drug costs.
2. Know the costs of commonly prescribed prescription medications.
3. Ensure that patients maximize their reimbursement potential through their insurance.
4. Maximize generic drug use.
5. Consider lower cost brand name medications.
6. Consider tablet splitting when appropriate.
7. Utilize all available assistance programs.
   a. Pharmaceutical industry–sponsored patient assistance programs
   b. Pharmaceutical industry–sponsored discount cards
8. Determine whether mail order can provide cost savings.
9. Periodically review all medications with the patient and whether each is necessary to maintain or improve the health of the patient

Because of this lack of coverage, the cost of prescription medications is often prohibitive in this vulnerable population, and adherence can be affected. Cost-containment strategies should not only be applied to the uninsured. Providers need to practice cost-effective prescribing for all patients to decrease overall health care expenditures and minimize patient out-of-pocket expenses (Table 5.8).

One of the most effective ways to reduce out-of-pocket spending is to maximize generic drug use. This strategy alone, however, will not ensure low drug costs for patients with multiple chronic diseases, as many drugs do not have generic equivalents. Thus, brand name medications cannot be avoided in many chronic conditions. It is important for providers to know the cost of brand-name-only drugs used to treat chronic conditions in order to comprehend the financial burden that is being placed on the patient.

Another less commonly used strategy involves tablet-splitting drugs that have flat pricing. A drug is considered to be flat priced when the cost of the medication remains the same regardless of the strength. For example, Lipitor 20mg, 40mg, and 80mg are all priced the same per tablet. If a patient is taking 20mg of Lipitor, the formulation and pharmacokinetics of this drug make it possible to cut the 40-mg tablet in half and dose one-half of a tablet per day, thereby cutting the cost of therapy in half. It is important to note that tablet splitting may not be appropriate for all flat-priced drugs. Some cannot or should not be split (e.g., sustained-release formulas, capsules, bitter-tasting drugs).

If generic drugs are maximized and the lowest cost brand name drugs are being used, and a patient is still unable to afford his or her medications, there are other programs that may be available to providers and patients. Most pharmaceutical companies have programs that provide free or low-cost brand name drugs to patients in need, and recently a program became available that also provides low-cost generic medications. These are often referred to as indigent programs or patient-assistance programs. Unfortunately, the programs can be confusing and difficult to use, as each company uses different forms, eligibility criteria, renewal processes, and mechanisms for the patient to obtain medications [31]. For these reasons, many of the programs are underutilized. There are, however, several useful Web sites to assist patients and providers in obtaining necessary information to successfully obtain medications (Table 5.9).

Another cost-saving option for those who need prescription drug assistance is pharmaceutical manufacturer-sponsored drug discount card programs. Drug discount card programs differ from patient-assistance programs. These discount card programs are intended for those patients whose income is above the levels necessary to qualify for patient-assistance programs. Many of these applications do not require a physician's signature

TABLE 5.9. Patient information: Useful patient-assistance Web sites and resources.

www.pparx.org
The Partnership for Prescription Assistance brings together America's pharmaceutical companies, doctors, other health care providers, patient advocacy organizations, and community groups to help qualifying patients who lack prescription coverage get the medicines they need through the public or private program that is right for them. Many can get their medicines free or nearly free. Among the organizations collaborating in this program are the American Academy of Family Physicians, the American Autoimmune Related Diseases Association, the Lupus Foundation of America, the NAACP, the National Alliance for Hispanic Health, and the National Medical Association. To access the Partnership for Prescription Assistance by phone, you can call toll free, 1-888-4PPA-NOW (1-888-477-2669).

www.rxassist.org
This Web site was created by Volunteers in Health Care to help physicians and other health care providers obtain the information they need to access pharmaceutical companies' patient-assistance programs. This site is very useful. It contains information about the federal poverty level, detailed information on individual patient-assistance programs (including eligibility, contact, and processing information, and forms that can be downloaded) This site also allows easy searching for patient-assistance programs by drug class, brand name, generic name, and company that manufactures the drug.

www.rxoutreach.com
Rx Outreach is an easy and affordable way for qualified people of all ages to get medicines they need. Through this program, people who qualify financially can get more than 55 generic medications that treat a wide range of conditions, including diabetes, asthma, heart disease, and depression. People may take advantage of the program even if they receive medicines through another discount program. The program is available to individuals and families with incomes of up to 250 percent of the federal poverty level. For a family of four, this figure is about $48,000 per year.

www.needymeds.com
This site provides another catalog of available programs listed according to drug name and the manufacturer. It also has some useful references to several information resources that could be convenient to use. Overall it has a similar format to rxassist.org, but it might be easier to navigate.

Rx Assist Plus
This is a useful patient-tracking device that interfaces with the Internet to quickly complete the appropriate patient-assistance forms. It also has a tickler feature, which reminds the advocate to provide the patient with timely refills and re-enrollment into programs when the patient is due.

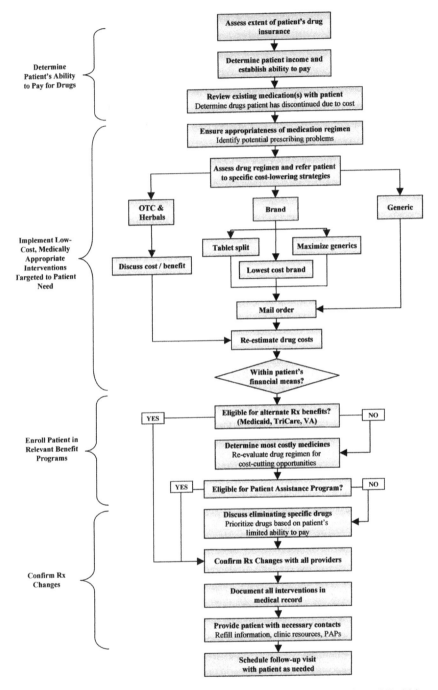

FIGURE 5.1. Price clinic cost containment algorithm. (By permission of Stebbins MR, Kaufman DJ, Lipton HL, J Managed Care Pharm 2005;11:333.)

and medications are obtained through the patient's pharmacy. Each company's program differs in qualifications and discounts, but they too can provide savings to the patient on brand name medications. Information on these discount cards may be found on pharmaceutical manufacturers' Web sites. Unfortunately, providers are faced with situations in which all cost-saving strategies have been exhausted and patients are still unable to afford their medications. It may become necessary to prioritize patients' medications based on their limited ability to pay and on their ability to stop taking certain medications. The cost-containment algorithm in Figure 5.1 is intended to provide a step-by-step approach to maximizing prescription cost savings while ensuring medically appropriate therapy.

Conclusion

Medication-related issues in chronic disease are complex and often inter-related. The topics discussed in this chapter are not all-inclusive but are intended to highlight common issues related to medication use in chronic disease. Polypharmacy, medication errors, and cost containment cannot be resolved independent of one another. Although time-consuming, addressing these issues will improve patient outcomes in the setting of chronic disease.

CASE STUDY

LF is a 68-year-old female with a history of hyperlipidemia, diabetes, depression, hypothyroidism, chronic pain, and obesity. She states that she has stopped her atorvastatin (Lipitor), sertraline (Zoloft), cetirizine (Zyrtec), and esomeprazole (Nexium) because she cannot afford to pay for them. She has a history of fatigue, dry mouth, difficulty waking in the morning, dizziness, reflux symptoms, and "sour sweat." She complains of fatigue and irritability associated with sweating episodes. She reports a pain score of 7/10. She has a total monthly income of $967 and no prescription coverage.

OBJECTIVE INFORMATION

The following information was obtained two weeks before the visit:

Total cholesterol, 216 mg/dL
Triglycerides, 577 mg/dL
LDL, 97 mg/dL
HDL, 34 mg/dL

TSH, 9.23
A1c, 6.1
FTs, wnl

She is currently being prescribed the following medications:

Levothyroxine 200 mcg once daily
Prazosin 10 mg twice daily
Methocarbamol 500 mg three times daily
Cyclobenzaprine 20 mg three times daily
Amitriptyline 50 mg once daily
Lisinopril 10 mg once daily
Glipizide 10 mg four times a day
Metformin 850 mg three times daily
Atorvastatin (Lipitor), 20 mg once daily (not currently taking)
Cetirizine (Zyrtec) 10 mg once daily (not currently taking)
Esomeprazole (Nexium) 40 mg once daily (not currently taking)
Sertraline (Zoloft), 200 mg once daily (not currently taking)

Polypharmacy Considerations

- Patient is taking multiple muscle relaxants at dosages that exceed maximum recommendations.
- Patient is taking two antihypertensives. Alpha-blockers (prazosin) are not recommended for patients with diabetes. Her lisinopril dosage was not maximized before the second agent was added.
- Glipizide is prescribed to be taken four times a day, which exceeds the recommended dosing.
- Patient is taking three medications concurrently that are considered inappropriate for the elderly (methocarbamol, cyclobenzaprine, amitriptyline).
- Patient is being treated for hypertriglyceridemia with a statin when a fibric acid derivative or niacin may be more appropriate.

Medication Errors

- Patient has a high TSH level, indicating of hypothyroidism that has not been adequately addressed.
- Patient is taking more than the maximum dose of glipizide and cyclobenzaprine, causing adverse events (hypoglycemia and anticholinergic toxicities, respectively).
- Patient is being treated for hypertriglyceridemia with a statin when a fibric acid or niacin may be more appropriate.
- The patient's chronic pain is not being treated adequately.

Cost Containment

- Patient is not taking four medications because of cost and lack of insurance coverage.

- Lipitor could be replaced with a less expensive generic (e.g., gemfibrozil).
- Nexium could be substituted with OTC Prilosec to save money.
- The excessive and duplicate dosing of medications can be reduced to save money.
- Zyrtec could be replaced by OTC loratidine.
- Zoloft could be replaced by a generic selective serotonin reuptake inhibitor.
- If brand name medications are medically necessary, the patient most likely qualifies for a patient-assistance program and a generic drug program.

References

1. Issues in Designing a Prescription Drug Benefit for Medicare. Washington, DC: Congressional Budget Office; 2002. Available at http://www.cbo.gov/showdoc.cfm?index=3960&sequence=0. Accessed July 20, 2005.
2. Medicare Prescription Drug, Improvement, and Modernization Act of 2003 (MMA). Public Law 108-173. Section 101, Subpart 2, Sec. 1860-D49(c); Cost and Utilization Management; Quality Assurance; Medication Therapy Management Program. Enacted December 8, 2003.
3. American Medical Association, Report 5 of the Council of Scientific Affairs (A-02), Improving the Quality of Geriatric Pharmacotherapy. 2002. http://www.ama-assn.org/ama/pub/category/13592.html. Accessed July 1, 2005.
4. Partnership for Solutions. Chronic Conditions. Making a Case for Care. September 2004 update. http://www.partnershipforsolutions.com/DMS/files/chronicbook2004.pdf. Accessed July 1, 2005.
5. Hunt SA, et al. ACC/AHA Guidelines for the Evaluation and Management of Heart Failure in the Adult. http://www.acc.org/clinical/guidelines/failure/pdfs/hf_fulltext.pdf. Accessed July 1, 2005.
6. Grundy SM, Cleeman JI, et al. Implications of recent clinical trials for the National Cholesterol Education Program Adult Treatment Panel III guidelines. Circulation 2004;110:227–239.
7. American Diabetes Association. Treatment of hypertension in adults with diabetes. Diabetes Care 2003;S26:S80–S82.
8. Hanlon JT, Schmader KE, Koronkowski MJ, et al. Adverse drug events in high risk older outpatients. J Am Geriatr Soc 1997;45(8):945–948.
9. World Health Organization. Adherence to Long-Term Therapies: Evidence for Action. 2003. http://www.who.int/chronic_conditions/en/adherence_report.pdf. Accessed July 1, 2005.
10. Ernst FR, Grizzle AJ. Drug-related morbidity and mortality: updating the cost-of-illness model. J Am Pharm Assoc 2001;41(2):156–157.
11. Lassila HC, Stoehr GP, Ganguli M, Seaberg EC, Gilby JE, Belle SH, Echement DA. Use of prescription medications in an elderly rural population: the MOVIES Project. Ann Pharmacother 1996;30(6):589–595.

12. Barat I, Andreasen F, Damsgaard EMS. The consumption of drugs by 75-year-old individuals living in their own homes. Eur J Clin Pharmacol 2000; 56(6–7):501–509.
13. American Society of Health System Pharmacists. Medication Use Among Older Americans. 2001. http://www.ashp.org/pr/over65.pdf. Accessed July 1, 2005.
14. Cutler TC, Mowers R, Mccloud M. Medication errors at an outpatient academic medical center. 2001. Poster Presentation, ASHP mid-year meeting, Las Vegas, Nevada.
15. Cornish PL, Knowles SR. Unintended medication discrepancies at the time of hospital admission. Arch Intern Med 2005;165(4):424–429.
16. Orchard TJ, Temprosa M, Golberg R, et al. The effect of metabolic syndrome: the diabetes prevention program randomization trial. Ann Intern Med 2005;142(8):611–619.
17. National Center for Chronic Disease Prevention and Health Promotion. http://www.cdc.gov/nccdphp/aag/aag_aging.htm. Accessed July 1, 2005.
18. Fick DM, Cooper JW, et al. Updating the Beers criteria for potentially inappropriate medication use in older adults. Arch Intern Med 2003; 163(22):2716–2724.
19. Aparasu RR, Mort JR. Inappropriate prescribing for the elderly: Beers criteria-based review. Ann Pharmacother 2000;34(3):338–346.
20. Curtis LH, Ostbye T, et al. Inappropriate prescribing for elderly Americans in a large outpatient population. Arch Intern Med 2004;164(15):1603–1604.
21. Institute for Safe Medication Practices. http://www.ismp.org. Accessed July 1, 2005.
22. Kaiser Family Foundation. http://www.kff.org/kaiserpolls/pomr111704nr.cfm. Accessed July 1, 2005.
23. Institute of Medicine. http://www.IOM.edu. Accessed July 1, 2005.
24. U.S. Agency for Healthcare Research and Quality (AHRQ). http://www.ahrq.gov/consumer/quicktips/tipprescrip.htm. Accessed July 1, 2005.
25. Joint Commission Accreditation of Hospital Organizations (JCAHO). http://www.JCAHO.org/accredited+organizations/patient+safety/dnu.htm. Accessed July 1, 2005.
26. Centers for Medicare and Medicaid Services. http://www.cms.hhs.gov/statistics/nhe/historical/highlights.asp. Accessed July 20, 2005.
27. Centers for Medicare and Medicaid Services. http://www.cms.hhs.gov/statistics/nhe/historical/t2.asp and http://www.cms.hhs.gov/statistics/nhe/historical/chart.asp. Accessed Aug 1, 2005.
28. Employee Benefit Research Institute. EBRI Notes, March 2004, table 3, p.11.
29. Poisal JA, Chulis GS. Medicare beneficiaries and drug coverage. Health Affairs 2000;19(2);248–256.
30. DeNavas-Walt C, Proctor BD, Mills RJ. Income, Poverty, and Health Insurance Coverage in the United States: 2003. Current Population Reports P60-226. Washington, DC: U.S. Department of Commerce, Economics and Statistics Administration, August 2004. www.census.gov/prod/2004pubs/p60-226.pdf. Accessed July 20, 2005; and Employee Benefit Research Institute, Estimates from the March Current Population Survey, 2004.
31. Duke KS, Raube K, Lipton HL. Patient-assistance programs: assessment of and use by safety-net clinics. Am J Health Syst Pharm 2005;62:726–731.

6
Providing Culturally Competent Chronic Disease Management: Diabetes Mellitus

DAVID STEMPEL AND BRUCE ALLEN CHERNOF

Summary

1. For disease management programs to succeed, they must acknowledge the potential impacts of culture within the treatment plan. They must be tailored to the needs of specific cultural communities or ethnic groups.
2. Even within broadly defined communities there can be great variation in expectations. Within the Latino and Asian communities, for example, there are significant differences in beliefs based on demographic characteristics, country of origin, and language.
3. Some of the challenges in providing culturally competent care include the following:
   a. Language, reading, and educational barriers
   b. Varying levels of acculturation within a family
   c. Use of traditional therapies and providers, side by side with Western therapies
   d. Expectations surrounding communication within the doctor–patient–family relationship
4. There are methods that you can use to develop a shared understanding of culture within the provider–patient relationship. You should explicitly acknowledge a diversity of cultural beliefs and the importance of these beliefs in decision making. You should ask questions such as the following:
   a. "For you and your family, how important are beliefs about . . . ?"
   b. "What are your concerns about . . . ?"
5. It is also extremely important to explicitly acknowledge potential differences among individual, family and community beliefs. You can begin such a discussion with, "I would like to ask you a few questions, just to make sure I have a clear understanding about what is important to you as we work together to manage your diabetes."
6. You should work to diminish the impact of literacy barriers. Patients with limited English proficiency will likely have problems reading

prescriptions and following medical recommendations. Techniques that you can use to overcome these literacy barriers include the following:

   a. Provide verbal education with concrete, simplified explanations of critical behaviors and goals.

   b. Ask your patients to repeat, in their own words, the information that they have just been given in order to assess their comprehension. If you are using an interpreter, make sure that the interpreter translates word for word what the patient and you say.

   c. Use picture-based education materials.

7. Common themes across cultures include the following:

   a. Determining who is the decision maker

   b. Understanding the cultural meaning of performing an examination or ordering a test

   c. Recognizing the significance of symptoms

   d. Recognizing that patients may be exceptionally deferential to your comments

8. It is important to consider using community resources to assist with your efforts in effective disease management. Effective community interventions have been described, mostly for the Latino population, and they include the use of community health workers (or promotores de salud), radio programs, public service announcements on Univison (the largest Spanish-language broadcast television network), community centers, and churches.

Background

Cultural belief systems have a profound impact on an individual's sense of wellness, illness, and approach to health care delivery. Chronic conditions are often highly culturally contextualized with respect to etiology, diagnosis, and treatment in terms that are quite different from those in traditional Western medicine. For disease management programs to succeed in these settings, the programs must be able to acknowledge the potential impact of culture within the treatment plan. The development of disease management programs for diverse populations must directly address these cultural challenges.

Cultural Challenges

The most obvious challenge is the diversity in the geographic region to be served. Disease management programs must be tailored to the needs of each cultural community or ethnic group. Even within broadly defined communities there can be great variations in expectations. Within the Latino and Asian communities, for example, there are significant differences in beliefs based on demographic characteristics, country of origin, and language. Diversity also plays a key role on the provider side of the equation. The demographic and cultural characteristics within a specific office or broader provider community often does not match the characteristics of the patients being served. Language, educational level, and reading ability present other key challenges. Written educational materials for non-English speaking or low-literacy populations should be kept at the fourth to sixth grade reading level. For those cultures that use characters as opposed to letters, written materials may be of little value. In many Asian cultures, it is not unusual for patients' primary language to be that of their country of origin, yet they may have very limited ability to read the written, character-based form. A recent study in a Cambodian community in Southern California demonstrated that more than two-thirds of individuals who identified themselves as primary Cambodian speakers were unable to read the written language. Another example are the Hmong, whose language did not have a written from until the early twentieth century when a Western cultural anthropologist created a written character-based alphabet.

A final set of challenges centers on the varying levels of acculturation that a provider may encounter among individuals as well as among families from the same cultural community. Multigenerational family structures are common in immigrant communities and this can result in widely varying levels of acculturation. Use of culturally traditional therapies and providers side by side with Western therapies is common. Expectations surrounding communication within the doctor–patient–family relationships can also very widely.

Methods to Enhance Cross-Cultural Understanding

It is neither possible nor reasonable to expect that any single provider or organization will have a nuanced understanding of every aspect of all the cultural communities and ethnic groups that they serve. There are methods, however, to develop a shared understanding of culture within provider–patient relationships that are also critical in the context of chronic disease management.

Keep Lines of Communication Open

Try to explicitly acknowledge the diversity of cultural beliefs and the importance of these beliefs in decision making. Cultural beliefs often frame expectations about causation, evaluation, and treatment. Try to ask questions, such as the following:

For you and your family, how important are beliefs about . . . ?
What are your concerns about . . . ?

Acknowledge Differences in Beliefs

It is also extremely important to explicitly acknowledge potential differences among individual, family, and community beliefs. Try to include statements that demonstrate your interest in understanding these beliefs. One way to do this is to say the following: "I would like to ask you a few questions, just to make sure I have a clear understanding about what is important to you as we work together to manage your diabetes."

Foster Self-Management

Work to foster the principles of self-management. The same techniques described in Chapter 2 can be used in shifting the locus of control to the patient. You can start this process by clarifying "importance" with the patient, for example, "How important is it to you to control your diabetes?" Clarifying "importance" and using the other techniques to promote self-management can help you develop a collaborative and culturally sensitive relationship with your patients.

Efforts to do this will not always be easy. Some patients will appear to expect an "authoritarian" approach. Use of an interpreter can also inadvertently aggravate communication asymmetry with the patient, particularly if the interpreter fails to provide an actual translation of the patient's response and instead provides summary statements. It is likely to take persistent efforts on your part to create the environment in which patients with limited English proficiency feel comfortable in taking part in setting goals and becoming "activated."

Diminish Literacy Barriers

Work to diminish literacy barriers. Language and literacy problems can have a substantial impact on the outcomes of your patients with chronic conditions. Patients with limited English proficiency will likely have problems reading prescriptions and following medical recommendations. Rothman and associates [1] provide good insights into these challenges. They studied the role of literacy on the effectiveness of a diabetes disease management program. For the patient group identified as having low literacy (less than sixth-grade reading level), they used the following techniques:

1. Verbal education with concrete, simplified explanations of critical behaviors and goals
2. A "teach-back" method to assess patient comprehension
3. Picture-based education materials

Over a one-year period, low-literacy patients working with these techniques were more likely to achieve goal HbA1c levels than those not using the techniques (42% versus 15%) [1].

The "teach-back" method to assess patient comprehension is similar to a communication method described in 1977 by Bertakis [2]. As the appointment comes to a close, ask your patients to repeat, in their own words, the information they had just been given. This method helps improve patient retention of information and provides greater satisfaction with their care.

Use Community Leaders and Peer Counselors

Consider using community resources to address the challenges of managing patients with chronic conditions. Effective community interventions have been described, mostly for the Latino population, including community health workers (or promotores de salud), radio programs, public service announcements on Univison (the largest Spanish-language broadcast television network), community centers, and churches [3].

Diabetes: General Education

For all patients there are critical elements that need to be covered, regardless of cultural or ethnic background. Probably the most important is to educate patients that diabetes is a chronic but manageable disease. For many patients diabetes may seem more like a clinical condition that is not dangerous if they do not have symptoms. Working with patients on diet planning consistent with their cultural background, as opposed to the standard Western-oriented food pyramid, is important. Also, developing a practical exercise plan that a patient can follow is an important, common cornerstone. Help patients develop a realistic walking program that they can share with family members. It is also critical to focus on obstacles to adherence to medication regimens. Medication regimens should take into account work and eating schedules as well as cultural concerns about injections. Many of these concerns also extend to concerns about venipuncture and other kinds of testing. Finally, encouraging all diabetics to perform careful foot examinations on a regular basis is critical.

Cultural Framing

Cultural beliefs at the patient, family, and community levels frame a patient's approach to adherence and self-management. Cultural framing helps physicians and patients focus on those elements of the clinical process and outcome that specific cultural beliefs directly impact. The culturally specific sections and tables that follow were developed as part of the Health Net of California, Inc., health insurance plan to help educate providers about cultural differences in the setting of diabetes. The generalized comments that follow will not apply to all patients in a particular ethnic group.

They are intended to provide background and insight into each group's culture and should be used in that spirit. The cultural issues presented were chosen specifically because they may be important to a patient's participation in the development of a genuinely shared treatment plan. By searching for and acknowledging critical cultural beliefs, physician and patient can work together to develop a treatment plan that is implementable.

Attitudes and Behaviors Regarding Diabetes Among Specific Cultural Groups

Latino beliefs come from a broad range of distinct cultures in Central and South America (Table 6.1). Family structure is very important; multigenerational and extended families within the same household are common, particularly among recently immigrated families. Patients may be deferential toward physicians' opinions, so it is important to work to gain trust and probe for problems with "compliance." Meals are an important time for socialization. Encourage patients to replace fats with canola or olive oils and to replace high-calorie drinks, such as soda, alcohol, and juices (e.g., jugo de savila or aloe juice), with lower carbohydrate alternatives. Suggesting an evening walk after the family meal is a good way to introduce a regular exercise program [4–7].

TABLE 6.1. Latino culture and diabetes care.

- **Family** is often involved in treatment and decision making. It is important to develop a personal relationship with Latino patients to develop trust.
- Often, Latino women place their needs beneath those of the family, and males may not assume personal responsibility for their diabetes care and management. **Involve both women and men**, as often as possible, in patient education.
- Latinos are often **deferential** toward physicians. Probe to ensure you are getting useful information about compliance.
- Some Latinos **distrust insulin** therapy, believing it causes blindness. Work sensitively to dispel this myth.
- Aloe juice (*jugo de savila*), a staple in some Latino households, is **contraindicated** for diabetes, as it is very high in carbohydrates. Suggest alternatives. Also, 7 Up® is a popular treatment for upset stomach. Suggest a sugar-free alternative, such as Diet 7 Up®.
- **Food** is an integral aspect of socialization among Latinos. Suggest incremental changes to diet:
  ▲ Eating earlier in the evening to avoid late-night suppers
  ▲ Taking a 15–30 minute walk after the evening meal
  ▲ Replacing fats, including lard, with more healthful choices, such as canola or olive oil
  ▲ Replacing corn tortillas with flour tortillas
  ▲ Switching from hard liquor to beer, from beer to light beer, from light beer to soda, and then from soda to diet soda—focus on small, achievable wins for patients and give positive encouragement when these changes are done successfully

Source: Data from references 4–7.

TABLE 6.2. Korean culture and diabetes care.

- Families of Korean descent are **egalitarian** in large part, although parents are closely involved in making decisions for their children. Women are often busy with work and childcare. As much as possible, confer with family members and check for understanding and agreement when delivering patient education.
- Many Koreans believe health to be the **equilibrium** between soul and physical being. They believe that illness is related to *karma* (past wrongdoing). Explain the chronic nature of diabetes. Encourage management through adherence to medical advice and family support.
- Patients will **avoid eye contact**, which is considered to be polite, and may refuse advice at first. Offer suggestions and advice numerous times, and allow ample time for questions, which may be slow in coming at first.
- **Do not point** to or beckon patients with the index finger. This is considered offensive. Diabetes is often treated in Korean households with **herbs and plants**, such as lychee fruit, cornelian cherry fruit, Chinese yam, and ginseng, as well as acupuncture and moxibustion. Recommend prescription medication as an essential supplement to more traditional remedies, and caution against treatments that break the skin and may spread infection.
- Explain the importance of **diet** and encourage patients of Korean descent to reduce reliance on high sodium foods such as Kimchee and miso, as well as red meat and fried foods. Suggest switching to lighter cooking methods using canola or olive oil.

Source: Data from references 8 and 9.

In Korean culture (Table 6.2), family structure is also important and tends to be egalitarian, so it important to check for understanding and agreement among family members. Patients may avoid eye contact and initially refuse advice as forms of cultural politeness. It is important to offer suggestions several times and to leave ample time for questions. Physicians should avoid pointing directly at the patient, particularly with the index finger. Health is often interpreted as equilibrium between spiritual and physical being. Traditional treatments, such as herbs, plants, and acupuncture, are commonly used, often in conjunction with Western therapies. The Korean diet is often high in sodium (e.g., in miso and Kimchee), red meat, and fried foods, so dietary suggestions might include low-salt alternatives and lighter oils [8,9].

Vietnamese culture (Table 6.3) centers on a family structure in which the father or eldest son is often the decision maker. Health is conceptualized as a balance between hot (*duong*) and cold (*am*). Injections and venipuncture may disturb this balance. Physicians are expected to perform an examination but should first seek permission to touch the patient. The examination should be done in order of head to toe, as the head is considered sacred and the feet profane. Meal planning is generally done by women. Important dietary changes include decreasing white flour and rice, red meat, nuoc mam (a fish sauce condiment consisting of salted and fermented anchovies), and coconut milk/oil and increasing brown rice, fish, lean white meat, fruits, and vegetables [10,11].

TABLE 6.3. Vietnamese culture and diabetes care.

- Many Vietnamese believe that **health maintenance** is the equilibrium of two natural forces—hot *(duong)* and cold *(am)*. Injections and venipuncture may be viewed as upsetting the hot and cold balance, as well as hurting the spirit. Explain that blood is necessary for laboratory testing and that the body will generate more.
- **Decisions** are made by the father or eldest son. Family is informed and part of the decision-making process. Encourage diabetes management through adherence to medical advice and family support.
- Your Vietnamese patients may expect any **examination** to be performed by you rather than by a nurse. Touching may be an issue, as the head is considered sacred (and the feet profane). Ask permission before touching your patient, especially on the head. To avoid bad feelings, begin a physical examination at the top of the body and move downward.
- Address **meal planning** to the female head of house. White flour, pastries, and white rice are popular elements of the Vietnamese diet. Suggest whole grain and reduced-sugar alternatives. Other dietary suggestions include the following:
  ▲ Reduce read meat in favor of lean white meat, fish, and more vegetables.
  ▲ Encourage eating fruit daily; many Vietnamese, especially seniors, do not consume fruit regularly.
  ▲ Reduce the use of sodium, monosodium glutamate, and fried foods.
  ▲ Decrease use of *nuoc man* (a fish sauce condiment consisting of salted and fermented anchovies).
  ▲ Limit use of coconut oil or coconut milk in foods; light coconut milk is preferable.

Source: Data from references 10 and 11.

In Cambodian culture (Table 6.4), health care is primarily sought in response to symptoms, so education about the chronic nature of diabetes is very important. Cambodian patients often have pronounced fears about Western health care. As in Vietnamese culture, examinations should be done in order from head to toe, and you should ask permission before starting the physical examinations. Patients may avoid eye contact with you as a sign of politeness. Older generations commonly use cupping, coining, pinching, and acupuncture, but these traditional therapies are far less common among younger or more acculturated patients. Meal planning is generally done by women. Rice and fish are staples, and sweet flavors are prevalent. Encourage whole grains, green vegetables (Chinese broccoli, bok choy, and mustard greens), and soaking dried fish to remove excess salt. Recommend fruit as a dessert substitute and use of light coconut milk in sweets [12].

In Filipino culture (Table 6.5), health is often viewed as a sense of balance. You should address both the patient and the eldest family member present at a visit as they may be the family decision maker. Encouraging discussion with family and friends is helpful in building trust. Filipinos commonly use spiritual healing techniques, and some patients have concerns about blood drawing. Families may consider overweight children to be healthy. Dietary staples include rice, noodles, and a wide range of meat,

TABLE 6.4. Cambodian culture and diabetes care.

- Although Cambodian culture is patriarchal, in the **family** husband and wife often share authority. Extended families, headed by an older parent or grandparent, are common.
- Many Cambodians **will not seek care** if they are asymptomatic. Explain the chronic nature of diabetes, and encourage diabetes management through family support and adherence to medical advice.
- An **older generation** of Cambodians is familiar with coining, cupping, and pinching as treatments for a variety of ailments. Educate your diabetic patients on the danger of procedures, such as acupuncture, that break the skin and may initiate infection.
- Patients will avoid **eye contact**. Physicians can show respect for Cambodian patients by avoiding eye contact with them.
- Your patients may expect any **examination** to be performed by you rather than by a nurse. Ask permission before touching your patient, especially on the head (which is considered sacred). Begin a physical examination at the top of the body and move downward.
- Many Cambodians have pronounced **fears** regarding medical care. Sensitive education will help your patients overcome these.
- Address **meal planning** with the female head of house. Rice and fish are common. Rice is fried, steamed, and used for noodles. Fish is served fresh, dried, or salted. Suggest increasing the use of whole-grain rice and soaking dried or salted fish in water to remove some salt. Encourage steaming vegetables, such as Chinese broccoli, bok choy, and mustard greens.
- Fruits in the Cambodian diet are generally **sweet**. Suggest alternatives, such as apples and oranges. Also encourage limiting desserts, such as coconut milk with banana, sugar, and tapioca and sticky rice.

Source: Data from reference 12.

TABLE 6.5. Filipino culture and diabetes care.

- When consulting with a member of a traditional Filipino **family**, speak to both the patient and the eldest family member, when possible, as this person is the family's chief spokesperson and caregiver. In the absence of parents, this will be the eldest child.
- **Encourage discussion** among the patient's family and community. This will build trust.
- Unless necessary, avoid direct eye contact, as this may make the patient uncomfortable.
- In **patient education**, be aware that many Filipinos have a fatalistic outlook on life and death. Health is balance; illness is imbalance. Because spiritual healing and related practices are a part of Filipino culture, explain the chronic nature of diabetes, and stress positive aspects of preventive care.
- Many Filipinos believe that an **overweight** child is a healthy child. Educate them on the connection between an overweight childhood and the development of diabetes.
- Your Filipino patient may believe that donating **blood** causes imbalance and anemia. Explain the importance of blood drawing for laboratory tests and that the body will make more blood.
- The traditional Filipino **diet** includes white rice and noodles, as well as seafood, vegetables, fruits, and meats. Canned and processed foods, e.g., corned beef, Spam®, and Vienna sausages, are common items. Alternatives you may suggest include the following:
  - ▲ Whole-grain rice and noodles
  - ▲ Canola and olive oil
  - ▲ Light coconut milk
  - ▲ Reduced-salt soy sauces, less fish sauce, and no monosodium glutamate

Source: Data from references 13 and 14.

seafood, and vegetables. Encourage the use of long grain rice, canola and olive oils, as well as light coconut milk, while decreasing intake of salty fish sauce and monosodium glutamate [13,14].

In African-American culture (Table 6.6) family structures are often extended and matriarchal, so physicians need to assess who is the decision maker. It is important to stress the chronic nature of diabetes and the importance of preventive care. Meal planning is generally done by women. Fried foods and gravies are common. Encourage the use of canola and olive oils, hotter frying, and not reusing oil. Reducing or substituting fatty gravies is also important. Eating lighter dinners and adding a walk after dinner is a good way to introduce regular exercise [15,16].

Extended, generally patriarchal families are common in Chinese culture (Table 6.7). Stress the chronic nature of diabetes and the value of preventive care. Disagreeing with physicians is considered disrespectful, and this can increase the difficulty in obtaining a complete history. Venipuncture is thought to weaken the body, and the removal of body parts (such as amputation of threatened/infected limbs or digits) is considered taboo. Traditional therapies, such as herbs, acupuncture, moxibustion (heart therapy), and massage, are commonly used, often in conjunction with Western therapies. Health is viewed as a sense of balance. Meal planning

TABLE 6.6. African-American culture and diabetes care.

- **African-American families** can include immediate, extended, and matriarchal (older female) members. The father or eldest male speaks for the family. Grandparents, especially grandmothers, play a crucial role. Stress that diabetes is a family issue. Encourage management of diabetes through support from the family and adherence to medical advice.
- African Americans often will not seek professional help until absolutely necessary. They may have little awareness of the value of **preventive health care** and take medication only when symptomatic. Explain the chronic nature of diabetes and the hazards of disease progression without proper medical intervention.
- Women prepare meals. Address **meal planning** with the female head of house. Food preparation methods include frying, barbecuing, and heavy use of gravy and sauces. Suggest a dietary consultation for alternative meal choices and preparation methods. Here are some suggestions:
  - Reduce intake of sodium, pork, red meats, and fried foods.
  - Avoid late, heavy dinners. Walk as a family after dinner. Start off with 5–10 minutes.
  - Switch to canola or olive oil.
  - Avoid reusing oil to fry foods. Reused oil is higher in fat.
  - Fry foods at proper (hotter) temperatures. Food will soak up oil at lower temperatures.
  - Reduce intake of corn meal, fatty gravies, and sauces. Prepare gravy with low-fat ingredients such as low-fat broth, low-fat milk and whole-grain flours.
  - Use artificial sweeteners and avoid diet and caffeine-free soda, as they are high in sodium.
  - Choose low-fat alternatives over sweets, such as fruit. Include fresh vegetables and fruits with each meal.

Source: Data from references 15 and 16.

TABLE 6.7. Chinese culture and diabetes care.

- The traditional Chinese family structure often includes extended family, with children, parents, and grandparents living together. Major decisions in this **patriarchal family** structure usually require input from the male head of household.
- Many Chinese do not believe in **preventive health care** measures, preferring to seek treatment, whether traditional Chinese or Western, when they are experiencing symptoms.
- You may encounter **difficulty** in obtaining full information, because it can be considered disrespectful to disagree with a physician. However, two beliefs are widespread: one is that venipuncture weakens the body; the other is that any removal of body parts is taboo.
- You may encounter **success** if you explain to your patients and their families the chronic nature of diabetes. Encourage family support to manage a patient's diabetes. Explain that blood is necessary only for laboratory tests and that the body will produce new blood.
- Emphasize proper foot care to avoid amputation.
- **Homeopathic therapies** include herbs, massage, acupuncture, and moxibustion. Advise your Chinese patients to avoid procedures that damage the skin. Explain that diabetes slows the body's healing process, and any breaking of the skin may initiate the spread of infection.
- Women prepare meals. Address **meal planning** with the female head of house. Explain the benefits of whole grains and fiber. Suggest increasing consumption of bok choy, Chinese broccoli, Chinese mustard greens, bitter melons, tangerines, and pumelo. Suggest eliminating or reducing pastries and sweet buns, especially those with fillings high in fat and sugar. Reduce high-sodium foods such as instant noodles. Suggest limiting oil in stir-fry, fried foods, and soy sauce and fish sauces and switching to canola or olive oil.

Source: Data from references 17 and 18.

is generally done by women. Families should be encouraged to decrease sweet pastries and sticky buns, sauces and instant noodles (high in salt), and high-fat oils used in stir-fry. Increasing whole grains and fiber, vegetables, and fruit, as well as using canola or olive oils, should be encouraged [17,18].

Hmong culture (Table 6.8) is generally patriarchal and includes the married sons' families in the extended family, and decision-making is done in a communal fashion. Illness is believed to result from soul wandering, angry ancestors, curses, or spells. Physicians should avoid direct eye contact, as this can be viewed as disrespectful. Common Hmong derm-abrasive medical techniques include cupping, coining, pinching, and ritual bleeding. Amputation procedures are thought to interfere with reincarnation, and venipuncture is feared because of a concern that the blood will not be replaced. Family members need to be instructed in care delivery, such as insulin injections. Meal planning is generally done by women, and staples include chicken, pork, rice, and vegetables. Physicians should encourage the use of canola or olive oil in stir frying and decreasing the use of salt (fish sauces) and monosodium glutamate [19].

TABLE 6.8. Hmong culture and diabetes care.

- **Family** is important to Hmong. Households often consist of married sons and their families. Family structure is patriarchal, and major decisions may take communal discussion.
- **Illness** is believed to be the result of the soul wandering from the body or caused by angry ancestors, hostile spirits, spells, curses, or the violation of taboos. Nonetheless, Hmong use a combination of Western medicine and Hmong shaman. Dermabrasive procedures such as cupping, coining, and pinching are common, as is pricking a finger with a needle to release blood into a bowl of water when ill. Counsel avoidance of procedures that break the skin because this could lead to infection. Explain that diabetics are slow to heal.
- Hmong resist the removal of body parts because it can affect the person's reincarnation and life in the afterworld. This is a good opportunity to recommend **compliance** with diabetes treatment to avoid possible foot amputation. Many Hmong also fear venipuncture out of the belief that blood is not replaced. Explain that blood is necessary only for laboratory tests and that the body will produce new blood.
- Many Hmong are resistant to, or uninformed about, self-care and preventive care. Family members will be expected to give **insulin injections**, so instruct family members on proper technique. Suggest that your patients take responsibility for their home foot examinations.
- Do not be concerned when Hmong patients **avoid eye contact**. They feel that direct and lengthy eye contact is rude.
- Address **meal planning** with the female head of house. Traditional diet includes chicken, pork, rice, and vegetables in a broth. Suggest that your patients reduce their use of monosodium glutamate and limit their use of oil in stir-fry and fried foods. Advise them to switch to canola oil, safflower oil, or olive oil. Suggest low-salt replacements for soy sauce and fish sauce.

Source: Data from reference 19.

Summary

To establish an effective disease management program, it is important to address culture-specific issues. You should work to find ways to address the unique communication "barriers" that may exist between you and patients of different cultures. This includes being willing to acknowledge the diversity of beliefs and the importance of these beliefs in decision making. You can do this by asking questions, such as "For you and your family, how important are beliefs about...?" Do not underestimate the significance of literacy barriers. Problems with limited English proficiency can often lead to misunderstandings on basic instructions such as how to take a medication. Some methods you can use to reduce the chance of a misunderstanding include the following:

1. Verbal education with concrete, simplified explanations of critical behaviors and goals
2. A "teach-back" method to assess patient comprehension, which involves asking patients, at the end of the visits, to repeat in their own words the instructions that you have given them
3. Picture-based education materials

It is not expected that all physicians will have a complete understanding of all the cultural nuances that they will face in the care of their patients. However, acknowledging the diversity and importance of cultural beliefs and working to reduce communication barriers will go a long way toward improving patient care.

Acknowledgments. The authors wish to acknowledge Tracy Vang and Diana Carr for their efforts to facilitate the community cultural stakeholder advisory boards that edited the content. The authors also wish to acknowledge Sandra Yates, Steven Owh, Peggy Haines, and Dr. Steven Raffin, who supported the development of this disease management program. This Diabetes Disease Management Program was developed as part of Medi-Cal Managed Care contracts through the California Department of Health Services. David Stempel's work was supported through a David Geffen School of Medicine Dean's Office Summer Administrative Fellowship Award.

References

1. Rothman RL, et al. Influence of patient literacy on the effectiveness of a primary care–based diabetes disease management program. JAMA 2004;292: 1711–1716.
2. Bertakis KD. The communication of information from physician to patient: A method for increasing patient retention and satisfaction. J Fam Pract 1977; 5:217–222.
3. Brown SA, Garcia AA, Kouzekanani K, Hanis CL. Culturally competent diabetes self-management education for Mexican Americans. Diabetes Care 2002;25:259–268.
4. Zoucha R, Purnell LD. People of Mexican Heritage. Purnell LD, Paulanka B. Transcultural Health Care: A Culturally Competent Approach. Philadelphia: F.A. Davis, 2003:264–278.
5. Boyle J. Central Americans. In Lipson J, Dibble S, Minarik P (eds). Culture and Nursing Care: A Pocket Guide. San Francisco: UCSF Nursing Press, 2004: 63–73.
6. Lagana K, Gonzalez-Ramirez L, de Paula T. Mexican Americans. In Lipson J, Dibble S, Minarik P (eds). Culture and Nursing Care: A Pocket Guide. San Francisco: UCSF Nursing Press, 2004:203–221.
7. de Pheils PB. Columbians. In Lipson J, Dibble S, Minarik P (eds). Culture and Nursing Care: A Pocket Guide. San Francisco: UCSF Nursing Press, 2004: 82–90.
8. Purnell LD, Kim S. People of Korean Heritage. In Purnell LD, Paulanka B (eds). Transcultural Health Care: A Culturally Competent Approach. Philadelphia: F.A. Davis, 2003:249–263.
9. Reardon T. Koreans. In Lipson J, Dibble S, Minarik P (eds). Culture and Nursing Care: A Pocket Guide. San Francisco: UCSF Nursing Press, 2004: 191–202.
10. Nowak T. People of Vietnamese Heritage. In Purnell LD, Paulanka B (eds). Transcultural Health Care: A Culturally Competent Approach. Philadelphia, F.A. Davis, 2003:327–343.

11. Farrales S. Vietnamese. In Lipson J, Dibble S, Minarik P (eds). Culture and Nursing Care: A Pocket Guide. San Francisco: UCSF Nursing Press, 2004: 280–290.

12. Kulig J. Cambodians (Khmer). In Lipson J, Dibble S, Minarik P (eds). Culture and Nursing Care: A Pocket Guide. San Francisco: UCSF Nursing Press, 2004: 55–63.

13. Pacquiao D. People of Filipino Heritage. In Purnell LD, Paulanka B (eds). Transcultural Health Care: A Culturally Competent Approach. Philadelphia: F.A. Davis, 2003:138–159.

14. Cantos A, Rivera E. Filipinos. In Lipson J, Dibble S, Minarik P (eds). Culture and Nursing Care: A Pocket Guide. San Francisco: UCSF Nursing Press, 2004: 115–125.

15. Glanville C. People of African American Heritage. In Purnell LD, Paulanka B (eds). Transcultural Health Care: A Culturally Competent Approach. Philadelphia: F.A. Davis, 2003:40–53.

16. Locks S, Boateng L. Black/African Americans. In Lipson J, Dibble S, Minarik P (eds). Culture and Nursing Care: A Pocket Guide. San Francisco: UCSF Nursing Press, 2004:37–43.

17. Wang Y. People of Chinese Heritage. In Purnell LD, Paulanka B (eds). Transcultural Health Care: A Culturally Competent Approach. Philadelphia: F.A. Davis, 2003:106–121.

18. Chin P. Chinese Americans. In Lipson J, Dibble S, Minarik P (eds). Culture and Nursing Care: A Pocket Guide. San Francisco: UCSF Nursing Press, 2004: 74–81.

19. Johnson S. Hmong. In Lipson J, Dibble S, Minarik P (eds). Culture and Nursing Care: A Pocket Guide. San Francisco: UCSF Nursing Press, 2004: 155–168.

Section II
Management of Specific Diseases

7
Type 2 Diabetes

Jim Nuovo

Summary

I. Management
  1. During the initial evaluation of a patient just diagnosed with type 2 diabetes mellitus (DM), you should include assessment of the following:
    a. Symptoms suggesting end-organ disease (e.g., paresthesias, visual impairment, and exertional chest pain or shortness of breath)
    b. Evidence of hypertension; use American Diabetes Association's definition of 130/85 mm Hg
    c. Physical examination findings suggesting end-organ disease (e.g., fundoscopic changes of retinopathy, distal sensation to monofilament or 125-Hz tuning fork, and foot hygiene)
    d. Laboratory evidence of glycemic control (HbA1c), associated risk factors for vascular disease (low-density lipoprotein [LDL] cholesterol), and end-organ disease (urine microalbumin)
    e. Evidence of cardiovascular disease, including ischemic heart disease and left ventricular hypertrophy, by electrocardiogram
    f. Comorbid conditions, particularly depression
  2. Your intake history should also include assessment of the following:
    a. Family history of DM and end-organ complications (e.g., blindness, renal failure, myocardial infarction, stroke, peripheral vascular disease, and amputation)
    b. Associated cardiovascular risk factors (i.e., sedentary lifestyle and tobacco use)
    c. Understanding of diabetes and its health effects
    d. Perception of barriers to lifestyle modification
  3. Self-management support is key to effective DM management. Techniques you can use to support self-management include the following:

a. Ask your patients about their readiness to change; only 20% of patients are ready to make a significant lifestyle change at the time of initial evaluation. This can be accomplished by asking, "How likely are you to pursue changing your diet at this point?" or "To help you understand more about diabetes, what type of information would be most helpful to you at this time: a pamphlet, a Web site, a class?"

b. Help your patients set goals. It is best if these goals are patient-generated, specific, short-term, achievable action plans, for example, "This week I will walk around the block before lunch on Monday, Tuesday, and Thursday."

c. Ask patients how confident they feel that they can make changes to achieve these goals. This can be done in the following way: "On a 10-point scale, how confident are you that you can start walking three times a week?" Patients who score their confidence level as less than 7 are unlikely to be successful for that goal. When this occurs, the goal should be changed to one that is more likely to be achieved.

d. Document patient-generated goals in the chart, and monitor for success in achieving these goals or in barriers encountered.

e. Have your office staff assist in reinforcing healthy behaviors and self-management goals (e.g., reinforce good foot care by asking patients to remove shoes and socks before you come in the room; prompt patients to discuss self-generated goals).

4. Provide educational resources that are culturally sensitive and tailored to a patient's specific needs, and goals. Resources available include the following:

a. The American Diabetes Association (ADA) is available at www.diabetes.org

b. The National Diabetes Information Clearinghouse is available at www.niddk.nih.gov/health/diabetes/ndic.htm

c. Diabetes Self-Management; available at www.DiabetesSelf-Management.com

5. Encourage your patients to learn the principles of healthy eating. Patients who adhere to an ideal meal plan can reduce their HA1c levels as effectively as those who take oral agents. General nutritional concepts to convey to patients include the following:

a. Weight loss is difficult; however, losing 10% of your body weight can have a big impact on blood glucose levels.

b. A weight loss of no more than 1 pound per week is recommended.

c. Emphasize fresh fruits, vegetables, and whole grains.

d. Limit calories from liquids.

e. Limit portion sizes.

   f. For those who eat when they are not hungry, look for other things to do instead: go for a walk, call a friend, drink water or diet soft drinks, chew sugarless gum.

6. Reinforce the value of an exercise program. The benefits of an exercise program can be substantial for patients ready to make lifestyle changes.

   a. Consider having your patients take an exercise treadmill test, particularly those with multiple cardiovascular risk factors, before starting an exercise program.

   b. A progressive walking program offers the best chance for long-term success.

   c. A pedometer can serve as an excellent means to help patients set reasonable goals and receive daily feedback.

7. Reinforce proper foot care to all patients. Advise your patients:

   a. To check their feet every day

   b. To always wear shoes that fit

   c. To keep the toenails properly trimmed

8. Depression is a common comorbid condition with all chronic diseases. Failing to treat depression often results in poor outcomes. Screen all patients with DM for symptoms of depression.

9. Oral agents are an important adjunct to the treatment of DM. Oral agents can achieve a 1% to 2% reduction in HA1c. Important principles to consider when prescribing these agents include the following:

   a. Sulfonylureas are considered the most effective oral agents in lowering blood glucose level.

   b. Two-drug regimens are common; it is important to consider complementary actions.

   c. Common comorbid conditions, such as renal impairment, heart failure, and hepatic disease, make it mandatory to assess and monitor the appropriateness of the oral agents.

   d. Triple-drug regimens are unlikely to achieve acceptable glucose control; most patients unable to achieve adequate control with two drugs should be considered for insulin therapy.

10. Areas of caution for the oral agents include the following:

   a. Metformin and lactic acidosis: Lactic acidosis is a rare complication, but you should use caution when prescribing metformin for patients with renal impairment and heart failure.

   b. Thiazolidinediones and congestive heart failure: These oral agents can cause fluid retention, which may exacerbate heart failure.

   c. Thiazolidinediones and hepatotoxicity: Patients may develop idiosyncratic hepatotoxicity. Liver function tests should be monitored.

      d. Glipizide and hypoglycemia in the elderly: Renal or hepatic insufficiency may cause elevated levels of glipizide and a prolonged episode of hypoglycemia.

   11. Insulin therapy should be considered for all patients who are unable to achieve adequate glycemic control with oral agents.

      a. Most patients and providers are hesitant to start insulin despite its known beneficial effects.

      b. More than 50% of patients believe that a recommendation to start insulin therapy means that they failed.

      c. You should:

         i. Avoid scare tactics

        ii. Solicit and address patient concerns

       iii. Discuss type 2 DM as a progressive disease that often will eventually require insulin therapy to maintain glycemic control

       iv. Explain the rationale for insulin therapy

        v. Recognize the importance of social support, emotional well-being, and patient acceptance of the use of insulin

      d. Most patients, once they receive training, adjust quickly to its use.

II. Monitoring

   1. Most providers fall short in meeting well-published consensus goals for management and monitoring of DM and its complications. To improve quality of care, consider developing a registry that includes the names of all patients with DM and facilitates access to the key monitoring parameters: weight, blood pressure, HbA1c, LDL cholesterol, renal function, urine microalbumin, fundoscopic examination for retinopathy, and foot examination for sensation and evidence of ulcers, calluses, and nail hygiene.

   2. If you do not have a registry, use monthly billing reports of patients with a 250.XX diagnosis as a proxy.

   3. The most effective intervention for a practice is to use templates for each office visit and to develop a system by which ongoing performance can be assessed for a particular patient and for the practice. While this can be facilitated with an electronic medical record, it can also be done with a standard paper checklist that includes an office visit template and flow sheet.

   4. Support self-management goals by including them in the medical record. Patient-generated goals should be documented in the record; ongoing assessments can be made regarding successes and barriers.

   5. Give all your patients an action plan (Table 7.1). The action plan should contain information that indicates when control is optimal and when interventions need to be made. This can be used to support self-management goals.

TABLE 7.1. Diabetes action plan.

Green zone: great control	Green zone means
Your goal HbA1c	Your blood sugars are under control
HbA1c is under 7%	Continue taking your medications as ordered
Average blood sugars typically under 150 mg/dL	Continue routine blood glucose monitoring
Most fasting blood sugars under 150 mg/dL	Follow healthy eating habits
	Keep all physician appointments

Yellow zone: caution	Yellow zone means
HbA1c between 7% and 9%	Your blood sugar may indicate that you need an adjustment of your medications
Average blood sugar between 150 and 210 mg/dL	Improve your eating habits
Most fasting blood glucose under 200 mg/dL	Increase your activity level
Work closely with your health care team if you are going into the YELLOW zone	Call your physician, nurse, or diabetes educator if changes in your activity level or eating habits don't decrease your fasting blood sugar levels
	Name: _____
	Number: _____

Red zone: stop and think	Red zone means
HbA1c greater than 9%	You need to be evaluated by a physician
Average blood sugars are over 210 mg/dL	If you have a blood glucose over ____, follow these instructions _____
Most fasting blood sugars are well over 200 mg/dL	**Call your physician**
	Physician: _____
	Number: _____
Call your physician if you are going into the RED zone	

Source: Courtesy of www.improvingchroniccare.org.

6. Specific targets for control, as recommended by the ADA, include the following:
   a. HbA1c <7.0%
   b. Preprandial glucose 90–130 mg/dL
   c. Peak postprandial glucose <180 mg/dL
   d. Systolic Blood Pressure <130 mm Hg
   e. Diastolic Blood Pressure <80 mm Hg
   f. LDL cholesterol <100 mg/dL
7. ADA-recommended frequency for monitoring tests are
   a. HbA1c: Quarterly if treatment changes or goals are not being met; at least twice a year if stable
   b. Dilated eye examination: Yearly
   c. Comprehensive foot examination: At least yearly

   d. Lipid profile: Yearly
   e. Microalbumin: Yearly
   f. Blood pressure: Each visit
   g. Weight: Each visit
8. You can use the registry to develop reports for the office, namely, how the practice is doing in achieving the recommended targets of control and monitoring tests (such as percentage of patients with DM who have had a HbA1c within the past year).
9. You can perform rapid-cycle Plan-Do-Study-Act interventions to help improve practice performance. They are the most effective means of improving outcomes in a practice. These are best when they are directed to one specific problem and involve participation from the practice team—provider and staff. For example, medical assistants can be trained to ask all patients with DM to remove their shoes and socks before the physician comes into the examination room. The performance of the practice can be measured before and after the intervention.

Background: Burden as a Chronic Disease

Summary

- Type 2 DM is the most prevalent form of diabetes. It is often asymptomatic in its early stages and can remain undiagnosed for years, long enough for patients to develop end-organ complications.
- About one-third of those with DM are undiagnosed.
- The prevalence of DM is approximately twofold greater for African Americans, Hispanic Americans, and Native Americans than for non-Hispanic whites.
- A substantial percentage of total health care costs come from the management of diabetes and its associated complications.

Prevalence

Approximately 95% of people with DM have the type 2 form. These patients are usually obese and have a relative insulin deficiency caused by insulin resistance. End-organ complications from the chronic effects of DM are a substantial source of morbidity and mortality. Patients with DM have 4 times the risk for blindness, 4 times the risk for myocardial infarction, 19 times the risk for end-stage renal disease, and 28 times the risk for lower extremity amputation. In the United States, DM is the leading cause of end-stage renal disease, nontraumatic lower extremity amputations, and adult blindness. With an increasing incidence worldwide, DM will continue to be a leading cause of morbidity and mortality for the foreseeable future. Approximately 18 million people in the United States have DM; one-third of these are undiagnosed. The total burden of DM represents ~6% of the population. The prevalence of DM is approximately twofold greater for African Americans, Hispanic Americans, and Native Americans than for non-Hispanic whites. The incidence of DM in these ethnic groups is rapidly increasing; and it is becoming more common to see this disease in younger age groups.

Costs

Several cost-of-illness studies related to DM have been performed over the last three decades. The findings all indicate that DM imposes a large economic burden on society. In the United States, the economic cost of diabetes was estimated to be as much as $100 billion per year in 1997 and may now approach $132 billion [1]. The total annual medical costs incurred by all payers in managing just one complication, diabetic nephropathy, was $15.0 billion [2]. According to a Veterans Administration (VA) study, the VA incurred $215 billion in outpatient expenditures and $1.45 billion in inpatient expenditures over a 4-year study period. The study found that hospitalization rates for patients with DM were approximately 1.65 admissions per year, and the average number of outpatient visits was 4.6 [3]. Rubin and associates [4] analyzed the annual medical costs of patients with DM. In a breakdown of how costs were distributed, they found that 63% went to inpatient hospital costs, 22% went to outpatient services, 9% to drugs and durable medical equipment, 4% to home health, 1% to emergency department services, and 1% to dental care [4].

Impact of Disease Management Programs

Summary

- Disease management programs have consistently been shown to have a positive impact on costs, utilization, patient outcomes, patient satisfaction, and provider satisfaction.
- Studies on cost savings suggest that a one percentage point reduction in HbA1c level results in 14% decrease in total mortality, 21% decrease in diabetes-related deaths, 14% decrease in myocardial infarction, 12% decrease in strokes, 43% decrease in amputations, and 24% decrease in renal failure.

One of the challenges of caring for patients with any chronic condition, including DM, has been to provide services that are recognized as having an impact on disease outcomes. Multiple studies of patients with DM have shown poor adherence to well-known markers for quality of care. For example, up to 30% of patients with DM go a least 1 year without seeing a doctor, 50% do not have an annual assessment of renal function, 60%

do not see an ophthalmologist each year, and 40% do not have an HbA1c test twice a year [5].

Disease management programs have been consistently shown to have a positive impact on costs, utilization, patient outcomes, patient satisfaction, and provider satisfaction. Bodenheimer and associates [5] reported on the impact of ambulatory care diabetes management programs. After implementation of the Chronic Care Model, outcomes for patients with DM demonstrated improvement. Some examples from their report included the following:

1. Premier Health Partners, Dayton, Illinois (100 physicians working in 36 private offices): Within 3 years of the intervention, the percentage of patients with DM with an HbA1c level below 7.0% increased from 42% to 70%. Similar improvements were recorded for documented foot examination, assessment of urine microalbumin levels, and use of angiotensin-converting enzyme (ACE) inhibitors.

2. Health Partners Medical Group, Minneapolis, Minnesota: The percentage of patients with DM with an HbA1c level below 8% increased from 60.5% to 68%.

3. Clinica Campesina, Denver, Colorado: Patients participating in this program had a reported decrease in HbA1c from 10.5% to 8.6% over a 2-year period. The percentage of patients with self-management goals increased from 3% to 65%. The percentage of patients having an eye examination increased from 7% to 51%.

In our own clinic we saw similar changes in these process outcomes. We care for approximately 700 patients with DM. Our population is very ethnically diverse, and many have limited English proficiency. Some of the outcome changes after 6 months of implementation of a disease management program included HbA1c level less than 7.0% increased from 25.2% to 35.3%; HbA1c level greater than 10.0% decreased from 19.3% to 12.6%; LDL cholesterol level under 100 gm/dL increased from 25% to 46%; LDL cholesterol above 130 mg/dL decreased from 38% to 25%.

Bodenheimer and associates [6] also reviewed 39 studies based on components of the Chronic Care Model. Overall, 32 of the 39 studies found that the intervention improved at least one process or outcome measure. An important question has been how disease management efforts, such as the ones described, affect total costs. Wagner and associates [7] studied two groups of patients at Group Health Cooperative in Puget Sound. Within 1 year, Group Health was saving between $685 and $950 per patient, per year. The savings came from fewer primary care and specialty visits. A similar analysis was done by Sidorov and associates [8] at the Geisinger clinic. They retrospectively examined paid health care claims over 2 years among 6,799 patients with DM; approximately one-half were enrolled in a disease management program. Their findings include the following: total costs per member, per month, were lower in the disease management group

($394 vs. $502); the lower costs were associated with reduced inpatient days and emergency room use. The group participating in the disease management program also had higher HEDIS performance scores for undergoing regular testing of HA1c, lipid, and urine microalbumin levels, as well as documented eye examinations.

The diabetes disease management program called Diabetes Decisions [9] also yielded cost savings. Started in 1998, the program grew to include 662 participants. Participants were entered into American Healthways' clinical information system and risk-stratified, and an individualized treatment plan was devised. Telephone case management by specially trained nurses was an important component of the intervention. Data were collected on key process measures, financial parameters, and participant satisfaction. By year 3, there were 422 continuously participating participants. From baseline to the third year of the program, significant increases in frequency of HbA1c testing (from 21.3% to 82.2%), dilated retinal examinations (from 17.2% to 70.7%), and foot examinations (from 2.0% to 75.6%) were observed. For 166 participants with five HbA1c determinations, their values dropped from 8.89% to 7.88%. Participants experienced a 36% drop in inpatient costs. Without adjustment for medical inflation, total medical costs decreased by 26.8% from the baseline period, lowering to $268.63 per diabetes participant per month (PDPPM) by year 3, a gross savings of $98.49 PDPPM. After subtracting the fees paid to Diabetes Decisions, a net savings of $986,538 was realized.

The National Coalition on Health Care and the Institute for Healthcare Improvement published a summary of the benefits of improved blood glucose control. They reported that a one percentage point reduction in HbA1c resulted in 14% decrease in total mortality, 21% decrease in diabetes-related deaths, 14% decrease in myocardial infarction, 12% decrease in strokes, 43% decrease in amputations, 24% decrease in renal failure— together representing a total of $800 million in health care costs [10].

Screening for Diabetes

Summary

- The ADA has recommended the Fasting Plasma Glucose (FPG) test for screening. Currently, an FPG level ≥126 mg/dL is the cut-off for an abnormal value.
- Patients with an impaired fasting glucose level (FPG ≥100 mg/dL but ≤126 mg/dL) are now referred to as having "pre-diabetes."
- It is unclear whether early treatment, as part of an aggressive screening program, will result in clinically important improvements in diabetes-related outcomes; however, the threshold for screening at-risk populations, and those with other cardiovascular risk factors, should be low.

Risk Factors

Type 2 DM frequently goes undiagnosed for many years, because the hyperglycemia develops gradually and in the early stages the symptoms are not specific. These patients are at increased risk of developing macrovascular and microvascular complications. It has been estimated that at the time the clinical diagnosis of DM is made, many patients have had the disease for 5 to 8 years—enough time to develop end-organ complications. Table 7.2 lists the risk factors for developing type 2 DM [11].

Impact of the Obesity Epidemic

The epidemic of obesity in the United States has an important role in the increasing incidence of type 2 DM. Figure 7.1 illustrates the relationship between increasing body weight and the risk of type 2 DM [12]. The data in Table 7.2 and Figure 7.1, together, indicate that an obese, sedentary patient who is over 45 years old has a high risk of developing type 2 DM; this risk increases if they are African American, Hispanic American, or Native American or if they have a positive family history of DM. Unfortunately, the profile of an obese, sedentary patient over 45 years old is common.

Screening Populations for DM

Because patients can have relatively long, asymptomatic periods, screening for earlier detection of DM is considered an important part of a disease management program [13]. In general, it is best to screen patients with significant risk factors: it remains unclear whether mass screening programs are of value in achieving this goal. Hoerger and associates [14] performed a cost-effectiveness analysis targeted toward the general primary

TABLE 7.2. Risk factors for type 2 DM.

Age >45 years
Overweight (BMI >25 kg/m^2)
Family history of diabetes
Sedentary lifestyle
Race/ethnicity (e.g., African American, Hispanic American, Native American, Asian American, and Pacific Islanders)
Impaired fasting glucose (IFG) level
History of gestational DM (GDM) or baby weighing >9 lbs
Hypertension (>140/90 mm Hg)
HDL cholesterol level <35 mg/dL
Polycystic ovarian syndrome (PCO)
History of vascular disease

Source: Data from American Diabetes Association [11].

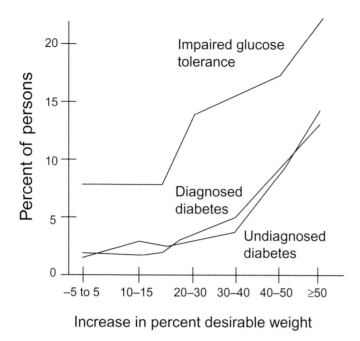

FIGURE 7.1. Relationship between body weight, impaired glucose tolerance (pre-diabetes), and the development of type 2 DM. (Data from Harris [12].)

care population in the United States [14]. They used data from the United Kingdom Prospective Diabetes Study (UKPDS) and the Hypertension Optimal Treatment (HOT) Trial. They found that diabetes screening targeted to people with hypertension, particularly those aged 55 to 75 years, is more cost-effective than universal screening.

Screening Tests

Three tests have been used for screening: FPG, 2-hour postload plasma glucose, and HbA1c. The ADA has recommended the FPG test for screening, because it is easier and faster to perform and it is less expensive [13]. Currently, an FPG level ≤126 mg/dL is the cut-off for an abnormal value. The HbA1c test is less sensitive in detecting lower levels of hyperglycemia and, therefore, is subject to false-negative results. Random capillary blood glucose tests have been shown to be reasonably sensitive in detecting persons who have either an FPG level >126 mg/dL or a 2-hour postload plasma glucose level >200 mg/dL if the results are interpreted according to time since last meal. Table 7.3 lists the ADA criteria for the diagnosis of DM.

TABLE 7.3. American Diabetes Association criteria for the diagnosis of DM.

1. Symptoms of diabetes plus casual plasma glucose concentration >200mg/dL. Casual is defined as any time of day, without regard to time, since last meal. The classic symptoms of diabetes include polyuria, polydipsia, and unexplained weight loss.
2. FPG level >126mg/dL. Fasting is defined as no caloric intake for at least 8 hours.
3. 2-hour postload glucose >200mg/dL during an oral glucose tolerance test. The test should be performed as described by the World Health Organization, using a glucose load containing the equivalent of 75g anhydrous glucose dissolved in water.

Source: Data from American Diabetes Association [13].

Impaired Fasting Glucose Condition (Pre-diabetes)

The Expert Committee of the ADA published guidelines for the identification of patients with impaired fasting glucose (IFG) but who do not meet the criteria for diabetes [13]. Impaired fasting glucose is defined as an FPG level >100mg/dL but <126mg/dL. Patients with IFG are now referred to as having pre-diabetes, indicating their relatively high risk for subsequently developing diabetes. Impaired fasting glucose is associated with metabolic syndrome, which includes obesity, dyslipidemia, and hypertension. Whether interventions such as lifestyle modification will have an impact on long-term health outcomes has been the subject of the Diabetes Prevention Program (DPP). Palmer and associates studied the impact of metformin plus standard lifestyle advise versus intensive lifestyle changes and the subsequent risk of developing DM [15]. They found that both regimens worked; metformin plus standard lifestyle advise reduced the risk by 31% and intensive lifestyle changes reduced the risk by 58%. Their analysis suggested that the savings (DM-free years of life, improvements in life expectancy, and other cost savings) outweighed the initial implementation costs.

Screening Recommendations

Given the prevalence of DM, the threshold for screening for DM should be relatively low. However, as mentioned earlier, there appears to be little to no benefit of mass screening programs. Two important organizations, the U.S. Preventive Services Task Force and the ADA, have published screening recommendations. The U.S. Preventive Service Task Force screening recommendations are listed in Table 7.4 [16], and the ADA screening recommendations are listed in Table 7.5 [17]. The U.S. Preventive Services Task Force endorses diabetes screening for those patients deemed at increased risk for cardiovascular disease (e.g., those with hypertension or hyperlipidemia). The ADA would extend screening recommendations to those deemed at high risk for developing DM (e.g., an obese patient more than 45 years old) and suggest that screening be performed every 3 years.

TABLE 7.4. Screening recommendations from the U.S. Preventive Services Task Force.

Background statements

1. There is good evidence that the available screening tests can accurately detect type 2 DM during the early, asymptomatic phase.
2. There is good evidence that intensive glycemic control in patients with clinically detected diabetes can reduce the progression of microvascular disease.
3. However, the benefits of tight glycemic control on microvascular complications takes years to become apparent.
4. Existing studies have not shown that tight glycemic control significantly reduces macrovascular complications, including myocardial infarction and stroke.
5. It has not been demonstrated that beginning diabetes control early as a result of screening provides an incremental benefit compared with initiating treatment after clinical diagnosis.

Screening recommendations

1. The decision to screen individual patients is a matter of clinical judgment.
2. Patients at increased risk for cardiovascular disease may benefit most from screening.
3. Screening for patients with hypertension or hyperlipidemia should be part of an integrated approach to reduce cardiovascular risk.

Source: Data from U.S. Preventive Services Task Force [16].

TABLE 7.5. Screening recommendations of the American Diabetes Association.

1. Evaluation for type 2 DM should be performed within the health care setting. Patients, particularly those with a BMI >25 kg/m^2, should be screened at 3-year intervals beginning at age 45 years; testing should be considered at an earlier age or be carried out more frequently for those who are overweight if additional diabetes risk factors are present.
2. The FPG is the recommended screening test. It is preferred because it is faster, easier to perform, more convenient and acceptable to patients, and less expensive.

Source: Data from Harris, et al. [17].

Initial Evaluation

Summary

- Given the relatively high incidence of end-organ complications discovered at the time of initial diagnosis, the initial evaluation should include a search for evidence of retinopathy, nephropathy, neuropathy, and ischemic heart disease.

Assessments

Once the diagnosis of DM is made, assessments should be made for end-organ disease, risk factors associated with metabolic syndrome, and the patient's understanding and awareness of the implications of DM to their health. When performing an initial assessment on a patient with DM, it is important to remember that many patients will have end-organ complications at the time of diagnosis. End-organ complications at the time of diagnosis have been estimated to be retinopathy, 20%; proteinuria, 10% to 37%; neuropathy, 9%; angina, 10%; and myocardial infarction, 5% [18].

Components recommended in the initial evaluation of a patient with DM are listed in Table 7.6. The intake history should focus on symptoms

TABLE 7.6. Initial evaluation of patients with newly diagnosed type 2 DM.

History	
Review of systems for indicators of end-organ disease or impact on quality of life Polyuria/nocturia Polydipsia Polyphagia Weight change Parasthesias Visual impairment Exertional chest pain or shortness of breath	

Focused physical examination	Ideal findings
Blood pressure	<130/85
Weight/BMI	<25 kg/m^2
Fundoscopic examination	No evidence of diabetic retinopathy
Monofilament test	Sensate
Foot examination	Good skin and nail hygiene; no calluses or ulcers

Laboratory evaluation	Ideal findings
HbA1c	<7.0%
Lipid panel	LDL <100 mg/dL; HDL >35 mg/dL
Microalbumin level	<300 mg/dL

Patient assessment	
Past medical history	History of ischemic heart disease, peripheral vascular disease, cerebrovascular disease, renal disease
Family history	Family history of DM and end-organ complications, (e.g., blindness, renal failure, myocardial infarction, stroke, peripheral vascular disease, amputation)
Allergies	Allergies to sulfonamides
Habits	Diet, alcohol intake, tobacco use, exercise
Personal/social	Understanding of diabetes and health effects; perception of barriers to lifestyle modification
Comorbid conditions	Assessment for presence of depression

suggestive of end-organ disease (e.g., parasthesias, visual impairment, or exertional chest pain or dyspnea) and those that impact quality of life (e.g., polyuria and polydipsia). The physical examination should target end-organ complications, such as diabetic retinopathy (fundoscopic examination), peripheral neuropathy (sensate to monofilament or 125-Hz tuning fork), peripheral vascular disease (distal pulses), and foot hygiene (presence of foot calluses, ulcers, and nail care). The examination should also assess for commonly associated comorbid conditions, such as hypertension. Laboratory evaluation should target the stated end-organ complications (e.g., nephropathy/microalbuminuria), associated comorbid conditions (e.g., hyperlipidemia), and measures of control (e.g., HbA1c level). Further history should target additional cardiovascular risk factors (family history and use of tobacco products), personal habits associated with control (diet and exercise), and common comorbid conditions associated with poor control (depression). Finally, it is always important to gauge a patient's understanding of the disease, their concerns associated with the diagnosis, and their willingness to make the necessary lifestyle changes in order to optimize their health.

Management

Summary

- Effective treatment of DM requires enhancing each patient's self-management skills. Perhaps the most critical component of this intervention is to appreciate the importance of "self-efficacy," the confidence to carry out a behavior necessary to reach a desired goal. On a 10-point scale, patients who rate their level of confidence under 7 are unlikely to be successful for that goal.
- Assessment of a patient's "readiness to change" is an important part of chronic disease management; approximately 20% of patients are ready for change at the time of initial evaluation. Failing to assess the patient's readiness often results in ineffective management, especially provider frustration, which often ends with the patient being labeled as "noncompliant."
- Self-management promotion represents a paradigm shift for most patients and providers; the key element to the paradigm shift is a patient-centered approach, with the provider functioning as a "health coach."
- Self-management can be promoted through patient-generated, specific, short-term, achievable action plans, for example, "This week, I will walk around the block before lunch on Monday, Tuesday, and Thursday."
- The glucometer can be used as an effective adjunct to a patient-centered approach that values the principles of self-management. Specifically, each patient is advised that the glucometer can be used to assess the impact of dietary and activity habits.

- Patients who adhere to an ideal meal plan can reduce their HbA1c levels as effectively as those who use oral agents.
- A pedometer can help patients set reasonable exercise goals and provide daily feedback.
- Depression is common among patients with any form of chronic disease. Failing to treat depression often results in poor outcomes.

Self-Management Support and Assessing Readiness to Change

The evidence strongly suggests that the key to effective disease management of any chronic condition, including DM, is to set an environment that promotes self-management. Self-management education includes information/instruction, counseling, and behavioral intervention. Although this book focuses on self-management training in the office setting, it is important to recognize that effective settings also include work sites, churches, senior centers, community centers, homes, and extended-care facilities. Two critical components can help support your patient's efforts in self-management:

1. Appreciating the importance of self-efficacy, the confidence to carry out a behavior necessary to reach a desired goal [19]
2. Assessing the patient's readiness to change, a component that has been associated with greater efforts with self-care and improved control and lifestyle modification [20]

Approximately 20% of patients at the time of initial diagnosis are ready to accept and act on necessary lifestyle changes. Failing to assess the patient's readiness often results in ineffective management, especially the frustration that we feel, which often ends with the patient being labeled as "noncompliant." An example of this includes sending patients to an education class on dietary change and lifestyle modification when they are not ready to make these changes. Assessment of readiness to change can be accomplished by asking the following types of questions:

1. "How likely are you to pursue changing your diet at this point?"
2. "To help you understand more about diabetes, which of the following information would be most helpful to you at this time: a pamphlet, a Web site, a class?"

More information on assessment of readiness to change can be found in the works listed in Table 7.7. Rollnick et al. [21] wrote for health care professionals, and their book contains much detail about specific methods to foster behavior change. Prochaska et al. [22] developed the model of the stages of change known as the transtheoretical model. In the process of investigating behavior change, they noted six stages of change (phases that

TABLE 7.7. Resources for health behavior change information.

For health professionals
Rollnick S, Mason P, Butler C. Health Behavior Change. A Guide for Practitioners.
Toronto: Churchill Livingstone, 1999
Prochaska JO, DiClemente CC, Norcross JC. In search of how people change:
applications to addictive behavior. Am Psychologist 1992;47:1102–1114
For patients
Diabetes Self-Management, a bimonthly magazine; call 1-800-234-0923

individuals go through) in order to address problematic behavior: Pre-contemplation (has no intention to take action within the next 6 months), Contemplation (intends to take action within the next 6 months), Preparation (intends to take action within the next 30 days and has taken some behavioral steps in this direction), Action (has changed behavior for less than 6 months), Maintenance (has changed behavior for more than 6 months), and Termination (adverse behavior will never return). The magazine *Diabetes Self-Management* is a bimonthly publication for patients and shows specific examples of behavioral change.

Self-Management Support and Training for Patients

Holman and Lorig [23] have done extensive work on self-management training for patients and have summarized the responsibilities of the patient in the presence of chronic disease:

1. Using medications properly
2. Changing behaviors to improve symptoms or slow disease progression
3. Adjusting to social and economic consequences
4. Coping with emotional consequences
5. Interpreting and reporting symptoms accurately

They also describe what patients with chronic conditions want but cannot typically get from their physicians:

1. Access to information concerning the diagnosis, its implications, and available treatments and their consequences
2. An understanding of the potential impact on their future
3. Continuity of care and ready access to it
4. Coordination of care, particularly with specialists
5. Infrastructure improvements (flexible scheduling, wait times, billing)
6. Ways to cope with symptoms, such as pain, fatigue, disability, and loss of independence, and ways to adjust to disease consequences, such as uncertainty, fear, depression, anger, loneliness, sleep disorders, memory loss, exercise needs, nocturia, sexual dysfunction, and stress

Self-Management Support/Promotion by Providers

Self-management promotion represents a paradigm shift for most patients and for most physicians and their practices. The key element to the paradigm shift is a patient-centered approach in which the physicians' role is, in part, to serve as a "health coach." This is an important shift, as many physicians feel helpless or ineffective in providing counseling for health promotion. Of physicians surveyed in 1991, less than 10% thought that they could be successful in modifying patients' behaviors [24].

Developing a Short-Term Action Plan

A key feature to self-management education is the patient-generated short-term action plan. As described by Bodenheimer et al. [19], this is "similar to a New Year's resolution, but of shorter duration, such as 1 to 2 weeks." It is also more specific, for example, "This week I will walk around the block before lunch on Monday, Tuesday, and Thursday." The action plan must be patient-generated and realistic and have reasonably high self-efficacy. Physicians should ask patients what they feel the likelihood is that they will be able to achieve their short-term action plan. This can be done by asking the following question: "On a scale of 0 to 10, how sure are you that you can accomplish this goal?" If the answer is 7 or greater, the action plan is likely to be accomplished. If the answer is below 7, it would be reasonable to reassess the plan and make it more realistic.

Based on our experience, we believe the following techniques will help promote self-management:

1. Elicit patient-generated goals for each visit, e.g., "What goal would you like to focus on in managing your diabetes?"

2. Assess self-efficacy for each goal. Provide patients with a 10-point response scale, with the following lead question: "How confident are you that you can achieve this goal?" A patient's self-efficacy rating of less than 7 is a strong indicator that the patient will be unlikely to achieve that particular goal.

3. Provide a means to document patient-generated goals and monitor success in achieving these goals or the barriers encountered. Recognize achievement in meeting self-generated goals.

4. Work with office staff to reinforce health behaviors and self-management goals, (e.g., reinforce good foot care by asking the patient to remove shoes and socks before the physician enters the room and prompting the patient to discuss self-generated goals).

Helping Patients Set Their Goals

How should we emphasize the patient's role? It begins with a simple message: "Diabetes is a serious condition. There are things you can do to live better with diabetes and things the medical team can do to assist you. We are going to work together on this." In setting goals, it is important for you to assist in helping to set realistic goals, understand and use an action plan, assess the barriers to achieving goals, make appropriate changes, and recognize achievement of objectives. You can support this in the following ways [25]:

1. Promote goal setting. This is best done by working toward one goal at a time, a goal that focuses on a behavior and not an outcome, a goal that is patient generated, and a goal that the patient feels is achievable.
2. Ensure that you have a system to help you keep track of the goals so that in follow-up visits you will remember to inquire about how the patient did.
3. Be nonjudgmental and nonfatalistic about "failures."
4. Remember to recognize success.

Motivational Interviewing

Motivational interviewing is a technique designed for providers as a tool for helping patients [26]. The mnemonics FRAMES and OARES describe the strategies: FRAMES—provide Feedback, understand that the Responsibility for change lies with the patient, give Advise, offer a Menu of change options, use an Empathic interview style (understanding the world through the patients' eyes), and enhance Self-efficacy (the confidence to carry out a behavior necessary to reach a desired goal); OARES—use Open-ended questions, Affirm (provide supporting statements), use Reflective listening, Elicit self-motivational statements, and Summarize.

A technique to facilitate setting goals, an action plan, and follow-up is outlined in Table 7.8. The following are key elements of the technique:

TABLE 7.8. Techniques to promote self-management.

1. Elicit patient-generated goals for each visit, for example, "What goal would you like to focus on in managing your diabetes?"
2. Assess self-efficacy for each goal. Provide patients with a 10-point response scale with the lead question "How confident are you that you can achieve this goal?" A patient's self-efficacy rating of 6 or less is a strong indicator that the patient is unlikely to achieve that particular goal.
3. Provide a means to document patient-generated goals and to monitor success in achieving these goals or the barriers encountered.
4. Work with office staff to reinforce healthy behaviors and self-management goals, for example, reinforcing good foot care by asking the patient to remove shoes and socks before the physician comes in the room; prompting the patient to discuss self-generated goals.

Source: Data from Lorig, et al. Outcome Measures for Health Education and Other Health Care Interventions. Thousand Oakes, CA: Sage Publications, 1996.

1. Assisting the patient in developing a plan
2. Clarifying the specific actions
3. Performing an assessment of barriers and the patient's confidence in meeting these challenges
4. Facilitating problem solving

A patient handout on setting goals is presented in Appendix A. This handout was designed to reinforce the message of self-management and to guide patients toward goals that may reduce adverse outcomes by addressing such areas as foot examinations, exercise, nutrition, use of tobacco, and blood glucose level monitoring.

Education Supporting Self-Management

Education is clearly important in promoting self-management. Key areas of understanding include monitoring blood glucose level, nutrition therapy, weight control, exercise, and stress reduction.

Monitoring Blood Glucose Level

Self-monitoring of blood glucose level has now become routine. Available meters are accurate, small, and less dependent on user technique. Many have memories that can store glucose values. One caveat is that the "halo effect" is an important issue for some patients, namely, being labeled a good patient. Some patients will report phantom values or downgrade readings from their machine into a personal log. An article that appeared in the *American Journal of Medicine* more than 20 years ago is still germane [27]. The study included 19 patients with diabetes. All were given new-generation glucose monitors. They were told to record their readings in a diary and to bring the information to the next visit. They were not told that there was a computer "chip" installed in the monitors that also was recording the dates, times, and levels of blood glucose. After comparing the results recorded in the patients' diaries with the machine records, investigators found a number of "phantom" values as well as a tendency to downgrade high numbers. Two-thirds of the patients reported values in such a manner as to obscure hyper- and hypoglycemia, creating misleading clinical impressions about fluctuations in metabolic control.

The glucometer can be an effective adjunct to a patient-centered approach that values the principles of self-management. Specifically, advise your patients that the glucometer can help assess the impacts of diet and exercise on blood glucose control. Encourage patients to test not exclusively on a regular schedule, but when they are interested in assessing the impacts of what they eat or what they do. This can help promote a sense of empowerment.

Nutrition Therapy

Without nutrition education and a change in eating behavior, it is unlikely that patients will achieve optimal management of their condition. Patients who adhere to an ideal meal plan can reduce their HbA1c levels as effectively as those who use medication. Patients who receive no dietary education usually show no change in their HbA1c.

To provide proper education on the necessary dietary changes, it is important to guide patients to resources such as dietitians, certified diabetic educators (CDEs), and information available on-line and in books and pamphlets. Excellent printed materials are available from the ADA (www.diabetes.org). Changing a lifelong pattern of eating is a substantial challenge for patients. Before referring patients to educational resources, we should do the following:

1. Assess the patient's readiness to change. If the patient is not yet ready to make dietary changes, it is better, initially, to provide the patient with printed or on-line educational resources.
2. Assist the patient in establishing reasonable nutritional goals.
3. Assess the patient's self-efficacy (the confidence to make changes).

TABLE 7.9. General nutritional concepts for weight management to convey to patients with diabetes.

1. Weight loss is difficult. Losing 10% to 20% of your body weight can have a big impact on blood glucose levels.
2. Fad diets and quick-loss programs can harm health and interfere with diabetes management. Weight loss of no more than 1 lb per week is recommended.
3. Awareness of the calorie content of foods can help patients choose foods to lose weight or to avoid weight gain.
4. To decrease calories: emphasize fresh fruits, vegetables, and whole grains; choose measured amounts of lean meat, fish, poultry, and skim milk; limit added-fat and high-fat foods; limit calories from liquids.
5. Do not give up your favorite foods; however, limit portion sizes; choose a low-fat version of the food; limit the number of portions per day or week; limit between-meal snacking; eat high-calorie foods less often.
6. If you tend to eat when you are not hungry, look for other things to do. Examples include going for a walk, calling a friend, drinking water or diet soft drinks, chewing sugarless gum.
7. Exercise, including walking, is an important component to any weight management program.

Set reasonable short-term and long-term goals; for example, for a short-term action plan, ask your patient: "What is one action you could take next week that would move you closer to your goal?"

Source: Data from Funnell, et al. [28].

General nutritional concepts are outlined in Table 7.9 [28]. Nutritional goals described by the ADA can be achieved by:

1. Following regular meal planning advise and guidelines and balancing food intake with drug therapy and exercise.

2. Maintaining reasonable weight by monitoring calorie consumption (10% to 20% of calories from protein; less than 10% of calories from saturated fat; less than 10% of calories from polyunsaturated fat; 60% to 70% of calories from monounsaturated fat and carbohydrates; and less than 300 mg of cholesterol per day).

Key features of a "diabetic diet" include carbohydrate management and reduced fat intake. Current recommendations are that carbohydrates and monounsaturated fatty acids, together, should comprise 60% to 70% of daily caloric intake. The exact proportions are not specified, and individualization is recommended. One of the reasons for this is a desire to move toward greater flexibility for the large, culturally diverse populations with DM.

Carbohydrate Counting

There have been different recommendations for medical nutrition therapy for DM over time, (e.g., the "exchange" program). Most dietary recommendations have emphasized the use of complex carbohydrates and the avoidance of simple carbohydrates, based on the belief that simple sugars would be digested more quickly and would lead to elevated postprandial blood glucose levels. Based on the results of a number of studies, this concept was challenged in that many starchy foods such as baked potatoes and white bread produced higher glycemic responses than simple sugars. In response, the concept of the glycemic index (GI) of food was developed. The GI of foods depends on the rate of digestion and the speed of absorption of the carbohydrate. The overall blood glucose response is determined not only by the GI value of a food but also by the amount of carbohydrate: the lower the GI, the less the impact on blood glucose levels. The product of the GI value and carbohydrate content (in grams) has been called the *glycemic load*. Glycemic load represents the quality and quantity of the carbohydrates consumed. Examples of the GI and glycemic load of common foods are presented in Table 7.10. Patients able to adhere to a diet with low GI foods have consistently shown improvement in glycemic control and lipid profiles.

The clinical utility of GI is controversial. The current trend is to recommend carbohydrate counting. Carbohydrate counting focuses on the total amount of carbohydrate rather than its source. One carbohydrate "source" is equal to 15 g of carbohydrate. The goal of carbohydrate counting is to allow patients to assess the "optimal" grams of carbohydrates needed in each meal to meet their goals for glycemic control. Patients are taught how to count carbohydrates by reading the labels of the foods they eat or referring to educational materials. This method allows more flexibility, parti-

TABLE 7.10. Glycemic index and glycemic load of common foods.

Food	Serving size	Glycemic index	Carbohydrates (g)	Glycemic load
White rice	1 cup	125	53	67
Baked potato	1	121	51	61
Doughnut	1	108	23	25
French fries	4 oz	107	35	37
Honey	1 tbsp	104	17	18
Bagel	1	102	38	39
Carrots	½ cup	101	8	8
White bread	1 slice	101	12	12
Wheat bread	1 slice	98	12	12
Ice cream	½ cup	87	16	14
Orange juice	6 oz	81	20	16
Popcorn	1 cup	78	6	5
Corn	½ cup	78	16	12
Banana	1	75	27	20
Grapes	½ cup	61	14	9
Orange	1	61	16	10
Bran cereal	½ cup	60	23	14
Apple	1	51	21	11
Whole milk	1 cup	38	12	5
Grapefruit	½	36	10	2
Peanuts	1 oz	20	5	1

cularly with culture-specific food choices. Examples of amounts of carbohydrates are listed in Table 7.10. Effective training in carbohydrate counting and other aspects of medical nutrition therapy for DM is best done in an interactive forum taught by a dietitian, a certified diabetic educator, or a community health promoter.

Reduction in Fat

Evidence from multiple studies corroborates the adverse impacts of saturated and polyunsaturated fats on glycemic control and cardiovascular health. Recent prospective and cross-sectional studies suggest that it is the specific type of fat, rather than the total fat content, that plays a role in the development of type 2 DM. In the Nurses' Health Study, a high intake of vegetable fat was inversely associated with the risk of type 2 DM during a 6-year follow-up period. This finding has been confirmed in other long-term studies [29]. Other fats of interest include long-chain n-3 fatty acids (in fish) and trans-fatty acids. Long-chain n-3 fatty acids are found in high concentration in fish oil. Although current studies are limited, there may be a beneficial effect in the risk of developing DM and glycemic and lipid control. Further work needs to be done to clarify the role of fish oils. Trans-fatty acids are formed when vegetable or fish oils are "hardened." Diets high in trans-fatty acids tend to increase the risk of DM and worsen glycemic control. As mentioned earlier, the ADA has established guidelines for the optimal amounts and ratios of dietary fats for patients with DM.

Patient education materials for medical nutrition therapy (including healthy eating rules, carbohydrate counting, low-fat eating, cook books, and a food diary) are presented in Appendix B.

Weight Control

There is a close relationship between obesity and type 2 DM. Most patients with DM have a body mass index (BMI) of >25 kg/m². A BMI <25 kg/m² is considered normal, 25 to 30 kg/m² is considered overweight, and >30 kg/m² is considered obese. Insulin resistance usually is seen with a BMI of 27 kg/m² or higher. Success in losing weight is problematic for most obese patients with DM. Again, weight loss programs should be tailored to patient-generated goals when the patient demonstrates a readiness to change. Long-term success in weight control is typically associated with lifestyle modification involving diet and an exercise program.

Exercise

Sixty percent of Americans do not engage in any form of moderate activity, and 30% do not exercise at all. Many patients with DM have comorbid conditions that add barriers to engaging in exercise. For those who can walk, a progressive walking program offers the best chance of long-term success. A pedometer can help patients set reasonable goals and receive daily feedback. A study by Tudor-Locke and Bell [30] studied the impact of this simple intervention. The group that used a pedometer had a significant increase in activity, by the end of the study equivalent to 3,000 steps per day (30 minutes of walking). Other studies of pedometer use show similar outcomes [31]. Patient education materials for the role of exercise in the treatment of DM are presented in Appendix C. It is important to encourage patients to:

1. Pick an exercise that they enjoy.
2. Start slowly, increasing length, frequency, and intensity gradually.
3. Set reasonable goals for their exercise program.

Before starting an exercise program, patients with DM should consider taking an exercise stress test.

Foot Care

The most common causes of amputations in the United States are the end-organ effects of DM. Maintaining good foot hygiene is the most effective way to prevent foot ulcers, osteomyelitis, and amputation. Self-care information for patients is presented in Appendix D. The patient information sheet lists some dos and don'ts of foot care.

At each visit, emphasize the need for good foot care and examine the feet for ulcers, calluses, skin cracking, and sensation. Assess sensation with a monofilament and a 125-Hz tuning fork.

Behavioral Concerns

Patients with DM have a twofold increase in the rate of depression. Depression is associated with suboptimal control and increased rates of end-organ complications. Williams and associates [32] studied the effectiveness of interventions to treat comorbid depression and to determine depression's impact on measures of diabetes control. They performed a randomized trial of 1,801 patients using focused management of depression. Their intervention improved measures of depression control and improved patients' overall functioning. However, overall control of HbA1c level was not affected. Given the rate of depression in this population and the impact on quality of life and control of the disease, all patients with DM should undergo periodic screening for signs of depression.

Education Resources

There are a number of resources available to assist patients in dealing with common barriers, including pain management, fatigue management, relaxation, achieving better emotional control, nutrition, exercise, medications, home glucose monitoring, insulin injection, foot care, and regular eye examinations. They are listed in Table 7.11. Another valuable resource is the "Control Your Diabetes for Life" Program, developed by the National

TABLE 7.11. Educational resources for patients with DM.

American Diabetes Association
1660 Duke Street
P.O. Box 25757
Alexandria, VA 22313
http://www.diabetes.org

National Diabetes Information Clearinghouse
One Information Way
Bethesda, MD 20892-3560
www.niddk.nih.gov/health/diabetes/ndic.htm
National Diabetes Education Program

National Institute of Diabetes & Digestive & Kidney Diseases
National Institutes of Health
Building 31, Room 9A04
31 Center Drive, MSC 2560
Bethesda, MD 20892-2560
www.ndep.nic.gov

Health Disparities Collaboratives (a program designed to reduce health outcome disparities for poor, minority, and other underserved people); see www.healthdisparities.net

Magazines
Diabetes Forecast, available from the American Diabetes Association; call 1-800-806-7801
Diabetes Self-Management, available from www.DiabetesSelfManagement.com or call 1-800-234-0923

Diabetes Education Program (a joint effort of the National Institutes of Health and the Centers for Disease Prevention and Control). It is available at http://www.cdc.gov/diabetes/ndep.

Some health plans offer personal health coaching and/or educational materials to help address a wide variety of DM health issues. An example of this is Health Net's Decision Power [33]. Using a shared decision-making technique, the plan offers health "coaching" to impart the skills necessary for patients to become more involved in their health decisions. The plan includes videos and printed materials produced in collaboration with the Foundation for Informed Medical Decision Making, the Health-wise Knowledgebase (a Web-based library of general health information), and Health Crossroads (a Web-based library of decision support modules for a number of serious conditions).

Medications

Summary

- Sulfonylureas are considered the most effective oral agents in lowering blood glucose level.
- Two-drug regimens are common; it is important to consider complementary actions.
- Common comorbid conditions, such as renal impairment, congestive heart failure, and hepatic disease, make it mandatory to assess and monitor the appropriateness of the oral agents.
- Triple-drug regimens are unlikely to achieve glucose control; most patients unable to achieve adequate control with two drugs should be considered for insulin therapy.

The medications used to treat type 2 DM are directed toward the main metabolic defects in the condition: insulin resistance and relative insulin deficiency. Because two-drug regimens are common, it is important to consider complementary actions. Medications to lower blood glucose level are no longer referred to as *oral hypoglycemic agents*; the preferred terminology is *oral agents* or *oral glucose-lowering agents* because the term *hypoglycemic* is not accurate. Table 7.12 summarizes the key features of each of these agents, including initial and maximum dosages, impact on HbA1c level, common adverse reactions, and costs.

The sulfonylureas, meglitinides, and d-phenylalanine derivatives are referred to as *secretagogues*, because they stimulate the beta cells of the pancreas to produce more insulin. Alpha-glucosidase inhibitors slow the absorption of glucose from the gut. The biguanides and thiazolidinediones (glitazones) act by different mechanisms, but both treat insulin resistance and are therefore referred to as *insulin sensitizers*.

TABLE 7.12. Oral agents for type 2 DM.

Drug	Initial dose/ maximum dose	Impact on HbA1c (range)	Adverse reactions/ cautions	Costs
Alpha-glucosidase inhibitors: delay carbohydrate absorption from the gastrointestinal tract				
Glyset/miglitol	25 mg TID at the start of each meal/100 mg TID	−0.26% to −0.81%	Abdominal pain, diarrhea, and flatulence/ avoid with inflammatory bowel disease	$56.67
Precose/acarbose	25 mg TID at the start of each meal/100 mg TID	−0.54% to −0.78%	Abdominal pain, diarrhea, and flatulence/ avoid with inflammatory bowel disease and cirrhosis. Caution with impaired renal function	$60.41
Biguanides: decrease hepatic glucose production/minor stimulation of insulin-mediated glucose transport into skeletal muscle				
Glucophage/Riomet/metformin	850 mg daily or 500 mg BID/ 2,550 mg daily		Diarrhea, nausea, flatulence/lactic acidosis. Caution for patients with impaired renal or hepatic function or with chronic heart failure and for the elderly	$46.99
Insulin secretagogues: Stimulate beta-cell insulin secretion				
Sulfonylureas: stimulate pancreatic islet beta-cell insulin release				
Amaryl/glimepiride	1 mg daily/8 mg daily, 1, 2, 4 mg daily	Up to 2.0%	Hypoglycemia, bone marrow suppression, dizziness, fatigue	$12.06
Diabinese/chlorpropamide	100 mg daily/750 mg daily	Up to 1.0%	Hypoglycemia, bone marrow suppression, cholestasis, hepatic dysfunction/ caution for patients with impaired renal or liver function and for the elderly	$7.50

TABLE 7.12. *Continued*

Drug	Initial dose/ maximum dose	Impact on HbA1c (range)	Adverse reactions/ cautions	Costs
DiaBeta/Micronase glyburide	2.5 mg daily/20 mg daily	Normal range	Hypoglycemia, bone marrow suppression/ caution with impaired renal function, e.g., creatinine clearance <50 Caution for the elderly	$13.76
Glucotrol/glipizide	5 mg daily/40 mg daily		Diarrhea, nausea, hypoglycemia/caution with impaired renal or hepatic function	$5.00
Orinase/tolbutamide	1,000 mg daily/3,000 mg daily		Hypoglycemia, bone marrow suppression, jaundice	n/a
Tolinase/tolazamide	100 mg daily/250 mg daily		None reported	$12.00
Meglitinides				
Prandin/repaglinide	0.5 mg daily/16 mg daily; take 15–30 min before meals/skip dose if meal skipped	−0.17% to −0.6%	Hypoglycemia, headache, upper respiratory infection/caution for patients with renal dysfunction	$30.00
Phenylalanine derivatives Starlix/nateglinide	60 mg TID/take 15–30 min before meals/skip dose if meal skipped	−0.50% to −0.7%	*Do not use in combination with sulfonylureas*/ hypoglycemia, nausea, dyspepsia/caution for patients with impaired hepatic function	$101.79
Thiazolidinediones: increase insulin sensitivity; may also inhibit hepatic glucose production				
Actos/pioglitazone	15 mg daily/45 mg daily	−0.3% to −1.0%	Hepatotoxicity, chronic heart failure, edema/monitor ALT at baseline and periodically thereafter	$90.99
Avandia/rosiglitazone	4 mg daily or 2 mg BID/8 mg daily	−0.8% to −1.5%	Hepatotoxicity, chronic heart failure, edema/monitor ALT at baseline and periodically thereafter	$114.46

Starting a Medication Regimen

When oral agents are prescribed, it is typical to start with metformin, a glitazone, or with an insulin secretagogue. Each of these agents will lower HbA1c level by 1% to 2%. Because each agent works by a different mechanism, drugs from different classes can be combined to achieve an additional glucose-lowering effect. Triple-drug regimens should be prescribed with caution. It is unlikely that a patient will achieve substantial improvement by taking three drugs.

Cost Considerations

Kabadi [34] recently reviewed the cost considerations of oral agents. His findings include the following: The most cost-effective drugs for type 2 DM tend to be the sulfonylureas. In combination therapy, the most effective, least costly, regimen was a sulfonylurea + metformin. This was followed by (in order of increased costs) sulfonylurea + glitazone; metformin + glitazone; sulfonylurea + alpha-glucosidase inhibitor; melglitinide + metformin; sulfonylurea + metformin + glitazone.

Areas of Caution

Weight Gain and Sulfonylureas

Weight gain is considered a significant drawback of sulfonylurea therapy, especially when metformin is thought to induce weight loss. In the U.K. Prospective Diabetes Study [35], however, gradual weight gain was noted in all patient groups regardless of therapeutic option, with the magnitude of weight gain being related to the degree of glycemic control.

Metformin and Lactic Acidosis

Lactic acidosis is a rare complication (reported rate of 0.03 cases per 1,000 patient years) associated with metformin use. There has been an excellent track record of safety with the use of metformin. Salpeter and associates [36] reviewed the literature and found no cases of lactic acidosis in 36,893 patient-years of use. Be cautious when prescribing for patients with renal impairment and heart failure.

Thiazolidinediones and Heart Failure

Thiazolidinediones, alone or in combination with other oral agents, can cause fluid retention, which can exacerbate or lead to heart failure. Patients should be monitored for signs and symptoms of heart failure, particularly those taking a thiazolidinedione and insulin [37].

Thiazolidinediones and Hepatotoxicity

Thiazolidinediones have been associated with idiosyncratic hepatotoxicity. Liver function tests should be monitored. Patients with abnormal liver function test results (e.g. ALT >2.5 times the upper limit of normal) should not take any of these drugs.

Glipizide and Hypoglycemia in the Elderly

Renal or hepatic insufficiency may cause elevated blood levels of glipizide and may increase the risk of serious hypoglycemic reactions. The elderly are particularly susceptible to this. The effect may take several days to wear off, necessitating a maintenance drip of intravenous glucose.

Triple-Drug Regimens

The use of three agents is becoming more common, especially when a patient's HbA1c level is well above the target range of 7%. Rather than add a third agent, it is advisable for patients with HbA1c levels >8% who are already taking two agents to consider using insulin therapy.

Alpha-Glucosidase Inhibitors and Hypoglycemia

When these medications are combined with other oral agents or insulin, hypoglycemia may occur and must be treated with pure glucose tablets/gel or milk in order to delay the absorption of other carbohydrates.

Insulin

At least 50% of patients with type 2 DM require insulin to maintain an HbA1c level below 7%. Many patients are hesitant to start. Some are afraid of giving an injection, some recall that a relative became seriously ill only after starting insulin, and some consider that the use of insulin implies failure [38].

The DAWN (Diabetes Attitudes, Wishes, and Needs) Study [39] included interviews with more than 5,000 patients and 3,000 health care providers. Findings include the following:

1. Very few patients had a positive attitude about insulin.
2. More than 50% of patients saw insulin therapy as meaning that they failed.

It is important to assess whether patients harbor these fears and to address them. The following are recommended to overcome this hesitancy:

1. Avoid scare tactics.
2. Solicit and address patient concerns.
3. Discuss type 2 DM as a progressive disease that often will eventually require insulin therapy to maintain glycemic control.

4. Explain the rationale for insulin therapy.
5. Recognize the importance of social support, emotional well-being, and patient acceptance of the use of insulin.

In our experience, most patients, once they receive training, adjust quickly to using insulin. Nevertheless, most physicians are hesitant to prescribe insulin, instead favoring ineffective triple-drug regimens or ignoring worsening glycemic control. Many physicians harbor beliefs about insulin therapy that are not accurate, (e.g., that insulin use raises blood pressure, increases the risk of atherosclerosis, and invariably results in weight gain). Although weight gain does occur with insulin therapy, there are interventions that can limit this effect. In the DAWN Study, provider barriers to starting insulin included the following:

1. Time required to teach patients about insulin and adjust therapy
2. Increased risk of hypoglycemia
3. Increased risk of weight gain
4. Increased risk of cardiovascular events
5. Lack of patient acceptance of insulin
6. Sense of failure for not being able to control DM

Insulin is available in rapid-, short-, intermediate-, and long-acting forms that may be injected separately or mixed in the same syringe. Insulin lispro (Humalog) and insulin aspart (NovoLog) are rapid acting. Regular (Humulin R, Novolin R) is a short-acting insulin. Intermediate-acting insulins include lente (Humulin L) and NPH (Humulin N). Ultralente (Humulin U) and insulin glargine (Lantus) are long-acting insulins. Insulin preparations with a predetermined proportion of intermediate-acting insulin mixed with short- or rapid-acting insulin (e.g., 70% NPH/30% regular, 50% NPH/50% regular, 75% NPL/25% insulin lispro, 70% NPL/30% insulin aspart) are available. The different forms of insulin available, along with suggested starting regimens, are listed in Table 7.13.

The ADA has prepared an Instructor's Guide to help providers educate patients about the use of insulin. This is available at www.diabetes.org. Despite the wide variety of choices available, it is typically best to start with a simple regimen and advance as the patient begins to understand how he or she can add flexibility with the different types of insulin.

In our clinic, the most common strategy that we use is to start with bedtime insulin in combination with an oral agent. We start with either NPH or Lantus, typically using 10 units as the initial dose. We instruct the patient that the first goal is to target the fasting blood glucose level. The rationale behind this method is that for patients who have an elevated HbA1c level, approximately 70% of the elevation comes from the fasting plasma glucose level. The fasting plasma glucose level is a reasonable first target, as there are less variables to contend with (i.e., meals and activity) and it gives the greatest chance for the patient to feel successful in the attempt to achieve better control.

TABLE 7.13. Types of insulin and common insulin regimens.

Type	Onset	Peak	End
Rapid-acting			
Lispro (Humalog)	5 min	1 hr	2–4 hr
Short-acting			
Regular (Humulin R, Novolin R)	½–1 hr	2–5 hr	6–16 hr
Intermediate-acting			
NPH (Humulin N)	1–1½ hr	4–12 hr	24+ hr
Lente (Humulin L)	1–2½ hr	6–15 hr	22+ hr
Long-acting			
Insulin glargine (Lantus)	2–4 hr	No peak	22–24 hr
Ultralente	4–6 hr	8–30 hr	24–36 hr
Mixtures			
NPH 70: regular 30	30 min	2–12 hr	24 hr

Common insulin regimens
One-shot regimen
Bedtime NPH (Humulin N) or Lantus (insulin glargine)
Two-shot regimens
Intermediate-acting insulin given at 6 am and 6 pm
Rapid- and intermediate-acting insulin given at 6 am and 6 pm
Short- and intermediate-acting insulin given at 6 am and 6 pm
Three-shot regimen
Short-acting insulin given at 6 am, 12 pm, and 6 pm; long-acting insulin given at 6 am

After starting the bedtime regimen, we instruct the patient to slowly increase the dose until a target of <120 mg/dL is achieved. If we are able to achieve adequate control of the fasting plasma glucose level and the HbA1c level is under 7%, we continue bedtime insulin. If the fasting plasma glucose level is controlled but the HbA1c level is above 7%, then we consider adding pre-meal insulin. For patients motivated to try multiple-injection therapy, we usually start with 10 units of regular or lispro insulin taken before each meal. This approach requires that a patient is willing to keep a blood glucose diary, is willing to learn about estimating the carbohydrate content of meals, is able to learn to recognize and manage hypoglycemia, and is willing to come to follow-up appointments to discuss the progress.

Monitoring

Summary

• Most providers fall short in meeting well-published consensus goals for management and monitoring of DM and its complications.

- A registry that includes information from visit-specific templates and monitoring flow sheets provides patients and physicians with the information needed to effectively manage DM.
- In support of an approach that enhances self-management, it is advisable to monitor patient-generated goals and action plans.
- Successful quality improvement interventions to impact outcomes in patients with DM require using at least two strategies.
- NCQA, in conjunction with the ADA, has established a provider recognition program that sets the benchmarks for clinical excellence. It is available at www.ncqa.org/dprp.
- A rapid-cycle Plan-Do-Study-Act (PDSA) intervention is the most effective means of improving process outcomes in a practice.

Evidence from studies show that many physicians fall short in meeting well-published goals for management of DM and its complications [40]. As mentioned earlier, disease management programs have consistently helped improve process outcomes, patient satisfaction, utilization of resources, and costs. The most effective intervention for a practice is to use templates for each office visit and to develop a system by which ongoing performance can be assessed for a particular patient and for the practice population. The means to achieve this level of documentation can be as sophisticated as an electronic medical record or a simple as a standard paper checklist.

Documentation

Ideally, a template should be used to monitor the key process outcomes for patients with DM. This should be available at the time of each visit, allowing the provider and the patient with the opportunity to review the most recent information, including the patient's self-generated goals. Figures 7.2 and 7.3 provide examples of a template for an office visit and a flow sheet to monitor process outcomes. These can be tailored to include patient-generated goals. We believe it is important to reinforce the principle of patient self-management and, therefore, include a summary of each patient's own data provided at the time of the office visit (Table 7.14). We also provide an action plan for each patient (see Table 7.1) to help detect warning signs of worsening control, and as a prompt to return to care before reaching a crisis.

Quality of Care

Despite established benefits of improved control of a number of process outcomes (e.g., HbA1c, lipid, and blood pressure levels), repeated studies show that many providers and practices fail to monitor and treat patients with DM in a manner consistent with national consensus guidelines. Over

UNIVERSITY OF CALIFORNIA DAVIS
HEALTH SYSTEM

UC DAVIS MEDICAL GROUP
DAVIS

PROGRESS NOTES
Diabetes

HT	WT	BP	T	P	R	Allergies: ☐ NONE KNOWN	Signature:

REASON FOR VISIT (CHIEF COMPLAINT) ☐ ADDITIONAL COMMENTS ON EXTRA PAGE	CURRENT MEDS: ☐ NONE ☐ SEE MED LIST	PAIN: YES ☐ NO ☐ LOCATION: _____
#1		
#2		INTENSITY: _____

THIS SECTION TO BE COMPLETED BY PATIENT

SINCE YOUR LAST ROUTINE DIABETES VISIT HAVE YOU HAD:	YES	NO	REMARKS
1. A diabetes-related ER or hospital visit?			
2. Excessive thirst, hunger, urination, blurred vision or blood sugar over 180?			
3. Shakiness, rapid heart, confusion, night sweats, headache or blood sugar below 70?			
4. Feet numbness, tingling, burning or cold sensation?			
5. Have you ever had a foot ulcer?			
6. Weight loss or gain of more than 10 pounds in last 6 months?			
7. Change or loss of vision?			
8. Skin problems or rashes?			
9. Female patients - Are you planning a pregnancy now or in the future?			
10. Are you feeling overwhelmed by your diabetes?			

11. How often do you check your blood sugar? _____   Highest blood sugar: _____   Lowest: _____

12. Which food affects your blood sugar the most?   ☐ Chicken breast   ☐ Salad   ☐ Rice or potato

☐ Cheese   ☐ Other _____   ☐ Don't know

13. Please list all "over the counter" medicines, vitamins, herbals and supplements you are using:

THIS SECTION TO BE COMPLETED BY PHYSICIAN

ETOH: ☐ Yes ☐ No   ☐ Cut down   ☐ Annoyed   ☐ Guilty   ☐ Eye opener

During the past month have you felt: ☐ Down, depressed or hopeless?   ☐ Little interest in doing things?

Home blood glucose monitoring assessed?   ☐ Yes ☐ No   Medication list reviewed?   ☐ Yes ☐ No

Other Complaints / Comments:

Page 1 of 2

FIGURE 7.2. Diabetes office visit form. (Courtesy of UC Davis Medical Group, Sacramento, CA.)

EXAM:	FOOT EXAM:	☐ Not assessed	
	A. PEDAL PULSES	☐ Yes	☐ No
	B. NAILS TOO THICK / LONG	☐ Yes	☐ No
	C. FOOT ABNORMAL SHAPE	☐ Yes	☐ No
	D. VIBRATORY SENSE OK	☐ Yes	☐ No

DRAW / LABEL FINDINGS

C = Callous, U = Ulcer, M = Maceration, R = Redness, S = Swelling

| Lab results reviewed   ☐ Yes   ☐ No | MONOFILAMENT EXAM (Draw in Circle): |
| | + = Positive sensation   − = Negative sensation |

ASSESSMENT

☐ TYPE 1 DM   ☐ TYPE 2 DM   ☐ ADEQUATE CONTROL - NO CHANGE IN TREATMENT   ☐ INADEQUATE CONTROL

WITH:

			WITH:	
1. DYSLIPIDEMIA	☐ YES ☐ NO		4. NEUROPATHY	☐ YES ☐ NO
2. HYPERTENSION	☐ YES ☐ NO		5. RETINOPATHY	☐ YES ☐ NO
3. NEPHROPATHY	☐ YES ☐ NO		6. _____	☐ YES ☐ NO

OTHER DX:

TREATMENT PLANS

RECOMMENDATIONS/PLAN:

☐ ASA   ☐ ANNUAL FLU   ☐ PNEUMOVAX   ☐ ACE INHIBITOR: _____

LABS: ☐ Hgb A1C   ☐ LIPIDS   ☐ MICRO A/CR RATIO   ☐ TSH   ☐ CHEM 7   ☐ OTHER: _____

REFERRALS – See flow sheet

FOLLOW UP APPOINTMENT: ☐ 1 MONTH   ☐ 3 MONTHS   ☐ 6 MONTHS   ☐ 9 MONTHS   ☐ OTHER: _____

PATIENT/FAMILY EDUCATION ASSESSMENT

Patient / Family Education Needs?   ☐ Yes   ☐ No

Barriers?   ☐ None   ☐ _____

Understanding?   ☐ Verbalized   ☐ Demonstrated

EDUCATIONAL MATERIALS PROVIDED:

SIGNATURE:

NAME LABEL HERE

Page 2 of 2

FIGURE 7.2. *Continued*

UCDMG - DAVIS   **DIABETES FLOW SHEET**

GOALS		DATE ↓	DATE ↓	DATE ↓	DATE ↓	Annual EXAMS	DATE ↓	ADA membership	
NONE	Tobacco use					Pneumovax		DATE ↓	DATE ↓
DAILY	Exercise					EYES			
DAILY EXAM	Foot counsel PATIENT					FLU SHOT			
	ERT					Sensory exam of FEET done			
If CV risk	ASA					Dietician appt			
125/75 ACE	HTN					Precon- ception counsel		CAD Hx	
	DATES →								
<6.5	HgbA1c QUARTERLY								
<125	FBS								
<140	ppGlucose								
<200	Cholesterol								
>40	HDL								
<100	LDL								
<4	Chol/HDL								
<160	TG								
0 - 1.8	Microalbuminuria								
neg	Proteinuria								

UCDMG - DAVIS   **DIABETES FLOW SHEET**

< 150 mg	24 hr Urine protein								
0.5 - 1.3	Creatinine								
	Cr clearance							sticker	here
	ECG						name		
	DM education						med rec #		
	Home glucose						DOB		

FIGURE 7.3. Diabetes flow sheet. (Courtesy of UC Davis Medical Group, Sacramento, CA.)

TABLE 7.14. Patient diabetes record.

My doctor is:

Blood Pressure:

My last blood pressure was:

The American Diabetes Association (ADA) recommends that blood pressures be less than 130/85. You can control Blood Pressure through diet, exercise, and blood pressure medication.

Blood Sugar Control:

This is measured by the hemoglobin A1C (HbA1c).

My last HbA1c was done on:
My last HbA1c measurement was:

The ADA recommends checking the A1c every 3–6 months. The ADA recommends keeping the A1c less than 7 to reduce the complications of diabetes. You can control blood sugar through diet, exercise, insulin, and oral diabetes medications.

Cholesterol:

This is measured by LDL (also known as the "bad cholesterol")

My last LDL was done on:
My last LDL measurement was:

The ADA recommends keeping LDL less than 100 to prevent heart attacks, stroke, circulation problems, and amputations. You can control cholesterol through diet, exercise, and cholesterol-lowering medications.

Foot Care:

Diabetes can cause foot problems, including nerve damage, ulcers, and infections. You should examine your feet every day, and your doctor should check them at every diabetes visit. Foot problems can be prevented by contacting your doctor if you should notice any changes.

My last foot exam was on:

Eye Care:

Diabetes can cause damage to your eyes. Patients who control their blood sugar and receive good eye care can prevent loss of vision and blindness. You can protect your eyes by seeing an eye doctor yearly.

My last diabetic eye exam was on:

Source: Courtesy of UC Davis Medical Group, Sacramento, CA.

one-half of patients with DM have poor glycemic control, with HbA1c levels >9.5%. A number of organizations have set standards for optimal management of DM and its complications. The National Center on Quality Assurance (NCQA), in conjunction with the ADA, has established standards consistent with excellence in the care of patients with DM. These are listed in Table 7.15.

There have been efforts by organizations interested in patient safety to provide disease-specific resources for quality improvement. The Leapfrog Group (www.leapfroggroup.org) has developed a Diabetes Health

TABLE 7.15. ADA clinical practice recommendations for glycemic control.

HbA1c	<7.0%
Preprandial plasma glucose	90–130 mg/dL
Peak postprandial plasma glucose	<180 mg/dL

Key concepts in setting glycemic goals
- Goals should be individualized
- Certain populations (children, pregnant women, and elderly) require special considerations
- Less intensive glycemic goals may be indicated for patients with severe or frequent hypoglycemia
- More intensive glycemic goals may further reduce microvascular complications at the cost of increasing hypoglycemia
- Postprandial glucose may be targeted if HbA1c goals are not met despite reaching preprandial glucose goals

Lipid and blood pressure goals			
Blood pressure (mmHg)		Lipids (mg/dL)	
Systolic	<130	LDL-C	<100
Diastolic	<80	HDL-C	>40
		Triglycerides	<150

Key tests/exams	
Test	Frequency
HbA1c	Quarterly if treatment changes or goals are not being met
	At least 2 times/year if stable
Dilated eye examination	Yearly
Comprehensive foot examination	At least yearly (more often for patients with high-risk foot conditions)
Lipid profile	Yearly (less frequently if normal)
Microalbumin measurement	Yearly
Blood pressure	Each visit
Weight	Each visit

Source: Data from American Diabetes Association [13].

Improvement (HIP) Program. This program offers education and diabetes management strategies. Health professionals provide members with a variety of health education resources, depending on their health status and condition. The health professionals serve as a "health coach," motivating and encouraging members to adopt behaviors that lead to a healthier lifestyle.

The Agency for Healthcare Research and Quality (AHRQ) commissioned a study in 2003 of the literature related to DM in an attempt to translate research into practice and to improve the overall standard of patient care [41]. Findings of the study are published in a new AHRQ Technical Review series, "Closing the Quality Gap: A Critical Analysis of Quality Improvement Strategies," as Volume 2, "Diabetes Mellitus Care."

Over 3,000 journal articles were initially considered for review. Researchers at Stanford University–University of California at San Francisco were asked to examine the results. They found that using at least two quality improvement strategies provides a greater chance for success in controlling blood sugar levels. Examples of quality improvement strategies include physician and patient reminder systems; telephone, fax, or e-mail transmissions of patient data from outpatient specialty clinics to the patient's primary care physician; and continuing education for physicians and patients.

The importance of meeting these "targets for control" is seen in the U.K. Prospective Diabetes Study (UKPDS). It was the largest and longest study of its kind for patients with type 2 DM. The study extended over a 15-year period. The 1% difference between conventional treatment and intensive treatment corresponded to a 25% reduction in the risk of complications of small vessel disease. Macrovascular disease was also reduced by intensive therapy.

Methods to Improve Outcomes

The most effective strategy to help a practice meet its targets for control is to use a registry as the basis for rapid-cycle Plan-Do-Study-Act (PDSA) interventions. In our disease management program, an example of this came from a review of our registry data. We started our process, much like most practices setting up a disease management program, with no registry. Once we set the registry up with relevant patient information, we were able to assess the practice and each provider for a specific outcome. For example, in our initial review we found that 32% of our patients with DM had not had an LDL cholesterol test within the past year. We developed a rapid-cycle PDSA intervention, which was designed to decrease the number of unscreened patients. This was a simple as doing a directed mailing to all of those patients who had not been screened, and offering a free "breakfast" on three separate dates, to be given after the fasting profile was done. The breakfast was available in our clinic, and nutrition education was offered when each patient arrived. We felt this was a relatively high-impact, low-cost intervention. Given the patient population differences among practice settings, it is likely that each practice site will have different effective interventions for a given problem.

The following points are essential elements toward care improvement for patients with DM:

1. Ensure every person with DM has a continuity physician. Start a registry, if one has not been used, and include documentation of the primary care provider. If you do not start a registry, use monthly billing reports of patients with a 250.XX diagnosis as a proxy.

2. Develop systems of team-based care with standing orders. Think of DM as a disease that requires a team for management. Members of the team can include nurses, clinic assistants, receptionists, educators, nutritionists, and pharmacists. Each member of the team can be responsible for a component of a comprehensive intervention. Standing orders can be adopted from evidence-based guidelines through the Institute for Clinical Systems Improvement's "Management of Type 2 Diabetes," September 2002 [42].

TABLE 7.16. NCQA recognition program: diabetes physician recognition program measures for adult patients.

Clinical measures (required)	Criteria	Points
HbA1c poor control, >9.0%	20% of patients in sample	10.0
HbA1c control, <7.0%	40% of patients in sample	5.0
Blood pressure control, <140/90 mm Hg	65% of patients in sample	10.0
Blood pressure control, <130/80 mm Hg	35% of patients in sample	5.0
Eye examination	60% of patients in sample	10.0
Smoking status and cessation advice or treatment	80% of patients in sample	5.0
Complete lipid profile	85% of patients in sample	5.0
LDL control, <130 mg/dL	63% of patients in sample	7.5
LDL control, <100 mg/dL	36% of patients in sample	2.5
Nephropathy assessment	80% of patients in sample	10.0
Foot examination	80% of patients in sample	10.0
Total points		80.0
Points needed to achieve recognition		60.0

Patient survey measures (optional)	Criteria	Points
Self-management education	90% of patients in sample	10.0
Medical nutrition therapy	90% of patients in sample	10.0
Self-monitoring of blood glucose		
• Non-insulin-treated patients	50% of patients in sample	1.0
• Insulin-treated patients	97% of patients in sample	4.0
Patient satisfaction with		
• Diabetes care overall	58% of patients in sample	1.0
• Answers to diabetes questions	56% of patients in sample	1.0
• Emergency access	46% of patients in sample	1.0
• Explanation of laboratory results	50% of patients in sample	1.0
• Courtesy/personal manner	77% of patients in sample	1.0
Total points (including required clinical measures)		110.0
Points needed to achieve recognition		80.0

Source: From NCQA (www.ncqa.org/dprp), with permission.

3. Measure performance at the level of the office practice. This can include summary performance data on the entire practice as well as generating a list of patients who need a specific service. For example, a "report card" can assess the percentage of patients who have had an HbA1c test within the last year and help generate a list of patients who have not.

As noted, the literature supports the use of disease management programs in an effort to improve these process outcomes. If you or your medical group is interested in setting up a disease management program and seek ongoing support, the Improving Chronic Illness Care Foundation provides the opportunity to participate through a "learning collaborative" (see www.improvingchronicillnesscare.org). There are also organizations that help providers assess their practice performance against consensus standards. The National Committee for Quality Assurance (NCQA) has a voluntary Diabetes Physician Recognition Program (see www.ncqa. org/dprp) co-sponsored by the ADA. Their standards are presented in Table 7.16.

Alternative Therapy

Summary

- Many patients use herbal, as well as traditional, therapies. It is important to ask about these and to be wary of potential drug–drug interactions.

It is important to appreciate that many patients use alternative medications in conjunction with traditional therapies, and many do not inform their providers. Studies show that up to 30% of patients use herbal remedies. It is important to inquire about these medications, particularly because drug–drug interactions are unknown. One example is the use of St. John's Wort to treat depression. As its use became more popular, a number of drug–drug interactions were noted associated with adverse events.

An interesting report by Wood and associates [43] gives an important message to providers whose patients use herbal remedies. They presented a case report of a patient who stopped traditional therapy after going to India and began using "three different herbal balls" each day. After starting this regimen, the patient experienced substantial improvement in control. Blood tests confirmed evidence of the oral agent chlorpropamide in the "herbal" regimen.

There are few well-conducted trials on the use of nontraditional treatments for DM. Patients who obtain information about diabetes from the Internet will find sites that advertise combinations of herbal preparations with testimonials on efficacy. These preparations are typically given names that sound similar to traditionally used oral agents. Table 7.17 summarizes some of the individual herbal remedies that have been used [44].

TABLE 7.17. Natural medicine/herbal remedies database.

Possibly Effective

Alpha-lipoic acid

Alpha-lipoic acid taken orally or intravenously seems to improve insulin sensitivity and glucose disposal for patients with type 2 diabetes. Patients who took alpha-lipoic acid 600–1,800 mg orally or 500–1,000 mg intravenously daily had significant improvement in insulin resistance and glucose effectiveness after 4 weeks of oral treatment or after 1 to 10 days of intravenous administration. However, alpha-lipoic acid does not seem to lower glycosylated hemoglobin (HbA1c) levels in patients with type 2 diabetes.

Beer

People who consume alcohol in moderate amounts seem to have a lower risk of developing type 2 diabetes. Diabetes patients who consume alcohol in moderate amounts seem to have a reduced risk of coronary heart disease compared with nondrinkers with type 2 diabetes. The risk reduction is similar to that found for healthy people who consume light to moderate amounts of alcohol.

Blond psyllium

There is some evidence that blond psyllium seed husk taken orally can significantly reduce postprandial serum glucose, insulin, serum total cholesterol, and low-density lipoprotein (LDL) cholesterol levels in patients with type 2 diabetes and hypercholesterolemia. Blond psyllium's maximum effect on the glycemic index occurs when psyllium is mixed and consumed with carbohydrate foods. However, blond psyllium does not lower postprandial glucose in people without diabetes.

Cassia cinnamon

Taking cassia cinnamon flower (the common type of cinnamon in U.S. grocery stores) orally seems to improve type 2 diabetes. Some research suggests that cassia cinnamon 1–6 g per day for 40 days can lower fasting serum glucose level by 18%–29%, triglycerides by 23%–30%, LDL cholesterol by 7%–27%, and total cholesterol by 12%–26%.

Chromium

There is some evidence that taking chromium picolinate orally can decrease fasting blood glucose and insulin levels and decrease glycosylated hemoglobin (HbA1c) in people with type 2 diabetes. Higher doses might be more effective and work more quickly. Taking 500 mcg twice daily significantly decreases HbA1c after 2 months of treatment. Taking 100 mcg twice daily can take up to 4 months to decrease HbA1c levels. Higher doses of 200 mcg three times daily or 500 mcg twice daily also seem to reduce triglyceride and total serum cholesterol levels after 2 to 4 months of treatment. This suggests that chromium might also benefit patients with metabolic syndrome (syndrome X), but there is speculation that chromium supplements might only help patients with low chromium levels. It does not seem to help all patients with type 2 diabetes. It only seems to have a blood glucose–lowering effect in 40%–80% of people with elevated blood glucose levels. Chromium levels are sometimes below normal in patients with diabetes. There is preliminary evidence that chromium picolinate might also have the same benefits for patients with type 1 diabetes or who have diabetes secondary to corticosteroid use. There is not enough evidence to recommend chromium for all diabetes patients. Consider trial use for interested patients to see if it helps. Use chromium picolinate preparations; chromium chloride may not be as effective. Remind patients that chromium is not an alternative to conventional medicines and should not be used in place of conventional treatments.

TABLE 7.17. *Continued*

Coffee

Long-term consumption of caffeinated coffee seems to significantly reduce the risk of developing type 2 diabetes. This effect seems to be dose dependent. Population research suggests that drinking 5–6 cups of coffee per day reduces diabetes risk by 61% for women and 30% for men. Drinking 10 or more cups of coffee per day reduces diabetes risk by 79% for women and 55% for men. This relationship persists regardless of age, weight, and tobacco or alcohol use.

Fenugreek

Consuming fenugreek, mixed with food during a meal, seems to reduce postprandial blood glucose levels in patients with diabetes. It may be consumed in combination with guar gum or by itself. Muffins made from a batter consisting of foxtail and barnyard millet, in combination with legumes and fenugreek, do not produce a substantial increase in postprandial blood glucose levels of diabetic patients.

Ginseng, American

Taking 3 g of American ginseng orally, up to 2 hours before a meal, can significantly reduce postprandial glucose levels in patients with type 2 diabetes. However, doses greater than 3 g do not seem to offer any additional benefit. The glucose-lowering effect may vary among preparations because of variations in the concentration of ginsenosides.

Ginseng, Panax

There is some evidence that taking Panax ginseng orally, 200 mg daily, can decrease fasting blood glucose and HbA1c levels in patients with type 2 diabetes.

Glucomannan

Taking glucomannan orally seems to reduce serum cholesterol and blood glucose levels in patients with type 2 diabetes. Glucomannan may improve serum total cholesterol and LDL levels, glycemic control, and systolic blood pressure in patients with type 2 diabetes and hyperlipidemia. Glucomannan also seems to improve insulin resistance syndrome, a pre-diabetic metabolic condition. The positive effect on insulin resistance syndrome appears to occur when glucomannan is mixed and consumed with carbohydrate foods.

Guar gum

Taking guar gum orally with meals seems to lower postprandial glucose levels in patients with type 1 diabetes.

Magnesium

Higher dietary magnesium intake seems to lower the risk of developing type 2 diabetes, especially in overweight middle-aged women. However, magnesium does not seem to improve glycemic control in type 2 diabetes.

Oat bran

Taking oat bran orally seems to reduce postprandial blood glucose level in people with diabetes. In a randomized cross-over study of 13 people with type 2 diabetes, a high-fiber diet that included oat bran was more effective than the standard ADA diet in lowering preprandial blood glucose level and the area under the curve for 24-hour plasma glucose and glucose (measured every 2 hours) and in improving cholesterol and triglyceride levels.

Oats

Consuming a high-fiber diet for 6 weeks significantly decreases preprandial blood glucose, 24-hour plasma glucose, and insulin levels in people with type 2 diabetes. There is some evidence that consuming 50 g daily, containing 25 g of soluble fiber, might be more effective than the moderate-fiber diet of 24 g daily recommended by the ADA.

TABLE 7.17. *Continued*

Prickly pear cactus
There is some preliminary clinical evidence that prickly pear cactus taken orally can decrease blood glucose levels in patients with type 2 diabetes. Single doses can decrease blood glucose levels by 17%–46% in some patient. However, it is not known if extended daily use can consistently lower blood glucose levels and decrease HbA1c levels. Only the broiled stems of the specific species *Opuntia streptacantha* seem to be beneficial. Raw or crude stems do not seem to decrease glucose levels. Other prickly pear cactus species also do not seem to significantly lower blood glucose levels.

Soy
In postmenopausal women with type 2 diabetes, treatment with a soy product containing 30g of soy protein and 132mg isoflavones daily for 12 weeks seems to lower fasting insulin levels, HbA1c level, insulin resistance, and LDL cholesterol. Preliminary clinical research suggests that an extract of the fermented soybean product, touchi, acts as an alpha-glucosidase inhibitor. It seems to modestly lower blood glucose, HbA1c, and triglyceride levels in patients with type 2 diabetes.

Vanadium
There is some evidence that high oral doses of vanadyl sulfate (100mg daily, 31mg elemental vanadium), can improve hepatic and peripheral insulin sensitivities in patients with type 2 diabetes and possibly reduce blood glucose levels; however, prolonged use of these high doses might not be safe. It is not known if lower doses have the same benefit. Until more is known, tell patients not to use vanadium for treating type 2 diabetes.

Wine
Light to moderate alcohol consumption in wine and other sources is associated with a reduced risk of type 2 diabetes in healthy men. Light to moderate alcohol consumption is also associated with a reduced risk of coronary heart disease (CHD) in men and women with type 2 diabetes compared with nondrinkers with type 2 diabetes. The risk reduction of CHD associated with light to moderate alcohol consumption in people with type 2 diabetes is similar to that for people without diabetes who consume light to moderate amounts of alcohol.

Xanthan gum
Taking xanthan gum orally seems to lower blood glucose and cholesterol in people with diabetes.

Possibly ineffective
Cranberry
Taking cranberry supplements orally does not seem to improve fasting serum glucose, HbA1c, fructosamine, triglyceride, HDL cholesterol, or LDL cholesterol levels in patients with type 2 diabetes.

DHA (docosahexaenoic acid)
Taking DHA orally does not substantially improve serum cholesterol or other lipid levels in patients with type 2 diabetes. DHA may worsen control of blood glucose.

EPA (eicosapentaenoic acid)
Taking EPA orally does not seem to substantially improve cholesterol or other serum lipid levels and may worsen blood glucose control in people with type 2 diabetes.

Garlic
Taking garlic orally has no significant effect on glucose in persons with or without diabetes.

TABLE 7.17. *Continued*

Wheat bran
Taking wheat bran orally does not seem to consistently improve indices of blood sugar control. It does not improve blood pressure, lipids, clotting factors, homocysteine, C-reactive protein, or other factors associated with cardiovascular disease in patients with type 2 diabetes.

Likely ineffective
Fish oils
Taking fish oils orally has no effect on fasting plasma glucose levels or serum HbA1c levels at doses less than 6g per day in people with type 2 diabetes. Several clinical studies have used fish oil products containing specific proportions of the fatty acids EPA and DHA. Most commonly used products have contained 35% EPA and 25% DHA.

Insufficient reliable evidence to rate
Bitter melon
Bitter melon fruit, fruit juice, and extract seem to improve glucose tolerance, reduce blood glucose levels, and lower HbA1c level in patients with type 2 diabetes. More evidence is needed to rate bitter melon for this use.

Branched-chain amino acids
There is some preliminary evidence that ingestion of carbohydrates with an amino acid/protein mixture consisting of leucine 25%, phenylalanine 25%, and a wheat protein hydrolysate 50% may increase the insulin response in patients with type 2 diabetes. Whether dietary supplementation of such a mixture can increase the efficacy of glucose-lowering medications or reduce dependency on insulin is unknown.

Buckwheat
Preliminary evidence suggests that consuming dietary buckwheat may improve long-term glucose tolerance in patients with diabetes.

Coenzyme Q-10
There is conflicting evidence about the effectiveness of coenzyme Q-10 for diabetes. Some research suggests that taking 200mg coenzyme Q-10 per day reduces HbA1c level in people with type 2 diabetes. However, other research in type 2 diabetes using the same dose shows no effect on HbA1c level. Some research involving people with type 1 diabetes also shows no effect. For patients with hypertension and coronary artery disease, there is evidence that coenzyme Q-10 might reduce insulin resistance.

Diacylglycerol
Some research suggests that diacylglycerol might be helpful for people with type 2 diabetes and hypertriglyceridemia. Diacylglycerol 10g per day in place of triglyceride fats seems to reduce triglycerides by about 40% and reduce HbA1c by about 10%. More evidence is needed to rate diacylglycerol for this use.

Gymnema
Preliminary clinical research suggests that taking a specific gymnema extract (GS4) orally in combination with insulin or oral hypoglycemics can further reduce blood glucose and glycosylated hemoglobin in patients with type 1 or type 2 diabetes. More evidence is needed to rate gymnema for this use.

Maitake mushroom
Preliminary clinical evidence suggests that maitake mushroom polysaccharides (MMPs) might lower blood glucose level in people with type 2 diabetes. More evidence is needed to rate maitake mushroom for this use.

TABLE 7.17. *Continued*

Milk thistle
Preliminary clinical evidence suggests that the milk thistle constituent silymarin can
reduce insulin resistance in people with coexisting diabetes and alcoholic cirrhosis.

Olive oil
Olive oil in a Mediterranean-type diet seems to reduce chylomicron remnant particles
compared with a polyunsaturated diet for diabetes patients, suggesting that it might
reduce the risk of atherosclerosis. Olive oil rather than polyunsaturated oils such as
sunflower oil might be a better choice for patients with diabetes. More evidence is needed
to rate olive oil for this use.

Stevia
Preliminary clinical research suggests that stevioside, a constituent of stevia, might reduce
postprandial glucose levels by 18% in people with type 2 diabetes. More evidence is
needed to rate stevia for this use.

Vitamin E
Vitamin E might be beneficial for diabetes and diabetic neuropathy, retinopathy, and
nephropathy. Some evidence suggests that it improves glucose disposal in type 2 diabetics,
improves monocyte function, which lessens atherogenesis, improves nerve conduction in
diabetic neuropathy, improves retinal blood flow, and decreases creatinine clearance.

Source: Excerpts in this table come from Natural Medicines Comprehensive Database.

Another resource for alternative medications is the "PDR for Herbal
Remedies."[45]

Given the frequent use of herbal remedies, it is important for providers
to determine whether their patients are taking them in addition to their
prescribed regimen or in place of it. Resources such as the PDR can be
used to help determine whether there is a potential for an adverse effect
or drug–drug interaction between the alternative therapy and conventional
treatment. However, in the absence of specific studies, providers will need
to rely on their clinical judgment.

Summary

It is fair to say that type 2 DM has become a worldwide epidemic. The
complications of the disease are well known. Its impact on the quality of
life of each patient and family affected are substantial. Type 2 DM can be
described as a disease of "self-management." A patient's ability to engage
in the lifestyle changes required to maintain adequate glycemic control can
be assessed with motivational interviewing techniques and by performing
an assessment for "readiness to change." Helping a patient set reasonable
goals and assessing their confidence in achieving these goals forms the
basis of a patient-centered approach. The current method of providing care
for patients with type 2 DM has consistently shown poor compliance with

consensus guidelines and benchmarks for quality care. A registry of patient information provides the best means to monitor how a patient or a practice is doing. Rapid-cycle PDSA interventions offer a specific means to improve quality of care and to adapt an intervention to the unique characteristics of a particular practice setting.

References

1. Ettaro L, Songer TJ, Zhang P, Engelgau MM. Cost-of-illness studies in diabetes mellitus. Pharmacoeconomics 2004;22:149–164.
2. Gordois A, Scuffham P, Shearer A, Oglesby A. The health care costs of diabetic nephropathy in the United States and the United Kingdom. J Diabetes Complications 2004;18:18–26.
3. Maciejewski ML, Maynard C. Diabetes-related utilization and costs for inpatient and outpatient services in the Veterans Administration. Diabetes Care 2004;27(Suppl 2):B69–B73.
4. Rubin RJ, Dietrich KA, Hawk AD. Clinical and economic impact of implementing a comprehensive diabetes management program in managed care. J Clin Endocrinol Metab 1998;83:2635–2642.
5. Bodenheimer T, Wagner EH, Grumbach K. Improving primary care for patients with chronic illness. The Chronic Care Model, part 2. JAMA 2002;288:1909–1914.
6. Bodenheimer T, Wagner EH, Grumbach K. Improving primary care for patients with chronic illness. JAMA 2002;288:1775–1779.
7. Wagner EH, Sandhu N, Newton KM, McCulloch DK, Ramsey SD, Grothaus LC. Effect of improved glycemic control on healthcare costs and utilization. JAMA 2001;285:1963–1964.
8. Sidorov J, Shull R, Tomcavage J, Girolami S, Lawton N, Harris R. Does diabetes disease management save money and improve outcomes? A report of simultaneous short-term savings and quality improvement associated with a health maintenance organization-sponsored disease management program among patients fulfilling health employer data and information set criteria. Diabetes Care 2002;25:684–689.
9. Snyder JW, Malaskovitz J, Griego J, Persson J, Flatt K. Quality improvement and cost reduction realized by a purchaser through diabetes disease management. Dis Manag 2003;6:233–241.
10. The National Coalition on Health Care and The Institute for Healthcare Improvement. Accelerating Change Today for America's Health. Limited distribution, May 2002.
11. American Diabetes Association. Screening for type 2 diabetes. Diabetes Care 2004;27(Suppl 1):S11–S14.
12. Harris MI. Impaired glucose tolerance in the U.S. population. Diabetes Care 1989;12:464–474.
13. American Diabetes Association. Diagnosis and classification of diabetes mellitus. Diabetes Care 2004;27(Suppl 1):S5–S10.
14. Hoerger TJ, Harris R, Hicks KA, Donahue K, Sorensen S, Engelgau M. Screening for type 2 diabetes mellitus: A cost-effectiveness analysis. Ann Intern Med 2004;140:689–700.

15. Palmer AJ, Roze S, Valentine WJ, Spinas GA, Shaw JE, Zimmet PZ. Intensive lifestyle changes or metformin in patients with impaired glucose tolerance: modeling the long-term health economic implications of the diabetes prevention program in Australia, France, Germany, Switzerland, and the United Kingdom. Clin Ther 2004;26:304–321.

16. U.S Preventive Services Task Force. Screening for type 2 diabetes mellitus in adults: recommendations and rationale. Ann Intern Med 2003;138:212–214.

17. Harris R, Konahue K, Rathore SS, Frame P, Woolf SH, Lohr KN. Screening for type 2 diabetes mellitus in adults: recommendations and rationale. Ann Intern Med 2003;138(3):215–219.

18. Engelgau MM, Geiss LS, Saaddine JB, et al. The evolving diabetes burden in the United States. Ann Intern Med 2004;140:945–950.

19. Bodenheimer T, Lorig K, Holman H, Grumbach K. Patient self-management of chronic disease in primary care. JAMA 2002;288:2469–2475.

20. Jones H, Edwards L, Vallis TM, et al. Change in diabetes self-care behaviors make a difference in glycemic control: the Diabetes Stage of Change (DiSC) Study. Diabetes Care 2003;26:732–737.

21. Rollnick S, Mason P, Chris Butler C. Health Behavior Change. A Guide for Practitioners. Toronto: Churchill Livingstone, 1999.

22. Prochaska JO, DiClemente CC, Norcross JC. In search of how people change: applications to addictive behavior. Am Psychologist 1992;47:1102–1114.

23. Holman H, Lorig K. Patient self-management: a key to effectiveness and efficiency in care of chronic disease. Public Health Rep 2004;119:239–243.

24. Yeager KK, Donehoo RS, Macera CA, Croft JB, Heath GW, Lane MJ. Health promotion practices among physicians. Am J Prev Med 1996;12:238–241.

25. Lorig K, Holman H, Sobel D, Laurent D, Gonzalez V, Minor M. Living a Healthy Life with Chronic Conditions. Self-Management of Heart Disease, Arthritis, Diabetes, Asthma, Bronchitis, Emphysema, 2nd ed. Palo Alto, CA: Bull Publishing, 2000.

26. Miller WR, Rollnick S. Teaching motivational interviewing. In Miller WR, Rollnick S (eds). Motivational Interviewing: Preparing People to Change Addictive Behavior. New York: Guilford, 1991:158–184.

27. Masse RS, Shamoon H, Pasmantier R, et al. Reliability of blood glucose monitoring by patients with diabetes mellitus. Am J Med 1984;77:211–217.

28. Funnell MM, Arnold MS, Lasichak AJ. Life with Diabetes, 2nd ed. Alexandria, VA: American Diabetes Association, 2000.

29. Hu FB, van Dam RM, Liu S. Diet and risk of type II diabetes: the role of types of fat and carbohydrate. Diabetologia 2001;44:805–817.

30. Tudor-Locke C, Bell RC. Controlled outcome evaluation of the First Step Program: a daily physical activity intervention for individuals with type II diabetes. Int J Obes Related Metab Disord 2004;28:113–119.

31. Yamanouchi K, Shinozaki T. Daily walking combined with diet therapy is a useful means for obese NIDDM patients not only to reduce weight but also to improve insulin sensitivity. Diabetes Care 1999;22:1754–1755.

32. Williams JW, et al. The effectiveness of depression care management on diabetes related outcomes in older patients. Ann Intern Med 2004; 140:1015–1024.

33. www.healthnet.com.

34. Kabadi UM. Cost-effective management of hyperglycemia in patients with type 2 diabetes using oral agents. Managed Care 2004;13:48–56.
35. Turner RC. The U.K. Prospective Diabetes Study. A review. Diabetes Care 1998;21(Suppl 3):C35–C38.
36. Salpeter SR, Greyber E, Pasternak GA, Salpeter EE. Risk of fatal and non-fatal lactic acidosis with metformin use in type 2 diabetes mellitus: systematic review and meta-analysis. Arch Intern Med 2003;163:2594–2602.
37. Nesto RW, et al. Aggravation of CHF with thiazolidiones. Thiazo use, fluid retention, and congestive heart failure, a consensus statement for the American Heart Association and the American Diabetes Association. October 7, 2003. Circulation 2003;108:2941–2948.
38. Mayfield JA, White RD. Insulin therapy for type 2 diabetes: rescue, augmentation, and replacement of beta-cell function. Am Fam Physician 2004;70:489–500.
39. Alberti SG. The DAWN (Diabetes Attitudes, Wishes and Needs) Study. Pract Diabetes Int 2002;19:22a–24a.
40. www.ncqa.org/communicatious/news/dprp.htm.
41. Closing the quality gap: a critical analysis of quality improvement strategies. Volume 2—Diabetes Mellitus Care. Stanford University—UCSR Evidence—based Fracture Center Markowitz AJ (managing editor) www.ahrq.gov/downloads/pub/evidence/pdf/qualgap2/qualgap2.pdf
42. www.icsi.org/knowledge/browse_bydate.asp?catID=298page=2
43. Wood DM, Athwal S, Panahloo A. The advantages and disadvantages of a "herbal" medicine in a patient with diabetes mellitus; a case report. Diabetes Med 2004;21:625–627.
44. Jepp M. Jellin Pharm D Therapeutic Research Faculty. Natural Medicines comprehensive database www.naturaldatabase.com
45. Gruenwald J. Brendles T, Jaenicke C. PDR® for Herbal Medicines. Montvale, NJ: Medical Economics, 1998.

Appendix A
Diabetes Self-Management: Setting Goals

You, the patient, are the most important person to manage your diabetes.

We will guide you and offer support as you manage your diabetes. Setting self-care goals will help you gain and maintain control of your diabetes to reduce damage to your blood vessels and nerves.
Choose goals that you are willing to work on to manage your diabetes.

Examples of Goals for diabetes care:

I will check my feet daily. If I notice a sore or irritation I will seek medical attention.
I will exercise (walk, run, bike, swim, etc.) _____ days per week.
I will follow my carbohydrate meal plan to lower my blood sugar.

or

I will eat a lower fat diet to reduce my risk for heart disease and stroke.
I will cut back on smoking or quit smoking.
I will check my blood sugar every day and bring my results with me to my medical appointments.
I will take an aspirin or enteric coated aspirin every day.

Selected Goal: _____

Action Plan: _____

_____

Barriers/ Solutions: _____

_____

Source: Courtesy of UC Davis Medical Group, Sacramento, CA.

Appendix B
Nutrition and Type 2 Diabetes

Blood Sugar Goals and Food:

Fasting and pre-meal	80–120 mg/dL
1 hour post-meal	<180 mg/dL
2 hours post-meal	<150 mg/dL

HEALTHFUL EATING

- Eat a variety of foods in controlled portions.
- Aim to eat 3 meals per day about 4–5 hours apart.
- If you are overweight, losing even 10% of your body weight or 10–20 pounds may bring your blood sugar down significantly.

GENERAL NUTRITION GUIDELINES

Moderation is the key to controlling blood sugar. Certain foods will cause your blood sugar to rise more than others. You need to know which foods will affect your blood sugar and how to balance your intake of these.

Calories. The number of calories you need depends on your current weight, activity level, and need to gain, maintain, or lose weight.

Carbohydrates. Food is made up of carbohydrate, protein, and fat. **Carbohydrate turns to sugar in your blood.** Learning which foods are "carbohydrate foods" and balancing your intake of carbohydrates are important.

Sugar. Sugar is a type of carbohydrate. Limit intake of sugar and high-sugar foods and liquids. Limit intake of sweetened beverages, such as Kool-aid®, regular soda, lemon-aide, Gatorade®, and chocolate milk, and high-sugar foods, such as icing, candy, ice cream, jam, pie, etc. If your intake of sugary foods is high, your blood sugar will also be high. (When you choose to have a food that is high in sugar, you must substitute it for another carbohydrate food at your meal. For example, if you want to have a small piece of birthday cake after a meal, eat less bread, rice, or pasta at that meal.)

Protein. You need a moderate amount of protein every day. Protein has little effect on blood sugar and is important to include in your diet, as it will help prevent hunger when you are making changes to your diet. Some examples of protein foods include meat, fish, eggs, cottage cheese, cheese, and tofu.

Fat. Following a diet low in saturated fat and total fat is important for preventing heart disease.

SERVING SIZES/PORTIONS

- Portion control is needed to control blood sugar and weight.
- It is important to control portions of all foods and particularly important to control the portions of carbohydrate foods you eat.

TIMING OF MEALS

- Aim to eat 3 meals every day, and limit snacks if you need to lose weight.
- Eat at almost the same time every day (it is best to space your meals no more than 4–5 hours apart).

ALCOHOL

- Alcohol contains calories and has little nutritional value, so avoid alcohol if you need to lose weight; if you do drink, limit it to 2 drinks per day (1 drink is 5 oz of wine, a 12-oz light beer, or 1½ oz of spirits).
- Alcohol also may raise triglycerides, which are a type of fat in your blood.
- If you are taking pills for diabetes, ask your doctor about drinking alcohol, as it is not recommended with some medications; if you take insulin, alcohol MUST be with a meal.

CALORIE-FREE SWEETENERS

- The use of these is acceptable, as they do not affect blood sugar (some examples of calorie-free sweeteners are aspartame, sucralose, acesulfame, and saccharine).
- *Use caution* with "sugar-free" products, as they are rarely carbohydrate free; check labels for **total carbohydrate** on these products.

FIBER

- Aim for 25–30 grams of fiber per day (check labels of some of the foods you commonly eat to see if they contain fiber); it can help you feel more full, which may help with weight loss.
- Foods that are high in fiber include whole-wheat breads, cereals and grains, and vegetables and fruit.

SODIUM

- Do not add salt during cooking or at the table.
- Avoid foods high in sodium.
- If you have high blood pressure, limit intake of sodium to less than 2,400 mg per day (read labels).
- To reduce sodium, read labels and keep in mind: a single serving of food should have less than 400 mg of sodium in it; entrees or convenience meals should have less than 800 mg of sodium in them.

Carbohydrate Counting

100% of carbohydrate eaten turns to sugar in the blood within about 2–3 hours of eating.

Balancing carbohydrate intake is critical to control diabetes.

Carbohydrate counting requires:

1. Knowing which foods have carbohydrate in them (for example: bread, fruit, milk)
2. Learning how much carbohydrate is in foods

Carbohydrate Counting

Carbohydrate is measured in terms of grams. You can find out the grams of carbohydrate there are in a food by reading the label or looking the food up in a carbohydrate resource book.

The average person with type 2 diabetes needs between <u>30 and 60 grams</u> of carbohydrate per meal and no more than <u>15 grams</u> per snack.

The best place to find out how much carbohydrate a food has is to go to the food label.

1) Check the **serving size**.   ━━━━━▶

If needed, use a measuring cup to measure the serving size.

2) Check the **grams** (g) of **Total Carbohydrate**.

━━━━━▶

This is the amount of carbohydrate **per serving**.

Nutrition Facts	
Serving Size 1 cup (253g)	
Servings Per Container 2	
Amount Per Serving	
Calories 260 Calories from Fat 72	
Total Fat 8g	
Saturated Fat 3g	
Cholesterol 120mg	
Sodium 1010mg	
Total Carbohydrate 22g	
Dietary Fiber 9g	
Sugars 4g	
Protein 25g	

If you have ½ of a serving, your total carbohydrate will be ½ of what is listed on the label (e.g., 11 grams). If you have 2 servings, your total carbohydrate will be doubled (e.g., 44 grams).

3) **Dietary Fiber**

Try to choose foods that have fiber. If the fiber is 5 or more grams per serving, subtract it from the total carbohydrate, as "Dietary Fiber" does not turn to sugar in your blood. In the example above, **the Total Carbohydrate** *would be 22 grams – 9 grams (dietary fiber) = 13 grams carbohydrate.*

Carbohydrate Food Groups (turn to sugar) Grams of Carbohydrate

Breads, Grains, Cereals, Starchy Vegetables

1 serving from this food group is:

1 sliced bread
½ small bagel or ¼ large bagel
½ hamburger or hotdog bun
1 tortilla (6 inch)
6 saltine crackers
½ of a 6-inch pita
½ cup pasta
½ cup cooked cereal
¾ cup unsweetened dry cereal
½ English muffin

1 waffle (4½ inch)
2 pancake (4 inches across)
15–20 tortilla or potato chips
   20 thin French fries
3 cups popcorn
¼ cup white or brown rice
½ cup cooked beans, lentils

Starchy Vegetables

½ cup corn or green peas
1 small potato
½ cup mashed potato, sweet
   potato or yam
1 cup winter squash

Each of the servings listed = 15 grams of carbohydrate

For example:

1 slice of bread = 15 grams of carbohydrate
½ cup pasta = 15 grams of carbohydrate
½ cup corn = 15 grams of carbohydrate

Fruits

1 serving from the fruit group is:

1 small fresh fruit (apples, small banana, orange, peach, etc.)
1¼ cup whole strawberries
½ cup canned fruit (canned in its own juice)
15 grapes
1 cup cubed melon

2 small tangerines
¾ cup blueberries
2 tbsp. raisins
¾ cup fresh pineapple
1 kiwi

Each of the servings listed = 15 grams of carbohydrate

For example:

1 small apple = 15 grams of carbohydrate
1 small orange = 15 grams of carbohydrate
¾ cup blueberries= 15 grams of carbohydrate

Milk

1 serving from the milk group is:

1 cup milk (choose nonfat or 1% unless your child is under 2 years)
1 cup soy milk
¾ cup plain yogurt
1 cup light (sugar free) yogurt

Each of the servings listed = 15 grams of carbohydrate

For example:

1 cup milk = 15 grams carbohydrate
1 cup light yogurt = 15 grams carbohydrate

Carbohydrate Food Groups (turn to sugar) Grams of Carbohydrate (*Continued*)

Low-Carbohydrate Food Groups

These foods contain some carbohydrate, but their impact on your blood sugar is minimal.

Vegetables

- Choose vegetables every day
- Be sure to check the carbohydrate food groups, as there are some "starchy vegetables" that do contain carbohydrate

(In large quantities, carrots may increase blood sugar.)

Other Foods

Free Foods

The following foods in the listed portions are considered "free foods." Limit your servings of these "free foods" to 3 per day.

1 tbsp. fat-free cream cheese

¼ cup salsa

1 tbsp. low-fat sour cream

2 tbsp. whipped topping

1 sugar-free hard candy

2 tsp. light jam or jelly

2 tbsp. sugar-free syrup

1 tbsp. mustard or ketchup

diet soda, diet beverages

1½ large dill pickle

vinegar

Meats and Other Protein Foods

- Lean beef, poultry, fish, pork
- Eggs
- Cottage cheese, cheese
- Peanut butter
- Tofu

Choose lean protein sources. Include protein in your daily intake.

Sugar and Sweets

Sugar and sweets convert into glucose in your blood. As with any other food, you need to know how much carbohydrate is in these foods. In moderation, sweets fit into a healthful diet.

If you are going to have something sweet, take some other carbohydrate out of your meal.

Fat

- Avocado
- Nuts
- Margarine
- Mayonnaise
- Oil

Bacon

- Cream cheese

Limit saturated fat.

Low-Fat Eating

USE LESS FAT IN COOKING

- Trim all visible fat off meat before cooking.
- Bake, broil, or roast meats.
- Steam vegetables.
- Do not fry or sauté foods.
- If you do fry, use a non-stick frying pan with no added fat or use non-stick cooking spray.

ADD LITTLE OR NO FAT TO FOODS

- Eat vegetables and breads without butter or margarine.
- Use lemon juice or vinegar on salads and cooked vegetables.

STAY AWAY FROM "FAST FOODS"

- These are almost always high in fat.

WATCH OUT FOR THESE FOODS THAT ARE HIGH IN FAT:

Avocados	Cream	Ham hocks	Salad dressings
Bacon	Cream cheese	Hot dogs	Salt pork
Butter	Cream sauces	Ice cream	Sandwich spreads
Cheese	Creamed soups	Margarine	(i.e., liverwurst,
Chocolate	Creamed vegetables	Mayonnaise	chicken spread, etc.)
"Cold cuts" (i.e., bologna, salami, etc.)	Croissants	Nuts	Sausages
	Donuts	Pastrami	Shortening
Corn chips	Fried foods	Potato Chips	Sour cream
Corned beef	Gravies		

USE "FREE FOODS"

These foods contain no fat and minimal or no calories:
  Broth
  Pickles (sour and dill)
  Bouillon (fat free)
  Salsa
  Catsup
  Soy sauce
  Coffee
  Tabasco sauce
  Herbs
  Tomato sauce
  Hot Sauce
  Vegetables (raw or cooked)
  Lemon juice
  Vinegar
  Mustard

READ LABELS FOR FAT CONTENT

Check the Serving Size
(2 "servings" would be 2 cups ½ "serving"
would be ½ cup)

Check Total Fat grams (g)
Check Saturated Fat grams (g)
Check Cholesterol milligrams (mg)

Nutrition Facts
Serving Size 1 cup (253g)
Servings Per Container 2
Amount Per Serving
Calories 260   Calories from Fat 72
Total Fat 8g
Saturated Fat 3g
Cholesterol 120mg
Sodium 1010mg
Total Carbohydrate 22g
Dietary Fiber 9g
Sugars 4g
Protein 25g

Daily limits for fat intake vary with the number of calories you need:

Calories	Total fat grams/day	Saturated fat grams/day
1,200	33–47	9
1,500	42–58	12
1,800	50–70	14
2,000	56–78	16

Cholesterol intake should be less than 200 mg/day.

Total fat is made up of saturated fat, monounsaturated fat, polyunsaturated fat, and trans fat (this one is not currently on labels). Monounsaturated fat and polyunsaturated fat do not raise cholesterol, but you still need to keep total fat intake within the guidelines regardless of what kind of fat you are eating.

DIABETES RESOURCE LIST

Resources for finding carbohydrate content of foods:
"The Doctor's Pocket Calorie, Fat and Carbohydrate Counter" (less than $10)
Allan Borushek
Family Health Publisher 2000
(949) 642–8500
www.calorieking.com or check local bookstores

"The Diabetes Carbohydrate and Fat Gram Guide" (less than $15)
LeaAnn Holzmeister, RD, CDE
American Diabetes Association, 2nd edition, 2000
1-800-DIABETES
www.diabetes.org

"Calories and Carbohydrates" (less than $10)
Barbara Kraus
Mass Market Paperback, 14th edition, 2001
Amazon.com or check local book stores

Cook books

Web sites:
www.diabetes.org
www.niddk.nih.gov

Cooking with the Diabetic Chef
Chris Smith

Diabetic Meals in 30 Minutes—Or Less!
Author(s): Robyn Webb, MS

The Great Chicken Cookbook for People with Diabetes
Author(s): Beryl M. Marton

Month of Meals: Classic Cooking
Author(s):   American   Diabetes
Association

Express Lane Diabetic Cooking
Author(s): Robyn Webb

Diabetes Meal Planning on $7 a Day
   or Less
Author(s): Patti B. Geil, MS, RD,
FADA, CDE

www.kraftdiabeticchoices.com
www.splenda.com
www.diabeticcooking.com

Tami A. Ross, RD, CDE

Food Diary

Write down all the foods and fluids you eat or drink in one day.

Time	Food	Amount	How prepared	Carbohydrate content (g)
For example: 8 am	Eggs Toast	2 2 slices (wheat)	Scrambled (no oil)	32 g

Source: Courtesy of UC Davis Medical Group, Sacramento, CA.

Appendix C
Exercise: Getting Started

- Talk to your health care professional, have tests done as recommended
- Wear proper shoes
- Pick an exercise you enjoy
- Exercise with a friend
- Start slow, increase length, frequency and intensity gradually
- Test blood sugar before and after exercise
- Let people know you have diabetes
- Have a fast-acting sugar for hypoglycemia
- *If you take insulin, talk to someone on your health care team — you may need to alter your regimen*
- *Stay hydrated*

Source: Courtesy of UC Davis Medical Group, Sacramento, CA.

Appendix D
Taking Care of Your Feet in Diabetes: Patient Education Sheet for UC Davis Health System

You *can* make a difference. This information will tell you how to take care of your feet if you have diabetes. It is important to take special care of your feet when you have diabetes. Poor care can lead to very serious complications.

Nerve damage can cause your feet to lose feeling. You will then not feel an injury that may need medical attention. Your feet can change shape, causing new pressure points that may lead to blisters, sores, ulcerations, infections, and loss of part of your foot. Blood flow may be poor to your feet. This causes injuries to heal more slowly.

What You Should DO to Take Care of Your Feet

- **Check your feet every day**. If you cannot see your feet, have a family member or friend check them. Check the tops, bottoms, and between the toes. Look for scratches, cuts, blisters, sores, and changes in color or shape. If you notice any of these problems, check with your primary care physician or podiatrist as soon as possible.
- **Wash your feet daily**. Use warm water and mild soap. If you can do this during bathing or showering, that will be fine. Make sure you dry your feet well, even between the toes. Then use a good **cream** to keep the skin on your feet and legs from becoming too dry and cracking. Do not apply the cream between your toes.
- **Toenails**. File them smooth. If you have good feeling in your feet, you can file your nails with an emery board to shorten and thin them.
- **Corns and Calluses**. Use soft, nonadhesive, nonmedicated pads between your toes. If they bother you, see your physician or podiatrist for treatment.
- **Shoes**. Good fitting shoes are very important. It is important to always wear some type of shoe to protect your feet. Purchase shoes in the afternoon, when your feet may be swollen. Break in new shoes slowly by wearing them for only 1 or 2 hours at a time and then checking your feet

for areas of irritation. Always wear socks or stockings with your shoes. Check the inside of your shoes for sharp or foreign objects before putting them on.

DO NOT DO THE FOLLOWING TO YOUR FEET

- **DO NOT SOAK YOUR FEET** unless instructed to by your physician. Soaking can cause your skin to get too dry and crack. That would open the skin to infection.
- **DO NOT GO BAREFOOT**. Shoes protect your feet from injury.
- **DO NOT WEAR TIGHT SHOES**. Do not wear shoes without socks or stockings.
- **DO NOT USE THE FOLLOWING ON YOUR FEET** unless instructed to by a physician or podiatrist: corn or callus removers, iodine preparations, razor blades, knives, or anything sharp.
- **DO NOT TRIM YOUR TOENAILS YOURSELF** if your feet are numb. You do not have any feeling in your feet, and you may cut yourself. File your nails to shorten and thin them.
- **DO NOT SMOKE**. This decreases the blood flow to your feet.
- **DO NOT WEAR TIGHT SOCKS**. This will cause swelling in your legs and feet.
- **AVOID EXTREMES OF TEMPERATURE. DO NO USE HEATING PADS, HOT WATER BOTTLES, OR PUT YOUR FEET NEXT TO A HEATER**. These can cause serious burns to your feet. Avoid extremes of temperature. Test water with your hand or elbow before bathing. Do not walk barefoot on hot surfaces, such as the cement on a hot day.

See your physician or podiatrist if you have any questions or concerns regarding the care of your feet.

Physician/Podiatrist name and phone number:

_____

Additional special instructions:

_____
_____
_____

Courtesy of UC Davis Medical Group, Sacramento, CA.

8
Asthma

SAMUEL LOUIE

Summary

Management

1. When managing a patient with asthma, the goal is asthma control. The NIH-NAEPP "Guidelines for the Diagnosis and Management of Asthma" are available for download to a Palm OS PDA device at http://hin.nhlbi.nih.gov/as_palm.htm.

    a. Reduction in health care utilization(s), patient safety, and improvement in quality of life are key outcome measures in chronic asthma management. The first step to successful management, however, is to correctly diagnose asthma and its severity.

    b. An accountability gap and/or achievement gap in asthma control frequently exists when a patient has uncontrolled asthma or difficult-to-control asthma. Rigorous clinical trials suggest asthma control can be achieved if patients and health care providers are accountable to each other and have defined goals of therapy to achieve. Although responsible for the problem, both hold the keys to the solution in a health care partnership.

    c. Performance measures and pay-for-performance strategies will be instituted by Medicare and private health care insurance companies to promote better quality of care by health care providers and better patient outcomes for a variety of chronic diseases, including asthma.

2. Successful asthma control prevents morbidity and mortality from asthma exacerbations that require health care resource utilizations (e.g., emergency room visits and lost days from work or school). Successful asthma control can only be achieved with competent self-management practices. A written asthma action plan can reduce mortality from asthma exacerbations, particularly when it incorporates prednisone for rescue. Train patients with the skills necessary to

control and monitor their symptoms, and provide educational materials and support (e.g., telephone service to help them build confidence in their problem-solving abilities). Consider quantifying asthma control with patient care tools (e.g., Asthma Control Test recommended by the American Lung Association, available at http://www.asthmacontrol.com).

3. The asthma patient must acquire self-management skills, including the abilities to:
   a. Follow a written asthma action plan
   b. Monitor peak expiratory flow rate measurements when symptoms or limitations appear
   c. Recognize the signs and symptoms of worsening asthma
   d. Take prescribed controller asthma medications daily or as directed
   e. Know who to call for help and who to seek immediate treatment from when asthma control is not achieved

4. Confirm the diagnosis of asthma when doubtful. Perform pulmonary function testing with spirometry to provide objective evidence of reversible airway obstruction (i.e., a $FEV_1 > 12\%$ after bronchodilator). Rule out asthma in uncertain cases with a methacholine challenge (PC20) test. Evaluate for other conditions that may mimic asthma and thwart asthma control. Most common are chronic obstructive pulmonary disease (COPD) from tobacco smoking, rhinosinusitis, gastroesophageal reflux disease (GERD), congestive heart failure (CHF), clinical depression, and barriers that might impact treatment plans. These often include difficulty with access to care, affording medications, family discord, and limited English skills (the ability to understand verbal and written instructions).

5. Consider uncommon presentations of common ailments and common presentations of uncommon disorders that cause episodic wheezing, cough, and dyspnea in patients who fail to respond to inhaled corticosteroids and bronchodilator therapy (e.g., rhinosinusitis, vocal cord dysfunction) or have other concerning symptoms not associated with asthma (e.g., hemoptysis, fever, night sweats, or weight loss, as in chronic bronchiectasis).

6. During your asthma control history, identify:
   a. Triggers that precipitate symptoms (look for poor adherence to the written asthma action plan)
   b. History of tobacco smoking or exposure to environmental tobacco smoke
   c. History of other allergic illnesses (i.e., atopic dermatitis or allergic rhinosinusitis)
   d. Medications that might precipitate cough or affect bronchospasm (e.g., use of an angiotensin-converting enzyme inhibitor or a beta-blocker)

7. Use the NIH-NAEPP Guidelines to initiate severity-specific treatment and chronic disease management. Determine if patients meet Mild, Moderate, or Severe Persistent category criteria. Recognize how clinical history, peak expiratory flow rate monitoring, and office spirometry can modify the written asthma action plan and chronic disease management. Whatever the disease severity, the goals of asthma treatment remain the same: asthma control and patient safety.

8. An assessment of the impact of asthma on the patient's quality of life can be measured accurately with the validated Asthma Quality of Life Questionnaire (AQLQ), which can be found on the American Thoracic Society website at www.atsqol.org/Juniper.asp.

9. Safety should be the foremost priority with any pharmacologic interventions designed to control asthma long term. The most effective controller medications in clinical trials are those that reduce airway inflammation (e.g., inhaled corticosteroids, antileukotriene drugs). For all inhaled medications delivered by metered dose inhaler (MDI) or dry powder inhaler (DPI), user technique is important.

10. Medicine is ever changing. Experienced health care providers and chronic disease management teams should incorporate periodic updates from the NIH-NAEPP and the medical literature, including guidelines on chronic disease management and drug treatment after thorough consideration of safety issues and predicted clinical outcomes.

    a. The accountability gap and achievement gap in chronic asthma management must be closed between patient and health care providers.

    b. Comparing fairly the quality of care provided by different managed-care health systems, when asthma severity in different patient populations varies geographically, will be a constant challenge.

    c. In the final analysis, we must do a clinical trial of one for every asthma patient.

Monitoring

1. Management requires frequent monitoring of clinical performance measures to be effective and to identify problems early to solve to improve quality of care. Look for gaps in accountability and achievement. Many health care providers do not achieve consensus goals for management and monitoring of asthma. Poor asthma control is epidemic. To improve the quality of care you provide for your practice or health system, consider creating an asthma registry or an electronic medical record database that includes the names of all patients with asthma and their written asthma action plans, which should include a medication list and best performance on peak flow.

2. Use asthma management templates for each office visit, and develop a system by which ongoing asthma control can be assessed for a particular patient and for the clinic practice.
3. Document self-management goals expected of the patient with the written asthma action plan and include them in the patient's medical record to help target person-specific asthma control goals and to identify barriers that may exacerbate accountability and achievement gaps.
4. The Physician Consortium for Performance Improvement has provided a series of tools that can be used to develop and measure quality improvement activities. To improve the quality of care for your patients with asthma, the Consortium recommends ongoing monitoring in the following areas, which echo NIH-NAEPP recommendations:
   a. Asthma assessment: Determine whether the goals of therapy are being met. Monitoring should be done in the following six areas:
      i. Signs and symptoms (daytime or nocturnal awakenings)
      ii. Pulmonary function (spirometry, peak expiratory flow rate monitoring)
      iii. Quality of life or functional status
      iv. History of asthma exacerbations
      v. Pharmacotherapeutic as-needed use of rescue inhaled short-acting beta-agonist or ipratropium bromide AND compliance or adherence to a regimen of long-term controller medications that aim to control airway inflammation and triggers of asthma exacerbations
      vi. Patient–provider communication and satisfaction (keeping the Asthma Control Test^{TM} score >19 is a helpful tool that can improve patient–provider communication; the test can be downloaded at http://www.asthmacontrol.com)
   b. Pharmacologic therapy: Demonstrate evidence of a stepwise approach that is severity-specific, keeping in mind the variable responses of asthma patients, to single-drug therapy or combinations of inhaled corticosteroids, leukotriene receptor antagonist or nedocromil, and long-acting beta-2-agonists, and the problem of compliance with taking daily medication regularly. The patient must take the prescribed medication as directed to properly evaluate the efficacy of any drug therapy.
5. The most effective strategy to help a practice or health care organization meet targets for chronic asthma management is to use an accurate asthma registry in conjunction with Plan-Do-Study-Act (PDSA) interventions employed by a health care team motivated to provide better health care. All of the aforementioned interventions can help close the large accountability gaps and achievement gaps that currently exist in asthma control.

Background

Summary

- Asthma is one of the most common chronic conditions in the United States.
- Approximately 26 million people have asthma, 8.6 million of whom are children.
- Lower socioeconomic groups and certain ethic groups (African Americans and Hispanic Americans, particularly Puerto Rican and Cuban Americans) suffer poorer asthma outcomes and experience higher mortality from asthma.
- The annual cost for asthma in the United States is $14.5 billion, coming mostly from hospitalizations and emergency room visits for asthma exacerbations.
- Eighty percent of the costs of asthma come from 20% of the patients with poor asthma control.
- For adults, asthma accounts for 13.9 million office visits, 400,000 hospitalizations, and 1 million emergency room visits each year.
- For children, asthma accounts for 5.8 million office visits, 89,000 hospitalizations, and 876,000 emergency room visits each year. Children miss school; parents miss work.

Prevalence and Impact on Society

Asthma is one of the most common chronic conditions in the United States; it is the sixth most common condition overall. It is a chronic respiratory syndrome characterized by remissions and exacerbations rather than by a distinct disease as taught to us by our mentors. Although determining the exact prevalence of this disease is challenging because of variations in reporting criteria, there is no question that the number of patients affected by asthma is on the rise [1]. The estimate that about 5% to 7% of the population is affected by this disease [2] may actually underestimate the true prevalence of asthma, which could be 10% or greater in certain regions and communities. Twenty-six million people have been diagnosed with asthma in the United States, 8.6 million of whom are children. In fact, asthma is the most common chronic disease in American children. More adult women suffer from asthma than men; women over age 55 years currently have the highest asthma mortality rate [3].

There is a disproportionate impact of asthma complications in patients from lower socioeconomic groups. Increased mortality in asthma is linked with ethnicity but may also be related to access to health care services. Age-adjusted death rates for asthma from 1990 to 1995 are reported higher for African Americans (38.1 deaths per million), Puerto Rican Americans (40.9 deaths per million) Cuban Americans (15.8 deaths per million),

TABLE 8.1. Key trends in asthma morbidity and mortality in the United States.

- Asthma mortality increased from 1980 to 1995, but declined from 1995 to 2002.
- Mortality is highest in African Americans; women and the elderly also have high mortality rates.
- The number of office visits for asthma continues to increase steadily; there were 13.9 million reported office visits in 2002.
- The number of emergency room visits continues to increase steadily; over the last 8 years, emergency room visits have increased 36%.
- Hospitalization rates for asthma are highest for African Americans, women, and children.

Source: From National Center for Health Statistics, Center for Disease Control and Prevention [3].

Mexican Americans (9.2 deaths per million), and non-Hispanic whites (14.7 deaths per million) [4]. In studies on children, there are also links between the high costs of care for asthma and poor psychological and family functioning. Some facts that highlight the trends of this disease are presented in Table 8.1 [3]. These trends demonstrate the challenges we face in dealing with this chronic disease: finding ways to lower mortality rates for high-risk groups and finding ways to deal with increasing utilization, particularly for emergency care.

Cost of Asthma Health Care

The costs associated with the treatment of asthma are substantial. Over the last several years, the annual cost for asthma care in the United States has been $14.5 billion, accounting for 1% of total health care costs [5]. As with most chronic conditions, a high percentage of the total costs are attributable to a small percentage of the patient population. Eighty percent of the costs of asthma come from 20% of the patients. This fact is important in developing effective disease management programs; it is smart to identify those who are having the most difficulty with symptoms from the disease and focus efforts on helping this group of patients. A substantial portion of these costs are from hospitalizations and visits to the emergency department, which are important clinical measures or activities to monitor in a chronic asthma management program. Asthma accounts for 13.9 million office visits, over 400,000 hospitalizations, and over 1 million emergency room visits. The cost of asthma-related hospitalizations is over $1 billion; the cost of asthma-related emergency room visits is almost $300 million. Asthmatic children costs are about $3 billion per year, with 5.8 million office visits, 89,000 hospitalizations, and 876,000 emergency room visits. Children with asthma have a high number of school absences (about 10 million missed school days each year), nighttime awakenings, and missed work days by their parents [6].

Public alarm is warranted because the incidence of asthma has increased by 60% since 1984. The need for asthma services (office visits, hospitalizations, emergency room use), has been increasing steadily. About 4,500 deaths per year are attributed to asthma [7]. Health care insurers have identified asthma most frequently as the disease for which integrated health care management ought to be devised. Given the number of patients affected, the burden of this disease on patients, especially the young and their families, and the burden on health systems, we must implement methods that are likely to improve the control of symptoms for our patients with asthma.

Chronic Disease Management Programs

Summary

- Disease management programs employing a team of motivated health care professionals reduce health care costs by decreasing resource utilization and improving patient outcomes.
- Interventions that target patients who are "high utilizers" or "frequent flyers" of health care resources provide the most marked improvement in outcomes.
- The National Institutes of Health–National Asthma Education and Prevention Program (NIH-NAEPP) Expert Guidelines for the Diagnosis and Management of Asthma remains the template for all chronic disease management programs.

Recent Studies

One of the greatest challenges in caring for patients with any chronic condition, including asthma, has been to provide services that are recognized as having a favorable impact on patient outcomes. Several investigations on the care provided to asthma patients have shown poor adherence to well-known markers for better care. Only 60% of all patients, regardless of age, in HEDIS-participating managed care plans receive appropriate asthma medications. There have been many different types of interventions studied: those that target high-risk patients in an asthma specialty clinic, those that target lower risk patients in a primary care practice, and those that are done in the community and in schools. Most of these disease management programs have shown a positive impact on health care costs, resource utilization, patient outcomes, patient satisfaction, and provider satisfaction. Interventions that target "high utilizers" or "frequent flyers" of health care resources provide the most marked improvement in outcomes and most clear-cut return on investment. Examples of chronic asthma management programs include the following:

Kelly and associates [8] assessed the impact of an intervention on 80 children with a history of frequent use of emergency services for asthma. Children in the intervention group received asthma education and medical treatment in a tertiary care pediatric allergy clinic. An outreach nurse maintained monthly contact with the families enrolled in the intervention group. During the study year emergency room use decreased from 3.5 to 1.7 visits per year. The need for hospitalizations decreased as well. Overall, average charges decreased by $721 per year.

Bratton and associates [5] looked at a multidisciplinary day program for children and adolescents with severe asthma. All of these patients prior to the intervention were frequent users of health care services. Their intervention included an intensive medical and psychological assessment using a "day treatment program" similar to that used for psychiatric therapy. Over a 2-year period the mean costs per patient decreased from $16,250 to $1,902.

Rossiter and associates [9] looked at the impact of disease management on outcomes and costs of care for low-income patients. They enrolled these patients in an educational intervention and found that the rate of emergency room use dropped an average of 41%, and use of controller medications increased by 25%. There was a return on investment to Medicaid of $3 to $4 for every incremental dollar spent on this intervention.

Beckham and associates [10] developed an integrated community-based asthma management program in an effort to reduce inappropriate utilization of urgent care services. Over a 3-year period 88 children participated in this program. There was a significant decrease in excessive utilization, with overall costs decreasing from $735 to $181 per year. Total visits to the emergency room for these patients decreased from 60 to 10.

Twiggs and associates [11] assessed the impact of an automated asthma Medication Management Information System (MMIS). The MMIS provided patient-specific guidance based on the NIH-NAEPP Guidelines. This system was implemented in primary care settings that had a centralized database with Internet access. Although the MMIS had a positive impact on the quality of care, the researchers found that physicians used severity-appropriate medications in only 60% of the cases. When they did not follow the guidelines, they tended to use too much medication rather than too little; this happened in 22% of cases.

The NIH-NAEPP Expert Panel Report 2, "Guidelines for the Diagnosis and Management of Asthma" [12], updated in 2002 [13], remains the template for all chronic disease management programs. These guidelines provide detailed management advice and advocate for patient education as a critical component of quality asthma care. An update of the NIH-NAEPP Expert Panel Report is expected in 2006.

University of California, Davis Asthma Network

In 1999, we developed our own program using the NIH-NAEPP recommendations (Tables 8.2, 8.3) that came to be known as the University of California, Davis Asthma Network (UCAN) to serve a large urban population in the Northern California Central Valley [14]. We describe our chronic asthma management program in this chapter, not with the intention of providing the reader a template for restructuring their health care organizations or clinical practices, but rather as an example of how nontraditional ideas, teamed with caring clinicians and administrators, helped difficult-to-control asthma patients find new hope and a better life.

We created UCAN as a resource for primary care providers to help manage poorly controlled, "high utilizer" asthma patients identified by primary care providers or administrative personnel who monitor health care resource utilization (e.g., emergency room [ER] visits). Our belief is that any ER visit, urgent care visit, or hospitalization represents a failure of outpatient asthma control and should prompt a patient referral for consultation to our program. High-cost patients defined by their ER and urgent clinic visit frequency account for 20% of the asthma population but 80% of the health care costs for asthma in the United States [15].

In the UCAN program, care is driven by two registered respiratory therapists (RRTs), who are certified asthma educators, under the direction

TABLE 8.2. Nine key clinical activities for quality asthma care.

1. Establish the diagnosis of asthma; remember to rule out other conditions.
2. Classify the severity of asthma.
3. Schedule routine follow-up care. See your patients every 1–6 months. In these visits:
   a. Review the goals of asthma therapy and administer the Asthma Control Test™
   b. Review the written action plan
   c. Perform spirometry every 1–2 years unless unstable
   d. Recommend influenza vaccine annually
4. Recommend measures to control asthma triggers: avoid tobacco smoke, and environmental and occupational triggers whenever possible.
5. Treat comorbid conditions, such as rhinosinusitis, GERD, COPD, and vocal cord dysfunction.
6. Prescribe medications according to the disease severity. Beware of variable responses to inhaled corticosteroids, beta-2-agonists, and leukotriene receptor antagonists.
7. Monitor use of beta-2-agonists; bring in the patient who uses one or more metered-dose inhalers of albuterol in a month.
8. Provide education on patient self-management. In our experience, repetition of the self-learning skills is an important key to success. This includes managing environmental triggers, inhaler, and peak flow techniques; understanding pharmacotherapy; and use of a written action plan.
9. Develop a written asthma action plan!

Source: Adapted from Centers for Disease Control and Prevention [1].

TABLE 8.3. NIH-NAEPP classification of asthma severity.

	Days with symptoms	Nights with symptoms	PEFR or FEV$_1$
Step 4 Severe Persistent	Continuous	Frequent	≤60% predicted
Step 3 Moderate Persistent	Daily	≥5/month	>60%, <80%
Step 2 Mild Persistent	3–6/week	3–4/month	≥80% predicted
Step 1 Mild Intermittent	≤2/week	≤2/month	≥80% predicted

Note: Assign the level of severity based on the step in which any feature appears.
Source: Adapted from National Asthma Education and Prevention Program [12].

of two asthmatologists (an allergist and a pulmonologist). Together, these four providers form the UCAN team. They have the responsibility to counsel and provide instructions to asthma patients, particularly those whose asthma is difficult to control. In the process, UCAN has established a uniform education model designed to help asthma patients acquire the knowledge and experience necessary for effective self-management skills. Clinical performance measures included assigning quality of life scores and tracking of asthma exacerbations, associated morbidities, and death.

A parallel purpose of our disease management program was to develop primary care expertise in asthma management, including familiarity with office spirometry and written asthma action plans. We believe that UCAN should not become a chronic asthma clinic, but should be an interim stop-over to help patients establish asthma control. Patients are released from UCAN after an average of four to five visits, generally accomplished over a period of two to three months. The primary care provider initiating the referral maintains principal responsibility and assumes management of asthma care when the patients depart UCAN Program.

Unfortunately, we found that few of the patients sent to our program received care consistent with the NIH-NAEPP recommendations. In particular, there was little evidence of efforts in primary care to support self-management. None of the patients possessed a written action plan. Only a few of the patients referred to our program had office spirometry done, and less than 50% had ever had formal pulmonary function testing. Approximately 30% of patients demonstrated adequate aerosol or dry powdered delivery device technique, and only 20% remembered to do a breath hold! None of the patients had had their quality of life objectively assessed with a validated measure, for example, the Asthma Quality of Life Questionnaire (AQLQ). These "real-world" deficiencies are very common in many health care organizations and have become important performance measures for clinical quality improvement interventions.

The UCAN RRTs assess the severity of the patients' asthma, perform office spirometry, and begin educating patients and formulating a plan of care that is approved and independently prescribed by the asthmatologists. Asthma education is provided utilizing an individualized written asthma action plan based on personal best peak flow rate (PEFR). Office spirometry, reinforcement of training to correctly use inhalation devices, and peak expiratory flow meter use are done by the RRTs during each visit. Patients return for additional visits until their asthma is controlled as measured by albuterol metered-dose inhaler (MDI) use (goal: less than one MDI canister a month), prednisone rescue (goal: no use), health care resource utilizations (goal: none), nocturnal awakenings (goal: less than two per month), and a better quality of life.

Between May 1999 and May 2004, we treated 309 patients by referral: 245 (79%) women and 64 (21%) men. The range in ages was from 8 to 86 years. Fifty-seven percent had Severe Persistent asthma, and 36% had Moderate Persistent asthma. Twenty-three of the 309 patients have been followed for six months, and 257 have been followed for one year or more. One hundred sixty patients incurred 574 ER visits and 178 hospitalizations in the year preceding the start of their first UCAN clinic visit. All new patients were provided with a written asthma action plan combining peak expiratory flow rate monitoring, allergy evaluation, and combination controller drug therapy. Perception of asthma control and anxiety in this group showed a mean change of 1.252 ($p = 0.0001$) as measured by the AQLQ and the State/Trait Anxiety Inventory (Juniper). No deaths occurred in the period of study or to date (2005). Outpatient education and combination controller therapy reduced the need for urgent care and for ER visits by 95% and hospitalizations by 97%. Direct cost savings from reduced health care resource utilization were $277,876 and $1,241,448 respectively.

Cost savings paralleled improved clinical outcomes, validating the important role RRTs have in primary care intervention in our health system. We believe this demonstrates that UCAN is a viable managed-care model for improving the quality and value of asthma care while achieving significant economic savings through improvement in health care navigation and utilization [14]. A chronic disease management program such as UCAN cannot hope to reach every asthma patient who is a member of a larger health care system, nor is it always necessary for every patient to consult an asthmatologist. This disease is simply too common to expect disease management programs to reach every patient. The responsibility for asthma chronic disease management resides with every primary health care provider.

Evaluation of Asthma: Initial and Subsequent

Summary

- No screening programs for the early detection of asthma in the general population are available.
- Asthma is a chronic respiratory *syndrome* characterized by remissions and exacerbations rather than a distinct disease.
- The most common criteria used to establish the clinical diagnosis of asthma are symptoms, namely, the occurrence of one or more of the "classic triad" of episodic wheezing, cough, and dyspnea.
- In the ongoing evaluation of asthma control, it is important that you do the following when asthma is difficult to control:
  - ▲ Confirm the diagnosis of asthma, generally based on clinical grounds.
  - ▲ Confirm that there is evidence of reversible airway obstruction.
  - ▲ Consider an evaluation for other conditions that may present with similar symptoms. Examples of common conditions include:
    - ◆ Rhinosinusitis
    - ◆ Gastroesophageal reflux disease
    - ◆ Chronic obstructive pulmonary disease
    - ◆ Congestive heart failure
    - ◆ Vocal cord dysfunction
    - ◆ *Do not forget depression*
- Pulmonary function testing, that is, peak expiratory flow rate (L/min) and spirometry (FEV_1, FVC, $FEV_1\%$), are valuable objective measures of expiratory flow limitation for use in the office.
- A negative methacholine challenge test rules out bronchial asthma.

Diagnosis

The first step to successful chronic asthma management is to correctly diagnose asthma and determine its severity (Table 8.4, Figure 8.1). Asthma is a chronic respiratory *syndrome* characterized by remissions and exacer-

TABLE 8.4. Six goals of asthma therapy.

1. Controlling of chronic asthma symptoms, day and night
2. Maintaining normal activity levels, including exercise and other physical activities
3. Maintaining normal or near-normal lung function as assessed by office spirometry
4. Prevention of recurrent exacerbations and minimizing need for emergency room visits and hospitalization
5. Avoiding adverse effects of drug treatment
6. Meeting expectations of patient and family with chronic asthma management

Source: Adapted from National Asthma Education and Prevention Program [12].

Stepwise Approach for Managing Asthma in Adults and Children Older Than 5 Years of Age: Treatment

Classify Severity: Clinical Features Before Treatment or Adequate Control			Medications Required To Maintain Long-Term Control
	Symptoms/Day — Symptoms/Night	PEF or FEV₁ — PEF Variability	Daily Medications
Step 4 Severe Persistent	Continual Frequent	≤ 60% > 30%	■ Preferred treatment: – High-dose inhaled corticosteroids AND – Long-acting inhaled beta₂-agonists AND, if needed, – Corticosteroid tablets or syrup long term (2 mg/kg/day, generally do not exceed 60 mg per day). (Make repeat attempts to reduce systemic corticosteroids and maintain control with high-dose inhaled corticosteroids.)
Step 3 Moderate Persistent	Daily > 1 night/week	> 60% – < 80% > 30%	■ Preferred treatment: – Low-to-medium dose inhaled corticosteroids and long-acting inhaled beta₂-agonists. ■ Alternative treatment (listed alphabetically): – Increase inhaled corticosteroids within medium-dose range OR – Low-to-medium dose inhaled corticosteroids and either leukotriene modifier or theophylline. If needed (particularly in patients with recurring severe exacerbations): ■ Preferred treatment: – Increase inhaled corticosteroids within medium-dose range and add long-acting inhaled beta₂-agonists. ■ Alternative treatment (listed alphabetically): – Increase inhaled corticosteroids within medium-dose range and add either leukotriene modifier or theophylline.
Step 2 Mild Persistent	> 2/week but < 1x/day > 2 nights/month	≥ 80% 20–30%	■ Preferred treatment: – Low-dose inhaled corticosteroids. ■ Alternative treatment (listed alphabetically): cromolyn, leukotriene modifier, nedocromil, OR sustained-release theophylline to serum concentration of 5–15 mcg/mL.
Step 1 Mild Intermittent	≤ 2 days/week ≤ 2 nights/month	≥ 80% < 20%	■ No daily medication needed. ■ Severe exacerbations may occur, separated by long periods of normal lung function and no symptoms. A course of systemic corticosteroids is recommended.

Quick Relief All Patients	■ Short-acting bronchodilator: 2–4 puffs short-acting inhaled beta₂-agonists as needed for symptoms. ■ Intensity of treatment will depend on severity of exacerbation; up to 3 treatments at 20-minute intervals or a single nebulizer treatment as needed. Course of systemic corticosteroids may be needed. ■ Use of short-acting beta₂-agonists >2 times a week in intermittent asthma (daily, or increasing use in persistent asthma) may indicate the need to initiate (increase) long-term-control therapy.

Note

Step down — Review treatment every 1 to 6 months; a gradual stepwise reduction in treatment may be possible.

Step up — If control is not maintained, consider step up. First, review patient medication technique, adherence, and environmental control.

- The stepwise approach is meant to assist, not replace, the clinical decisionmaking required to meet individual patient needs.
- Classify severity: assign patient to most severe step in which any feature occurs (PEF is % of personal best; FEV₁ is % predicted).
- Gain control as quickly as possible (consider a short course of systemic corticosteroids); then step down to the least medication necessary to maintain control.
- Minimize use of short-acting inhaled beta₂-agonists. Overreliance on short-acting inhaled beta₂-agonists (e.g., use of approximately one canister a month even if not using it every day) indicates inadequate control of asthma and the need to initiate or intensify long-term-control therapy.
- Provide education on self-management and controlling environmental factors that make asthma worse (e.g., allergens and irritants).
- Refer to an asthma specialist if there are difficulties controlling asthma or if step 4 care is required. Referral may be considered if step 3 care is required.

Goals of Therapy: Asthma Control

- Minimal or no chronic symptoms day or night
- Minimal or no exacerbations
- No limitations on activities; no school/work missed
- Maintain (near) normal pulmonary function
- Minimal use of short-acting inhaled beta₂-agonist
- Minimal or no adverse effects from medications

FIGURE 8.1. NIH-NAEPP stepwise approach for managing asthma. (From the National Institutes of Health, http://www.nhlbi.nih.gov/guidelines/asthma/execsumm.pdf.)

bations rather than a distinct disease. Despite public concern and prevalence of asthma in the United States, there are no screening programs for the early detection of asthma in the general population, although spirometry, according to the criteria established by the American Thoracic Society,

Usual Dosages for Long-Term-Control Medications

Medication	Dosage Form	Adult Dose	Child Dose*
Inhaled Corticosteroids *(See Estimated Comparative Daily Dosages for Inhaled Corticosteroids.)*			
Systemic Corticosteroids		*(Applies to all three corticosteroids.)*	
Methylprednisolone	2, 4, 8, 16, 32 mg tablets	■ 7.5–60 mg daily in a single dose in a.m. or qod as needed for control	■ 0.25–2 mg/kg daily in single dose in a.m. or qod as needed for control
Prednisolone	5 mg tablets, 5 mg/5 cc, 15 mg/5 cc	■ Short-course "burst" to achieve control: 40–60 mg per day	■ Short-course "burst": 1–2 mg/kg/day, maximum
Prednisone	1, 2.5, 5, 10, 20, 50 mg tablets; 5 mg/cc, 5 mg/5 cc	as single or 2 divided doses for 3–10 days	60 mg/day for 3–10 days
Long-Acting Inhaled Beta₂-Agonists *(Should not be used for symptom relief or for exacerbations. Use with inhaled corticosteroids.)*			
Salmeterol	MDI 21 mcg/puff	2 puffs q 12 hours	1–2 puffs q 12 hours
	DPI 50 mcg/blister	1 blister q 12 hours	1 blister q 12 hours
Formoterol	DPI 12 mcg/single-use capsule	1 capsule q 12 hours	1 capsule q 12 hours
Combined Medication			
Fluticasone/Salmeterol	DPI 100, 250, or 500 mcg/50 mcg	1 inhalation bid; dose depends on severity of asthma	1 inhalation bid; dose depends on severity of asthma
Cromolyn and Nedocromil			
Cromolyn	MDI 1 mg/puff	2–4 puffs tid-qid	1–2 puffs tid-qid
	Nebulizer 20 mg/ampule	1 ampule tid-qid	1 ampule tid-qid
Nedocromil	MDI 1.75 mg/puff	2–4 puffs bid-qid	1–2 puffs bid-qid
Leukotriene Modifiers			
Montelukast	4 or 5 mg chewable tablet	10 mg qhs	4 mg qhs (2–5 yrs)
	10 mg tablet		5 mg qhs (6–14 yrs)
			10 mg qhs (> 14 yrs)
Zafirlukast	10 or 20 mg tablet	40 mg daily (20 mg tablet bid)	20 mg daily (7–11 yrs) (10 mg tablet bid)
Zileuton	300 or 600 mg tablet	2,400 mg daily (give tablets qid)	
Methylxanthines *(Serum monitoring is important [serum concentration of 5–15 mcg/mL at steady state]).*			
Theophylline	Liquids, sustained-release tablets, and capsules	Starting dose 10 mg/kg/day up to 300 mg max; usual max 800 mg/day	Starting dose 10 mg/kg/day; usual max: ■ < 1 year of age: 0.2 (age in weeks) + 5 = mg/kg/day ■ ≥ 1 year of age: 16 mg/kg/day

Estimated Comparative Daily Dosages for Inhaled Corticosteroids

Drug	Low Daily Dose Adult	Low Daily Dose Child*	Medium Daily Dose Adult	Medium Daily Dose Child*	High Daily Dose Adult	High Daily Dose Child*
Beclomethasone CFC 42 or 84 mcg/puff	168–504 mcg	84–336 mcg	504–840 mcg	336–672 mcg	> 840 mcg	> 672 mcg
Beclomethasone HFA 40 or 80 mcg/puff	80–240 mcg	80–160 mcg	240–480 mcg	160–320 mcg	> 480 mcg	> 320 mcg
Budesonide DPI 200 mcg/inhalation	200–600 mcg	200–400 mcg	600–1,200 mcg	400–800 mcg	> 1,200 mcg	> 800 mcg
Inhalation suspension for nebulization (child dose)		0.5 mg		1.0 mg		2.0 mg
Flunisolide 250 mcg/puff	500–1,000 mcg	500–750 mcg	1,000–2,000 mcg	1,000–1,250 mcg	> 2,000 mcg	> 1,250 mcg
Fluticasone MDI: 44, 110, or 220 mcg/puff	88–264 mcg	88–176 mcg	264–660 mcg	176–440 mcg	> 660 mcg	> 440 mcg
DPI: 50, 100, or 250 mcg/inhalation	100–300 mcg	100–200 mcg	300–600 mcg	200–400 mcg	> 600 mcg	> 400 mcg
Triamcinolone acetonide 100 mcg/puff	400–1,000 mcg	400–800 mcg	1,000–2,000 mcg	800–1,200 mcg	> 2,000 mcg	> 1,200 mcg

* Children ≤ 12 years of age

FIGURE 8.1. *Continued*

may be performed for any cooperative child older than 5 years of age and for virtually any adult man or woman. The problem inherent in asthma is that FEV₁, FVC, and FEV₁% are very often within the predicted normal range in between asthma attacks.

The risk factors for the development of asthma syndromes are complex. Although several gene sites have been associated with the susceptibility to asthma and allergy, complex gene–environmental interactions also play a role in the development of the syndrome. Early life sensitization to allergens, the presence of atopic dermatitis or allergic rhinitis, maternal smoking during pregnancy, environmental exposure to tobacco smoke, lower respiratory tract infections with respiratory syncytial virus, exposure to air pollutants, and estrogen replacement in women are among the factors associated with an increased risk for development of chronic asthma. Estimates vary, but up to 40% of patients with allergic rhinosinusitis have associated bronchial asthma, and up to 78% of asthma patients have allergic rhinosinusitis.

The diagnosis of asthma is most commonly established on clinical grounds. We have all been taught the pathologic changes that occur in the respiratory tract that constitute the syndrome of asthma, from presenting with the nonspecific symptoms of wheezing or cough occurring during the day or waking the patient from sleep, to dyspnea or exercise limitation. An allergen or other type of stimulus initiates a cascade of events in respiratory epithelial cells, alveolar macrophages, dendritic cells, T-helper $CD4^+$ lymphocytes, mast cells, and eosinophils that cause airway inflammation and intermittent bronchospasm. All current therapies aim to modulate airway inflammation caused by the aforementioned cells and bronchoconstriction by airway smooth muscle. Control of symptoms and exacerbation can be achieved, but there is no cure yet available for asthma.

Other common symptoms of the asthma syndrome include nighttime cough, exercise-related cough, and, in children, post-tussive emesis. The reliability of any one of these symptoms in establishing the diagnosis (particularly for mild disease) is problematic. Any of these symptoms alone may be present in only one-quarter to one-third of patients with asthma. However, the occurrence of multiple symptoms with recurrent episodes, particularly when there is a rapid response to bronchodilator therapy, is generally sufficient diagnostic evidence.

The two most commonly used pulmonary function tests to corroborate the clinical diagnosis of asthma by documenting decreased expiratory flow rates are:

1. Peak expiratory flow rate (PEFR), measured in L/min
2. Spirometry: forced expiratory volume in 1 second (FEV_1), measured in L/sec

Peak expiratory flow rate is an easy test to perform; however, it is very dependent on the effort of the patient and is not reliably reproducible. The patient is asked to exhale with maximum effort through the peak flow device immediately after taking a maximum deep breath. With repeated trials the patient's "best" value can be compared with their values during an exacerbation. This value can be used as a guide to determine severity of symptoms and subsequent treatment recommendations.

The FEV_1 test is more reproducible than PEFR and considered the better test of airway expiratory flow rate. It can also be used to determine disease severity, again, with results compared to a table of predicted values. In general, classification of severity is as follows:

1. FEV_1 > 80% predicted (normal)
2. 60% to 80% (mild)
3. 40% to 60% (moderate)
4. FEV_1 < 40% (severe)

The FEV_1 response to bronchodilator therapy can also help confirm the diagnosis. Specifically, an increase of ≥12% after the use of a short-acting bronchodilator (e.g., albuterol) is compatible with asthma. Indications for more sophisticated testing, such as bronchoprovocative testing (i.e., methacholine challenge test), should be considered for patients whose diagnosis is uncertain, particularly those who fail to respond to a trial of asthma management. A negative test is confirmed if the patient's baseline FEV_1 does not fall more than 20% at a methacholine dose of 8 mg/mL or lower. The methacholine challenge test is the best to rule out asthma, but there are a few asthma centers that use low doses of methacholine (4 mg/mL or less) to detect asthma in the elderly.

A chest x-ray (posteroanterior and lateral projections) and laboratory blood tests (e.g., serum IgE and RAST panel against commonly encountered antigens) are generally not indicated in the initial evaluation of patients with asthma. Neither normal spirometry nor a normal chest x-ray can rule out asthma. A chest x-ray should be considered for patients with persistent cough, wheezing, or dyspnea despite a reasonable period of treatment (e.g., two to three weeks) or for those who have developed additional symptoms, such as hemoptysis, fever, or weight loss. Tests such as serum IgE and RAST panel should be considered when patients fail to respond to therapy, for severe persistent asthma cases, and/or in consultation with an asthma specialist. Information from the RAST panel can help in educating patients to better control their environment if they have specific allergic triggers, such as cat dander.

Other conditions can occur with asthma (e.g., GERD, COPD). The NIH-NAEPP report has established a series of practical guidelines for the evaluation and management of patients with asthma [12]:

1. Confirm the diagnosis of asthma. Again, the diagnosis of asthma is, for the most part, a clinical diagnosis based on recurrent symptoms of shortness of breath, wheezing, or cough, often worse at night, and often associated with precipitating "triggers."
2. Confirm that there is objective evidence of reversible airway obstruction, for example >12% improvement in FEV_1 after bronchodilator challenge.
3. Consider an evaluation for other conditions that may present with similar symptoms.

Always suspect COPD when there is a tobacco smoking history. Smoking cessation, exercise, and use of cholinergic receptor blockers and beta-2-agonists are the cornerstones of COPD management. Gastro-esophageal reflux disease is often silent in poorly controlled asthma and can be treated effectively with proton pump inhibitors. Allergic rhinosi-nusitis is a difficult problem, beyond the scope of this chapter, but often requires various combinations of antihistamines, leukotriene receptor antagonists, nasal antihistamines, nasal corticosteroids, and/or immuno-therapy. Asthma control is often difficult to achieve until rhinosinusitis or GERD is controlled first. Cardiac asthma or CHF should not be diffi-cult to diagnose but assay for beta-natriuretic peptide (BNP), a marker of stress or damage to the ventricular muscle, may be helpful. Vocal cord dysfunction may be suspected with a flow-volume loop demonstrating a variable extrathoracic upper airway obstruction or require further diag-nostic studies.

When gathering asthma control history from a patient with asthma, focus on the following:

1. Triggers that precipitate symptoms. This may include exercise, sea-sonal exposure to plant allergens, episodic exposure to pets, episodic expo-sure to lung irritants at work or at home, and hobbies that include activities that produce lung irritants.

2. History of exposure to tobacco smoke. All patients should be asked whether they smoke, have a history of smoking, or have ongoing exposure to second-hand smoke.

3. History of other atopic illnesses. Patients with atopic dermatitis or allergic rhinitis have a higher frequency of asthma.

4. Symptoms that suggest other diagnostic possibilities, including chronic bronchiectasis, acute pulmonary embolism, acute or chronic pneumonia, and CHF. Perform a review of systems to assess for concerning symptoms that warrant additional evaluation. Examples of these symptoms include hemoptysis, fever, chills, night sweats, weight loss, chest pain, leg edema, orthopnea, and paroxysmal nocturnal dyspnea.

5. Medications that might precipitate cough or affect bronchospasm. Examples include an angiotensin-converting enzyme inhibitor and a beta-blocker.

Additional information that you should consider obtaining includes the following:

1. Immunization history, particularly whether the patient receives the influenza vaccine
2. Social history, particularly with regard to barriers that might impact treatment plans, including difficulty with access to care, affording medi-cations, and understanding written instructions

Patients with two or more asthma exacerbations per week tend to have Moderate-to-Severe Persistent asthma (Table 8.4). The current reported frequencies of each asthma severity category in the United States are the following:

1. 75% have Moderate-to-Severe Persistent disease
2. 15% have Mild Persistent disease
3. 10% have Mild Intermittent disease

These figures are a dramatic departure from the generally accepted opinion of health care agencies (since 1992) that 60% to 70% of asthma patients have Mild-to-Moderate Persistent asthma [16].

Patients typically overestimate their asthma control. Health care providers underestimate disease severity. In the Asthma in America Survey, completed in 1998 and available at http://www.asthmainamerica. com, 61% of patients meeting NIH-NAEPP criteria for Moderate Persistent asthma considered their asthma as being "well controlled" or "completely controlled." Thirty-two percent of patients who meet the criteria for Severe Persistent asthma considered their asthma as being "well controlled" or "completely controlled." The inability to recognize poor asthma control is a major safety issue because acute asthma exacerbations occur frequently and place patients at risk for greater morbidities and even death.

Although a thorough physical examination is reasonable in the initial and subsequent evaluations of patients with asthma, it must be recognized that many patients will have normal findings. However, once asthma control becomes the problem, look for evidence of rhinosinusitis, GERD, COPD, and CHF.

Evidence for other atopic diseases include the following:

1. Nasal polyps or significant nasal congestion
2. Atopic dermatitis, often appearing as a dry, papular eruption in the flexor creases of the arms and legs

Evidence for alternative explanations include for COPD, the tell-tale signs of cigarette smoking; for GERD, the Trudeau sign; and for CHF, peripheral edema, hepatojugular reflux, lung crackles, and an S3 gallop. Remember that a normal lung examination does not exclude the diagnosis of asthma!

Quality of Life Assessment

After the patient's history and physical examination have been completed, you should assess how asthma has affected his or her quality of life. There are many different quality of life instruments available, including the Asthma Quality of Life Questionnaire (AQLQ), which can be found at the American Thoracic Society website (www.atsqol.org/Juniper.asp). If you are not inclined to use the AQLA, then probably the easiest approach is to ask the following questions to assess quality of life:

1. How has asthma affected the quality of your life?
2. How has it affected your ability to do the things you enjoy?
3. What are you unable to do because of your asthma?
4. Are there any activities that you would do if your asthma was under better control?

Answers to these questions should give you better insight into how patients are affected by their asthma and what "outcomes" they would consider to be important. These, in turn, become personal goals or expectations with chronic asthma management.

Closely linked to quality of life is the common problem seen in higher frequency in all chronic disorders: *depression*. People with asthma report depression at a rate of 20% to 50%, with higher numbers frequently occurring among inner city residents, including children. Missing school days, not being able to play with other children, waking up in the middle of the night with an asthma attack, and going to the emergency room can lead to feelings of helplessness in children with asthma. People with asthma may have poor self-esteem, which can cause them to blame themselves for asthma attacks and never attempt to get better. This type of "learned helplessness" can negatively affect self-efficacy, problem-solving skills, and family interactions and can lead to depression. Patients with asthma and depression are less likely to follow their asthma management plan, and they may have difficulty adjusting their behaviors overall. The result of this can be asthma symptoms prompting feelings of helplessness and depression, which then lead to poor self-management of asthma, resulting in worsening of asthma symptoms [13].

In your initial evaluation of patients with asthma, you should always include questions to assess their understanding of their disease. However, it is a good idea to start with basic questions. These can include the following:

1. What is your understanding about what causes asthma and what can be done to treat it?
2. What have you been told by family and friends about asthma?
3. What are your expectations about treatment?
4. What format would be most useful to you in order to get a better understanding of asthma and what you can do to control the symptoms? A class? A pamphlet? A Web site?

In our experience, patients with asthma are seldom, if ever, interested in the pathobiological aspects of their syndrome and the actions of different drug therapies which underlie much of the current prescribed asthma care. They are keenly interested in living a normal life, as defined by personal expectations, and reducing their need to see health care providers.

This type of understanding, along with appropriate education and self-management support, usually leads to improved patient satisfaction and measures of control.

Management

Summary

- The goals of chronic asthma management are asthma control and patient safety.
- The written asthma action plan can anchor chronic asthma management and provide a contract for asthma care to be followed by the patient and the health care provider.
- The asthma patient or designated provider must acquire self-management skills, including the ability to:
  - ▲ Follow a written asthma action plan
  - ▲ Monitor peak expiratory flow rate measurements when symptoms or limitations appear
  - ▲ Recognize the signs and symptoms of worsening asthma
  - ▲ Take prescribed controller asthma medications daily or as directed
  - ▲ Know who to call for help and to seek immediate treatment early
- The general goals health care providers should use for managing patients with asthma are:
  - ▲ Preventing chronic asthma symptoms and asthma exacerbations during the day and night (help your patient avoid problems such as sleep disruption, missed work or school days, urgent care/emergency department visits, and hospitalizations; these are all markers for inadequate management)
  - ▲ Maintaining normal activity levels, including exercise and other physical activities
  - ▲ Achieving normal or near-normal lung function
  - ▲ Being satisfied with the asthma care received
  - ▲ Having no or minimal side effects while receiving optimal medications
- Major recommendations from the NIH-NAEPP you should incorporate into your practice include the following:
  - ▲ Ensure that the diagnosis of asthma is correct.
  - ▲ Establish a patient–clinician partnership, that is, address the patient's concerns, agree upon the goals of asthma therapy, and agree upon a written action plan for self-management.
  - ▲ Reduce inflammation, symptoms, and exacerbations (e.g., prescribe anti-inflammatory medications for patients with mild, moderate, or severe persistent asthma and reduce exposures to precipitants of asthma symptoms).

▲ Monitor and manage asthma over time.
  ◆ Train all patients to monitor their symptoms; those with Moderate-to-Severe asthma should monitor their PEFRs and use the values as a guide to what action to take.
  ◆ Ensure that patients are seen at least every one to six months.
  ◆ Perform ongoing reassessments of goals of therapy and patients' concerns.
  ◆ Review the action plan; make sure that patients understand how to use them.
  ◆ Check inhaler and peak flow technique.
  ◆ Ensure that medication therapy is "severity specific."
▲ Treat asthma episodes promptly (e.g., prompt use of inhaled short-acting beta-agonists; if the episode is moderate to severe, prescribe a 10- to 12-day course of oral steroids).
• Poor adherence with prescribed treatments over time by asthma patients is perhaps the most important barrier to asthma control and better asthma outcomes.

Asthma Control

When managing a patient with asthma, the goal is asthma control. Every asthma patient and health care provider can achieve a better quality of life and clinical outcomes by:

1. Recognizing the burden of poor asthma control on the patient and health care provider, the highly variable response to asthma drug therapy, and the vital need to identify and expertly manage difficult to control cases
2. Implementing key clinical activities (see Table 8.2), including a written asthma action plan, to ensure patient safety and attain the goals of asthma care (action plans also provide health care organizations opportunities to continuously track clinical performance measures over time)
3. Closing the achievement and accountability gaps that will persist between the patient and health care provider without a joint partnership for asthma care

Reduction in health care utilization(s) and improvement in quality of life are key outcome measures in chronic asthma management. The first step to successful management, however, is to correctly diagnose asthma and determine its severity (see Table 8.4 Figure 8.1). The subsequent steps are much more difficult to take.

An accountability gap or achievement gap in asthma control frequently exists when a patient has uncontrolled asthma or difficult-to-control asthma. Rigorous clinical trials suggest that asthma control can be achieved at http://www.aafp.org/fpm/20041000/43asth.html. Reinforce the principle of self-management with every visit. The record should include documentation of self-management skills, for example, mastering MDI and PEFR monitoring technique, use of a written action plan as prompted by symptoms, and PEFR measurement. Document self-management goals expected of the patient with the written asthma action plan and include them in the patient's medical record to help target person-specific asthma control goals and to identify barriers that may exacerbate accountability and achievement gaps.

Performance measures and pay-for-performance strategies will be instituted by Medicare and private health care insurance companies to promote better quality of care by health care providers and better patient outcomes for a variety of chronic diseases, including asthma.

Successful asthma control prevents morbidity and mortality from asthma exacerbations that require health care resource utilizations (e.g., emergency room visits) and lost days from work or school. Successful asthma control can only be achieved with competent self-management practices. A written asthma action plan can reduce mortality from asthma exacerbations, particularly when it incorporates prednisone for rescue [18]. You can assess asthma control in each patient by asking about the following:

1. Frequency during the past week of waking up at night because of asthma symptoms
2. Frequency during the past month of use of urgent care and emergency room services or hospitalization for asthma
3. Number of times a week or day during the past week that a rescue inhaler of albuterol was needed
4. Number of missed days of school or work or inability to do work at home due to asthma during the past month

Consider quantifying asthma control with patient care tools, for example, the Asthma Control Test™ developed by QualityMetric Incorporated and recommended by the American Lung Association to alert patients when asthma is not controlled (Figure 8.2). The Asthma Control Test™ is available at http://www.asthmacontrol.com. A score of 19 or less suggests that your patient's asthma may not be controlled as well as it could be. It is an excellent learning tool and monitoring tool for chronic asthma management.

Use the following procedure when asthma control is not achieved:

1. Confirm the diagnosis of asthma when doubtful. Asthma is often diagnosed based on history of episodic wheezing, cough, and dyspnea. Perform pulmonary function testing with spirometry to provide objective evidence of reversible airway obstruction (i.e., an $FEV_1 > 12\%$ after bronchodilator). Rule out asthma in uncertain cases with a methacholine challenge (PC20) test.

if patients and health care providers are accountable to each other a
defined goals of therapy. Although responsible for the problem, bo
the keys to the solution in a health care partnership. Poor adherenc.
prescribed treatments over time by asthma patients is perhaps the
important barrier to better health care outcomes, with less than ?
adherence to inhaled corticosteroids and long-acting beta-agonists, a
less than 50% adherence to leukotriene receptor antagonists [17].

Concerns for the quality of care delivered to patients with chronic cond
tions, including asthma, are expressed by a number of organizations. These
include the National Institutes of Health, Centers for Disease Control and
Prevention, the National Heart, Lung, and Blood Institute, the Institute of
Medicine, the National Committee on Quality Assurance (NCQA), the
Centers for Medicare & Medicaid Services, the Agency for Healthcare
Research and Quality (AHRQ), and the Physician Consortium for Performance Improvement. Evidence demonstrating the importance of setting
up an effective monitoring system includes the following:

1. High rates of suboptimal treatment for asthma
2. High utilization of albuterol/urgent care/emergency room services
3. High utilization of hospital bed days
4. High rates of missed school days and work days
5. Noncompliance or poor adherence with prescribed treatment(s)

Albuterol should not be used to control asthma, and a reduction in
albuterol use usually correlates well with improving asthma control. It is
properly used as a rescue medication in a written asthma action plan, but
many asthma patients continue to use this and other short-acting beta-2-
agonists in lieu of controller therapies. Albuterol is typically supplied in
6.8 g MDI canisters containing 80 metered inhalations or 17 g canisters
containing 200 metered inhalations. Frequent pharmacy refills of albuterol
can help identify the poorly controlled asthma patient. The underutilization or ineffective use of appropriate medications and other evidence-
based, guideline-recommended therapies contribute to poor asthma control
and poor patient outcomes.

Disease management programs have consistently led to improvements
in process outcomes, patient satisfaction, utilization of resources, and costs.
Although there are multiple components in setting up an effective disease
management program, as described in the Chronic Care Model at www.
improvingchroniccare.org, a key feature is the ability to adequately document and monitor the outcomes of interest, to maintain this information
in the form of a registry, to retrieve relevant data, to analyze these data in
the form of practice reports, and to implement practice changes that are
aimed at improving outcomes for all patients.

One method to improve documentation is to use a template for each
office visit and a flow sheet to monitor outcomes that can assess quality of
care. An example of an asthma management encounter form can be found

Take the Asthma Control Test™ and Know Your Asthma Score

1. In the past **4 weeks**, how much of the time did your **asthma** keep you from getting as much done at work, school or at home?

   All of the time ○ Most of the time ○ Some of the time ○ A little of the time ○ None of the time ○ ☐

2. During the past **4 weeks**, how often have you had shortness of breath?

   More than once a day ○ Once a day ○ 3 to 6 times a week ○ Once or twice a week ○ Not at all ○ ☐

3. During the past **4 weeks**, how often did your **asthma** symptoms (wheezing, coughing, shortness of breath, chest tightness or pain) wake you up at night or earlier than usual in the morning?

   4 or more nights a week ○ 2 or 3 nights a week ○ Once a week ○ Once or twice ○ Not at all ○ ☐

4. During the past **4 weeks**, how often have you used your rescue inhaler or nebulizer medication (such as albuterol)?

   3 or more times per day ○ 1 or 2 times per day ○ 2 or 3 times per week ○ Once a week or less ○ Not at all ○ ☐

5. How would you rate your **asthma** control during the **past 4 weeks**?

   Not controlled at all ○ Poorly controlled ○ Somewhat controlled ○ Well controlled ○ Completely controlled ○ ☐

AMERICAN LUNG ASSOCIATION. The American Lung Association supports the Asthma Control Test.

print results close window

FIGURE 8.2. Asthma control test. (Copyright 2002 by QualityMetric Incorporated.)

2. Evaluate for other conditions that can mimic asthma and thwart asthma control. Most common are COPD from tobacco smoking, rhinosinusitis, GERD, and CHF.

3. Consider uncommon presentations of common ailments and common presentations of uncommon disorders that cause episodic wheezing, cough, and dyspnea in patients who fail to respond to inhaled corticosteroids and bronchodilator therapy, including rhinosinusitis and vocal cord dysfunction, or who have other concerning symptoms not associated with asthma, including hemoptysis, fever, night sweats, and weight loss, as in chronic bronchiectasis.

When obtaining the asthma control history, identify the following:

1. Triggers that precipitate symptoms, such as poor adherence to the written asthma action plan, exercise, seasonal exposure to environmental allergens, episodic exposure to pet animals, lung irritants at work or at home, and hobbies that may involve activities that produce lung irritants
2. History of exposure to tobacco smoke, whether they smoke or have ongoing exposure to second-hand smoke
3. History of other allergic illnesses, such as atopic dermatitis or allergic rhinosinusitis
4. Medications that might precipitate cough or affect bronchospasm, such as an angiotensin-converting inhibitor or a beta-blocker

A thorough initial physical examination is reasonable for patients with asthma, but subsequent visits should focus on the causes of poor asthma control. Direct your examination to look for comorbid conditions:

1. Evidence of other allergic diseases or disorders (e.g., nasal polyps or significant nasal congestion and skin findings of atopic dermatitis, such as a dry papular eruption in the flexor creases of the arms and legs)
2. Evidence of alternative explanations for cough, wheezing, and dyspnea especially in adults (lung crackles or a significant heart murmur or evidence of an S3 or S4 as signs of heart failure; gastroesophageal reflux, e.g., a positive Trudeau sign or subxiphisternal tenderness elicited on firm palpation using thumb or index finger)
3. Absence of wheezes, rhonchi, or a normal chest examination (however, do not exclude the diagnosis of asthma and may be a sign of status asthmaticus in the patient with acute respiratory distress, manifested by severe tachypnea).

The NIH-NAEPP recommends a stepwise approach to pharmacotherapy for asthma (see Figure 8.1) Medications for asthma can be divided into "rescue" and "controller " drugs and organized in a written asthma action plan (Figure 8.3). The rescue medications are short-acting beta-2-agonists (e.g., albuterol), anticholinergics (e.g., ipratropium bromide), and oral corticosteroids (e.g., prednisone). Controller medications include inhaled corticosteroids, long-acting beta-2-agonist bronchodilators, and anti-leukotriene drugs.

Safety should be the first priority with any drug interventions designed to control asthma, whether they include rescue or controller drugs. The most effective long-term controllers in clinical trials are those that reduce airway inflammation (e.g., inhaled corticosteroids, anti-leukotriene drugs). The NIH-NAEPP recommends a stepwise approach that is severity specific, keeping in mind the variable responses of asthma patients to single-drug therapy or combinations of inhaled corticosteroids, leukotriene receptor antagonist or nedocromil, and beta-2-agonists, and the problem of compliance with taking daily medication regularly. The patient

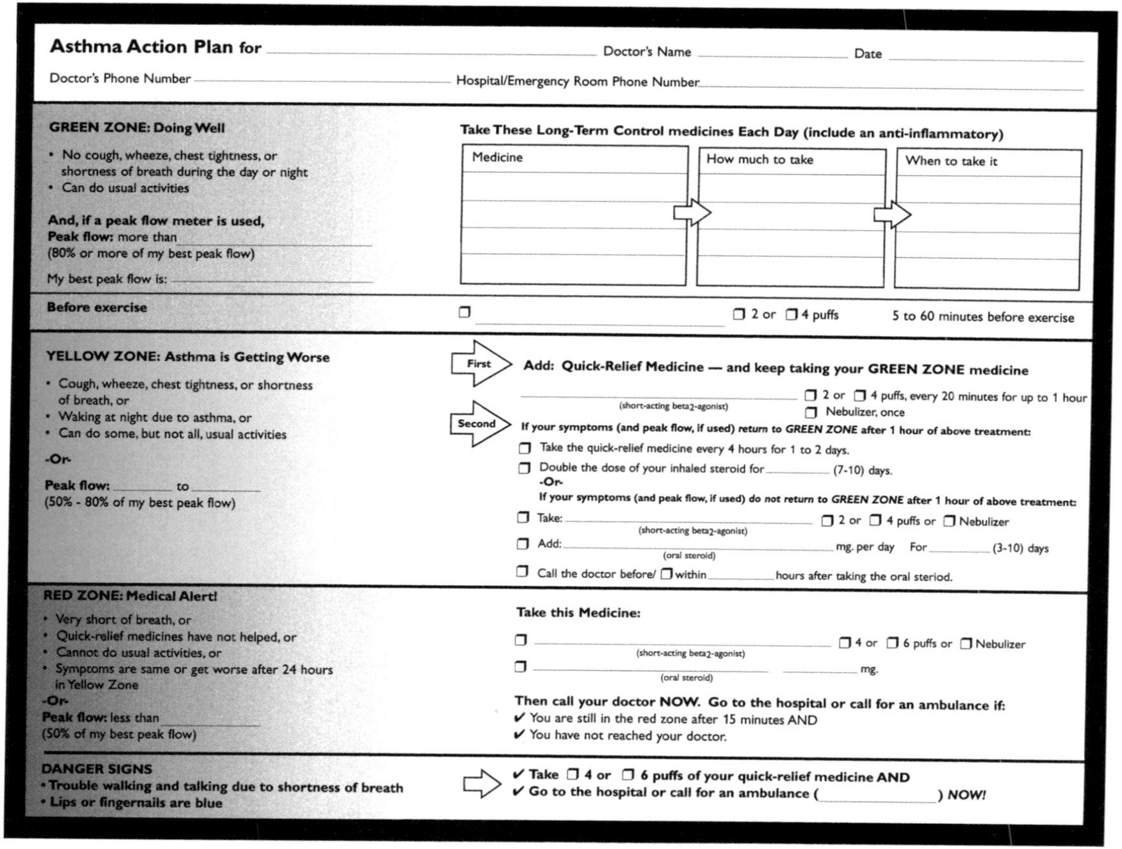

Asthma Action Plan for ______ Doctor's Name ______ Date ______

Doctor's Phone Number ______ Hospital/Emergency Room Phone Number ______

GREEN ZONE: Doing Well

- No cough, wheeze, chest tightness, or shortness of breath during the day or night
- Can do usual activities

And, if a peak flow meter is used,
Peak flow: more than ______
(80% or more of my best peak flow)

My best peak flow is: ______

Take These Long-Term Control medicines Each Day (include an anti-inflammatory)

Medicine	How much to take	When to take it

Before exercise ❐ ______ ❐ 2 or ❐ 4 puffs 5 to 60 minutes before exercise

YELLOW ZONE: Asthma is Getting Worse

- Cough, wheeze, chest tightness, or shortness of breath, or
- Waking at night due to asthma, or
- Can do some, but not all, usual activities

-Or-

Peak flow: ______ to ______
(50% - 80% of my best peak flow)

First: **Add: Quick-Relief Medicine — and keep taking your GREEN ZONE medicine**

______ (short-acting beta2-agonist) ❐ 2 or ❐ 4 puffs, every 20 minutes for up to 1 hour
❐ Nebulizer, once

Second: **If your symptoms (and peak flow, if used) *return to GREEN ZONE* after 1 hour of above treatment:**

❐ Take the quick-relief medicine every 4 hours for 1 to 2 days.
❐ Double the dose of your inhaled steroid for ______ (7-10) days.
-Or-
If your symptoms (and peak flow, if used) *do not return to GREEN ZONE* after 1 hour of above treatment:
❐ Take: ______ (short-acting beta2-agonist) ❐ 2 or ❐ 4 puffs or ❐ Nebulizer
❐ Add: ______ (oral steroid) mg. per day For ______ (3-10) days
❐ Call the doctor before/ ❐ within ______ hours after taking the oral steriod.

RED ZONE: Medical Alert!

- Very short of breath, or
- Quick-relief medicines have not helped, or
- Cannot do usual activities, or
- Symptoms are same or get worse after 24 hours in Yellow Zone

-Or-

Peak flow: less than ______
(50% of my best peak flow)

Take this Medicine:

❐ ______ (short-acting beta2-agonist) ❐ 4 or ❐ 6 puffs or ❐ Nebulizer
❐ ______ (oral steroid) ______ mg.

Then call your doctor NOW. Go to the hospital or call for an ambulance if:
✔ You are still in the red zone after 15 minutes AND
✔ You have not reached your doctor.

DANGER SIGNS
- **Trouble walking and talking due to shortness of breath**
- **Lips or fingernails are blue**

✔ Take ❐ 4 or ❐ 6 puffs of your quick-relief medicine AND
✔ Go to the hospital or call for an ambulance (______) *NOW!*

FIGURE 8.3. Asthma action plan. (From the National Institutes of Health, http://www.nhlbi.nih.gov/guidelines/asthma/execsumm.pdf.)

must take the prescribed medication as directed to properly evaluate the efficacy of any drug therapy.

Currently, Moderate and Severe persistent asthma patients should be treated with combination therapy (see Figure 8.1). Mild Persistent asthma cases will benefit from low-dose inhaled corticosteroids or anti-leukotriene drugs, or intermittent corticosteroid treatments. Inhaled corticosteroids are the most potent inhaled anti-inflammatory medications for asthma. Anti-leukotriene drugs are effective but less potent than inhaled corticosteroids. Long-acting beta-2-agonists, although classed as a controller, are not anti-inflammatory drugs and can actually worsen asthma control when used alone as a controller.

The FDA has issued important safety information (see http://www.fda.gov/cder/drug/infopage/LABA/default.htm) warning asthma patients and health care providers that long-acting beta-2-agonists may increase the risk of asthma-related deaths. When treating patients with asthma, health care providers should only prescribe long-acting beta-2-agonists or multiple drug delivery devices containing a long-acting beta-2-agonist and inhaled corticosteroid for patients not adequately controlled with other asthma controllers (e.g., low- to medium-dose inhaled corticosteroids) or whose disease severity clearly warrants initiation of treatment with two mainte-nance therapies. This uncommon adverse effect from long-acting beta-2-agonists should be considered for any patient with worsening asthma control despite apparent compliance with an asthma action plan and com-bination controller therapy. The use of a combination long-acting beta-2-agonist and inhaled corticosteroid is not indicated for patients whose asthma can be successfully managed by inhaled corticosteroids along with occasional use of inhaled short-acting beta-2-agonists.

For all inhaled medications delivered by MDI or dry powder inhaler (DPI), user technique is important. Always try to observe your patients' technique in the office, especially if they are having problems with asthma control. Take the time to teach them in the clinic until they can return the demonstration correctly.

The asthma patient or designated provider must acquire self-management skills, including the following abilities:

1. Follow a written asthma action plan
2. Monitor peak expiratory flow rate measurements when symptoms or limitations appear
3. Recognize the signs and symptoms of worsening asthma
4. Take prescribed controller asthma medications daily or as directed
5. Know who to call for help and where to seek immediate treatment early

It is vital to help patients acquire the skills necessary to control and monitor their symptoms, and to provide educational materials to help them build their confidence and problem-solving abilities.

As part of the initial assessment for an educational intervention, you should include questions that help determine your patients' understanding of their disease. It is a good idea to start with questions such as the following:

1. What is your understanding about what causes asthma and what can be done to treat it?
2. What are your expectations and your family's expectations about asthma care and treatment?
3. What type of information would be most useful to you in order to get a better understanding of asthma and what you can do to control symptoms?

Assessing Importance

For any self-management intervention, you must determine if your patient is ready to engage in the activity. This is done by evaluating "importance." Ask your patients the following question: "How important to you is getting control of your asthma symptoms?" Have them rate the importance on a scale of 1 to 10, where 10 is very important. A score of less than 7 may indicate substantial barriers to adequate asthma control. These are often social or behavioral issues, such as depression, family conflict, and financial issues. Failing to address these barriers will usually result in poor control of asthma.

Education is the key to changing patient behavior. If lifestyle changes would be beneficial to your patient (e.g., stop smoking), ask your patients about their readiness to change; only 20% of patients are ready to make significant lifestyle changes at the time of the initial evaluation. Your assessment can be accomplished by asking: "How likely are you to try to stop smoking at this point." Again, use the 10-point scale, where 10 is very likely and 1 is very unlikely. Those who say less than 7 are unlikely to make the behavior change. It is important to help these patients address the barriers that keep them in this situation. Help them set goals that they feel are achievable, even if the short-term goal is not "ideal health." It is best if these goals are incorporated into a patient-generated, specific, short-term, achievable action plan (see Chapter 2 for more information on self-management).

Try to set up a system that allows you to review the goals of asthma therapy as often as is feasible, preferably during an office visit. This can be facilitated by a form that includes questions such as:

1. Has your asthma disrupted your sleep? Caused you to miss work? Caused you to miss school?
2. Have you had to go to an urgent care clinic or emergency room since your last appointment because of a problem with your asthma?
3. Has your asthma limited your ability to do things you want to do?

4. Are you satisfied with the control you have over your asthma?
5. Are you having any side effects from your medications?

You can have the patient complete this form before the appointment.

Have your clinic staff (e.g., registered nurse or registered respiratory therapist who is a certified asthma educator) help reinforce healthy behaviors, self-management goals, and emergency action plans. For example, have the clinic staff remind patients that it is important to have an emergency action plan posted in an accessible place, such as on the refrigerator. Ensure that your patients with moderate to severe persistent symptoms can demonstrate how to use a peak flow meter and how to use the readings in a written asthma action plan.

Provide user-friendly educational resources that are culturally sensitive and tailored to a patient's specific needs and goals. There are several resources available on the Internet:

1. The American College of Allergy & Asthma Immunology, available at http://www.aaaai.org/patients.stm
2. The Centers for Disease Control and Prevention, available at http://www.cdc.gov/health/asthma.htm
3. The Allergy and Asthma Foundation of America, available at http://www.aafa.org
4. The National Heart, Lung & Blood Institute (NHLBI), available at http://www.nhlbi.nih.gov/health/public/lung/index.htm

The NHLBI Web site has the following forms you can give to your patients:

1. *What Everyone Should Know About Asthma*: A summary of what patients can do to get and keep control of their asthma
2. *How to Control Things That Make Your Asthma Worse*: A guide to environmental changes that may help control or prevent symptoms
3. *How to Use Your Metered-Dose Inhaler the Right Way*: A guide to the proper technique in using an MDI
4. *An Asthma Action Plan*: A specific plan to guide patients toward severity-specific interventions (Levels of severity are identified as Green Zone—Doing Well, Yellow Zone—Asthma Getting Worse, and Red Zone—Medical Alert! Recommendations for interventions are given for each level.)
5. *School Self-Management Plan*: A page that can be used for children to help prevent unnecessary missed school days
6. *How to Use Your Peak Flow Meter*: Describes the purpose of a peak flow meter linking the results with the action plan "zones" of control
7. *Patient Self-Assessment Form for Environmental and Other Factors that Can Make Asthma Worse*: A self-assessment form to assess environmental factors
8. *Patient Self-Assessment Form for Follow-Up Visits*: A quick summary of how the patient has been doing since the last visit

The interventions discussed earlier are a reflection of a philosophy of care as much as a call to specific actions. Set up an environment to initiate a partnership with the asthma patient. Provide the patient with the tools that support self-management (e.g., writing an action plan, training patients to monitor symptoms, training for optimal inhaler technique, and assessing and managing triggers). Provide severity-specific treatment, help manage exacerbations, and monitor the patient's progress in reaching their goals.

Medicine is ever changing. Experienced health care providers and chronic disease management teams should incorporate periodic updates from the NIH-NAEPP and the medical literature, including guidelines on chronic disease management and drug treatment after thorough consideration of safety issues and predicted clinical outcomes. The accountability gap and achievement gap in chronic asthma management must be closed between patient and health care providers. Knowing how to compare fairly the quality of care provided by different managed care health systems, when asthma severity in different patient populations vary geographically, will be a constant challenge. To paraphase Eugene Robin, MD, Professor of Medicine at Stanford, In the final analysis, for every patient, we must do a clinical trial of one.

Management Key Points

"There was never yet an uninteresting life. Such a thing is impossibility. Inside of the dullest exterior there is a drama, a comedy, and a tragedy."
—Mark Twain, *The Wit and Wisdom of Mark Twain*

The first priority in providing effective asthma care is to get to know the patient. An informed, motivated patient is the key to dealing successfully with this disease. Every patient should be taught and then asked to demonstrate vital self-management skills. These include the following abilities:

1. Follow a written action plan.
2. Recognize signs and symptoms of worsening asthma.
3. Monitor peak flow readings when symptoms worsen.
4. Take prescribed medications that match the severity of symptoms.
5. Use the correct technique when using inhaled medications.
6. Know how to use the action plan; who to call for help and when it is necessary to seek immediate treatment.

Your ability to develop a partnership with your patients that fosters their self-care abilities is key to success in managing asthma. Our experience is that every patient is unique and every patient has his or her own challenges in gaining optimal control. Rarely do we ever find an asthma patient unable to learn self-management skills over time. Each patient, however, must value and use the management skills, which coincidentally will improve self-respect. That being said, some patients are not ready to focus on self-management, often because of life "stressors." For these patients, it is important that you do not give in to the urge to label them as noncompliant; rather, help guide them to the resources they need to deal with the barriers to control.

The next step is to help keep your patient from suffering preventable complications. You should recognize and accept that every asthma patient can run afoul with an exacerbation. Hence it is imperative that you anticipate these problems and adopt an aggressive preventive and caring position to help patients recognize trouble early and be able to access help promptly. In our UCAN™ Clinics we do this by consistently reviewing the NIH-NAEPP goals of asthma therapy, as presented in Table 8.3, at every visit to help identify areas for improvement.

Next is to assess your practice for its ability to support quality asthma care. The key clinical activities are presented in Table 8.2. None of the activities requires sophisticated technologies or interventions. Finally, ensure that your practice follows the four essential components of asthma care as presented in Table 8.5.

Limited English proficiency hampers communication only when health care providers permit it to. Patients can benefit from other ways to receive self-management education (see Chapter 6 on cultural competence). An example of an intervention for these patients is the instructional DVD produced by Health Net of California, Inc., 21281 Burbank Boulevard,

TABLE 8.5. Four major components of asthma care.

1. Diagnose asthma and initiate a partnership with the patient.
   a. Diagnose asthma by establishing a history of recurrent symptoms and reversible airflow obstruction with spirometry and excluding alternative diagnoses.
   b. Establish patient–clinician partnership: address patient's concerns, agree on the goals of asthma therapy, and agree on a written action plan for patient self-management.
2. Reduce inflammation, symptoms, and exacerbations.
   a. Prescribe anti-inflammatory medications to patients with mild, moderate, or severe persistent asthma.
   b. Reduce exposures to precipitants of asthma symptoms: assess patient's exposure and sensitivity to individual precipitants (allergens and irritants), and provide written and verbal instructions on how to avoid or reduce factors that make the patient's asthma worse.
3. Monitor and manage asthma over time.
   a. Train all patients to monitor their asthma: all patients should monitor their symptoms; patients with Moderate-to-Severe Persistent asthma should also monitor their peak flow. The Asthma Control Test™ may be a helpful adjunct in discussion of asthma action plan changes if needed.
   b. See patients at least every 1–6 months: assess attainment of goals of asthma therapy and patient's concerns, adjust treatment if needed, review the action plan with the patient, and check the patient's inhaler and peak flow technique.
4. Treat asthma episodes quickly: Encourage prompt use of short-acting inhaled beta-2-agonists; if episode is moderate to severe, institute a 10–12-day course of oral steroids and prompt communication and follow-up.

Source: Adapted from National Asthma Education and Prevention Program [12].

Woodland Hills, CA 91367. The DVD is titled *How to Control Your Asthma* and is available in English, Spanish, Chinese, Hmong, Khmer, Lao, Vietnamese, Armenian, and Russian. Another resource is the monograph *Culturally-Competent Asthma Education*, available through the Association of Asthma Educators at http://www.asthmaeducators.org/web_resources.htm. While posing additional challenges, it is clear that providing culturally sensitive asthma education provides benefits to patients. Liu and associates [19] studied interventions designed to provide culturally appropriate materials to children and their families. They found that this intervention improved quality indicators for asthma care.

How effective are interventions that target self-management? There are a number of studies that have looked at this:

1. Wilson and associates [20] conducted a study with Kaiser Permanente patients in Northern California. Those with Moderate-to-Severe asthma were randomly assigned to small group education, individual teaching, or "usual care" (an information workbook). Data on 323 patients were obtained over 2 years. Self-management education programs were found to be associated with significant improvements in control of asthma symptoms and MDI technique. Small group education was also associated with significant improvement in physician evaluation of patients' asthma status and in patients' levels of physical activity. The small group program was simpler and less costly, and better received by patients and educators.

2. Gallefoss and Bakke [21] conducted a randomized trial with 78 patients with asthma. The intervention consisted of two 2-hour group sessions followed by one or two individual sessions administered by a nurse and a physiotherapist. Self-management was emphasized in all of the sessions. There were improvements in symptoms, measures of lung function, and costs. An interesting finding was the "number needed to educate." They found that it took training "2.2" patients to make one person symptom-free.

3. Krishna and associates [22] assessed the impact of an interactive, Internet-enabled multimedia education program with 228 children. The study was based on NIH-NAEPP education. The intervention group received additional self-management education through the interactive multimedia program. The interactive program increased knowledge of asthma for children and their caregivers, decreased asthma symptom days, and decreased emergency department visits.

4. Tinkelman and Schwartz [23] studied a school-based asthma program. School nurses recruited parents or caregivers. Parents were invited to attend an educational class. Children received peak flow meters and training and access to a diary of peak flow results. They had monthly asthma education at school and access to an online asthma education program. By 6 months, missed school days and doctor visits were reduced by two-thirds. Symptom frequency decreased as well.

Assessing Self-Efficacy and Confidence

Perhaps the most critical component of chronic asthma management intervention is to appreciate the importance of self-efficacy, the confidence to carry out a behavior necessary to reach a desired goal. Just as you can assess importance, you can measure your patient's confidence in carrying out specific self-management skills. You can do this by asking a very direct question for any of the targeted skills. For example, in determining confidence in following an action plan, you could ask: "How confident are you that you can use an action plan to help guide your treatment? On a 10-point scale, patients who rate their confidence under 7 are unlikely to be successful with that task. "See one, do one, teach one" also applies. Take the time to have patients return a demonstration of their understanding, which is equally important as demonstration of proper inhaler techniques in an asthma visit.

Barriers to Self-Management

Fast Facts

- The following are common barriers in asthma care:
  - Absence of communication with the physician or health care provider
  - Absence of a written asthma action plan incorporating appropriate drug therapy
  - Absence of drug delivery device competencies
  - Absence of periodic spirometry and formal pulmonary function testing
  - Absence of allergy testing (e.g., RAST panel, total IgE)
  - Absence of quality of life evaluations
- The following factors contribute to poor patient adherence in asthma care:
  - Patient underestimation of the problem or overestimation of asthma control
  - Provider underestimation of the problem or overestimation of asthma control
  - Controller regimen containing multiple medications and drug delivery devices
  - Different dosing schedules and methods of drug delivery (i.e., oral versus inhaled)
  - Adverse effects of drugs
  - Effects of daily treatments on activities of daily living and quality of life
  - Rising cost of asthma drugs and co-pays

Overcoming Barriers

An emphasis on self-management support represents a paradigm shift for most health care providers and most of our patients. We value our problem-solving skills. We are used to giving advise to our patients in the hopes of solving the problem for them. The paradigm shift is to act in a coaching role to guide patients to develop their own problem-solving skill and to help them gain the skills and confidence to manage the common problems associated with asthma.

It must be understood that, even under optimal conditions, a delay in action in a response to symptoms often results in an urgent care or emergency room visit for most asthma patients. Use these events, not as evidence of failure for you or your patient, but as an opportunity to understand the barriers to continuing control. We recommend that you do the following in searching for barriers:

1. Assess what your patient perceives as causative factors for clinical deterioration.

2. Revisit the written asthma action plan: Was it used? Does it need to be modified?

3. Review the patient's technique for use of inhalers.

4. Review the patient's severity of asthma and determine whether he or she is receiving severity-specific treatment.

5. Determine whether there are literacy barriers; patients with limited English proficiency may simply not be able to read the instructions on the medication bottles or on the emergency action plan. Determine whether there are socioeconomic barriers contributing to poor outcomes. Socioeconomic barriers are recognized as contributing to poor outcomes in patients with asthma.

6. Determine whether affordability of medications is posing a barrier.

7. Review the issues of "importance" and "confidence"—"How important is it for you to gain control of your asthma? How confident are you in your skills to control your asthma?"

The Agency for Healthcare Research and Quality (AHRQ) released the results of a study on medication usage by patients with chronic illnesses. About two-thirds of chronically ill adults do not tell their physicians when they have to cut back on their medications because of the cost. The AHRQ surveyed more than 4,000 adults with chronic disease. Over 600 patients said that they had stopped taking some medication in the past year because of the cost, and two-thirds of the group said they did not tell their physician in advance. Of those who did not tell their physician, 58% said they did not believe their physician could help them with the problem. Patients who did talk to their physician said that their medications were not changed to less expensive alternatives, and few reported getting any assistance such as information about programs that can help pay drug costs or about where to buy cheaper drugs [24]. Many patients have taken action by receiving their medications though pharmacies in Canada. Other resources are NeedyMeds.com and BenefitsCheckUp.org.

Role for Respiratory Therapists

"It is the friend you can call at 4 a.m. that matters."
—Marlene Dietrich, ongraving on address book

A basic truth of disease management programs is that "it takes a team." You cannot expect to accomplish all the goals of an asthma disease management program without help. One person who can offer a great deal of help is the registered respiratory therapist (RRT).

With written asthma action plans and the NAEPP guidelines, RRTs have been able to expand their skills by providing assessments and assisting with treatment plans for patients. Registered respiratory therapists have evolved into a highly trained group of health care specialists. The advances in the role of the RRT are presented in Table 8.6. Registered respiratory therapists can trace their origin to the modern use of supplemental oxygen and the need for experienced individuals who could administer this treatment. At the time, these professionals were called "oxygen technicians." Advances in respiratory care technology, particularly in the field of pulmonary function testing and mechanical ventilation, has demanded a corresponding increase in the skills and caliber of RRTs (i.e., technical training and experience in clinical decision making designed to meet the needs of patients with all forms of lung disease). Professional and personal skills change from health care setting to setting, requiring flexibility in problem-solving skills and communication.

Registered respiratory therapists may represent the best alternative for physicians and asthma specialists who have a large population of patients with chronic lung disease and who recognize that enhancing patient education and self-management support will improve outcomes. They can reduce the overall cost of caring for patients with chronic lung diseases in the hospital and in the clinic, but only if given the opportunity.

TABLE 8.6. Evolution of respiratory therapy.

- Its roots can be traced to the use of oxygen therapy in the early 20th century.
- A professional organization was established in 1946 called the Inhalation Therapy Association and later renamed the American Association of Inhalation Therapists.
- The first certification examination for inhalation therapy was offered in 1969.
- Entry-level standards were established in 1978.
- Protocol-based therapies are begun in the early 1980s.
- Registered respiratory therapy was recognized as a profession by the national government in 1990.
- The registered respiratory therapist's role continues to evolve; these therapists are currently underutilized, often because of unfortunate stereotyping.

Their participation in chronic disease management is logical and should be welcomed.

The UCAN™ Program's RRTs are the only two nationally certified asthma educators (AE-C) in our health system—a large urban university medical center. The RRTs are expert in providing NAEPP asthma education about self-management, goals of asthma therapy, the common triggers of acute exacerbation, and the correct use of medicinal delivery systems. Our UCAN™ RRTs take telephone calls day and night, even at 4 o'clock in the morning, to help our asthma patients in trouble. They are supported by a physician who is consulted and directs the immediate care needed. The RRTs perform the task of telephone "case management," answering patient questions about their disease. These calls are mostly answering questions about use of the action plan and management of an acute attack and handling refill requests and authorization requests— based on health plan requirements. In the past 5 years, the UCAN™ RRTs have become health care provider icons in their own right at our facility.

Certification of qualified asthma health care providers (e.g., RRTs, nurses, nurse practitioners, pharmacists, and physician assistants) by the National Asthma Educator Certification Board (NAECB; see http://www.naecb.org) is also a necessary requirement for reimbursement of time spent educating asthma patients. The NAECB examination is currently voluntary but may soon be required by law for employment in the field. Only 70% of those who have taken the test passed it. It is the policy in our program that AE-C certification is a necessary requirement for employment and promotion.

There is no question in our minds that an RRT improves the quality of care to our patients with asthma. Of course, before having an RRT join the asthma team, it is always necessary to convince the leadership of an institution of the added value. In the past, respiratory care practitioners were hospital employed and hospital based. The real change has been in using the services of an RRT in the outpatient setting. Registered respiratory therapists can increase the productivity of a pulmonary/asthma clinic. They can perform the roles typically assumed by registered nurses, including coordinating patient care efforts among other team members, ensuring quality of care, carrying out a physician's or nurse practitioner's orders, and documenting services or treatment in the medical records. Registered respiratory therapists can assist the asthma or COPD patient's need for respiratory care, evaluate and modify care to maximize therapeutic benefit, and, very importantly, calibrate, service, clean, and repair respiratory care equipment.

Several studies have shown that RRTs are better in the delivery of respiratory treatments, in the assessment of patients, and in the education of patients with lung disorders than other health care providers (i.e., nurses and physicians). Traditional roles and career expectations for RRTs will continue to change, coinciding with changes in health care delivery. Registered respiratory therapists must continue to diversify their responsibilities and work across numerous health care settings outside the hospital and ICU setting.

Regarding the costs, the average hourly rate in California for an entry-level RRT is $23.70/hr. This compares with an LVN at $17.30/hr, nurse at $28.12/hr, nurse practitioner at $34.45/hr, and physician assistant at $34.17/hr.

Difficult-to-Control Asthma

"Nothing clears up a case so much as stating it to another person."
—Sherlock Holmes, *Silver Blaze*

We have all experienced patients whose asthma seems particularly difficult to control. These patients' asthma may demand repeated hospitalizations, emergency room/urgent care visits, or excessive use of beta-2-agonist therapy. Difficult-to-control asthma may also cause repeated absences from school or work despite apparent adherence to a written asthma action plan. It is important to check that every step to provide care recommended by the NIH-NAEPP Guidelines has been tried before patients are labeled "difficult to treat." Helpful questions to ask in these patients are listed in Table 8.7. Difficult-to-control asthma is the most common reason for referral to our UCAN^{TM} program.

There have been studies of patients whose asthma is difficult to control. Szefler and associates [25] found that approximately 30% of asthma patients do not respond favorably to inhaled corticosteroids. Specifically, they found lack of improvement in FEV_1 with low, medium, and high doses of fluticasone or beclomethasone. There was significant variability in response to inhaled corticosteroid in approximately one-third of their patients with Mild-to-Moderate Persistent asthma. Approximately one-third experienced a >15% improvement in FEV_1, but one-third of the patients had <5% improvement after treatment with inhaled corticosteroids. There was no difference between inhaled fluticasone or inhaled

TABLE 8.7. Questions to consider for difficult-to-control asthma.

- Is it definitely asthma?
- Is there an improvement in FEV_1 after albuterol?
- Has there been a trial of prednisone for 2 weeks with repeat PFTs?
- Is a methacholine bronchial challenge test positive?
- Could it be COPD, GERD, rhinosinusitis, heart failure, or another syndrome?
- Is the patient's technique in using an MDI/DPI correct?
- Is there continued exposure to a known allergen/trigger?
- Is bronchoscopy needed to evaluate the larynx and vocal cords on inspiration and expiration?
- Is there evidence of tumor or bronchiectasis?

TABLE 8.8. Comparative dosing of inhaled corticosteroids for adults.

Drug	Form	Low	Medium	High
Beclomethasone	40 mcg/puff	2–6	6–12	>12
(QVAR)	80 mcg/puff	1–3	3–6	>6
Budesonide	200 mcg/dose	1–3	3–6	>6
(Pulmicort)				
Flunisolide	250 mcg/puff	2–4	4–8	>8
(AeroBid)				
Fluticasone MDI	44 mcg/puff	2–6	6–15	>15
(Flovent)	110 mcg/puff	1–2	3–6	>6
	220 mcg/puff	1	2–3	>3
Triamcinolone	100 mcg/puff	4–10	10–20	>20
(Azmacort)				

Source: Data from references 12 and 13.

beclomethasone when pharmacologically equivalent doses were used (Table 8.8). In summary, the NIH-NAEPP Guidelines may not bring asthma under control in approximately 30% of asthma patients! The variable response to inhaled corticosteroids was previously observed in asthma patients treated with the leukotriene receptor antagonist montelukast compared with inhaled belcomethasone [25].

Continued requirement for high-dose corticosteroids in combination controller therapy, or reliance on systemic corticosteroids without achieving asthma control, should prompt referral to an asthmatologist. Between 15% and 25% of asthma patients may have the Beta-Adrenergic Response by Genotype (BARGE) phenomenon. These patients will not respond to short- and long-acting beta-2-agonist bronchodilators in the manner expected by the NIH-NAEPP guidelines [26]. Blacks are more often affected by this phenomenon, but it also occurs in whites. For poor responders, anticholinergic bronchodilators, such as ipratropium bromide, can be used in acute exacerbations in place of short-acting beta-2-agonists.

Regular use of short- and long-acting beta-2-agonists may be associated with adverse outcomes and desensitization of the beta-2-adrenergic receptors, resulting in loss of asthma control, decline in morning peak flow, longer duration of asthma exacerbations, and rebound airway hyperresponsiveness. Persistent high-level activation of beta-2-adrenergic receptors in vitro increases expression of phospholipase C-beta in airway bronchial smooth muscle. Inflammatory mediators such as acetylcholine, histamine, and leukotrienes cause bronchoconstriction by acting on receptors coupled with phospholipase C-beta [27]. Chronic beta-2-agonist therapy may augment the effects of these bronchoconstrictors [28]. Reducing the chronic use of short- or long-acting beta-2-agonists may actually contribute to better asthma control! The current controversies surrounding inhaled corticosteroids and beta-2-agonists should not, however, prevent health care providers from prescribing them, particularly inhaled corticosteroids, which remain the most effective controller drug in asthma care.

Assuming a motivated patient with self-management skills, questions can be asked to determine whether there is need for further investigation or for discussing the case with an asthma specialist or asthmatologist [29]. The kinds of questions that come up are presented in Table 8.6. Control of rhinosinusitis, GERD, obstructive sleep apnea, tobacco smoking, or environmental tobacco smoke exposure may dramatically improve asthma control. Failure of the patient to improve after 2 to 3 months of asthma care should definitely trigger a patient referral to the asthmatologist. New pharmacotherapy may help to better manage difficult-to-control asthma and reduce the risk of long-term corticosteroid toxicities. Omalizumab or anti-IgE is an important, albeit expensive, therapy that can improve the control of allergen-mediated asthma, reduce the need for corticosteroid consumption (both inhaled and systemic), and lead to reductions in asthma exacerbation [30]. The indications for a 4- to 6-month trial of anti-IgE therapy for difficult-to-control asthma are clinical in nature and require further investigation. Other new therapeutics include the once-daily long-acting anticholinergic drug tiotropium [31], peptide immunotherapy against house dust-mite allergen, leukotriene 5-LO inhibitors (zileuton), novel corticosteroids (ciclesonide), and phosphodiesterase-4 inhibitors (roflumilast) [32]. However, new therapeutics will never obviate the need for regular primary care visits, patient education, testing self-management skills, and a written asthma action plan.

Clinical Performance Measures

As important as the NIH-NAEPP Guidelines have been for the diagnosis and management of asthma, the Physician Consortium for Performance Improvement has provided the tools necessary to develop and measure quality improvement activities. The Physician Consortium represents 50 national medical specialty societies and includes The Agency for Healthcare Research Quality and the Centers for Medicare and Medicaid Services. A full report of the consortium is available at on the Internet at www. ama-assn.org/go/quality.

A major part of the recommendations was the Asthma Core Physician Performance Measurement Set. This measurement set provides clinical recommendations for asthma assessment and pharmacologic therapies. These are presented in Figure 8.4. Along with these recommendations are Clinical Performance Measures that health care providers and administrators should regularly employ to determine quality of care and identify areas for quality improvement activities. The Consortium recommends ongoing monitoring in the following areas.

Physician Consortium for Performance Improvement
Asthma Core Physician Performance Measurement Set[a]

	Clinical Recommendations [10,11]	Clinical Performance Measures Per Reporting Year
Asthma Assessment	To determine whether the goals of therapy are being met, monitoring is recommended in the 6 areas listed below: • Signs and symptoms (daytime; nocturnal awakening) of asthma • Pulmonary function (spirometry; peak flow monitoring) • Quality of life/functional status • History of asthma exacerbations • Pharmacotherapy (as-needed use of inhaled short-acting beta$_2$-agonist, adherence to regimen of long-term-control medications) • Patient-provider communication and patient satisfaction (NAEPP EPR-2 recommendations are based on the opinion of the Expert Panel)	Percentage of patients who were evaluated during at least one office visit during the reporting year for the frequency (numeric) of daytime and nocturnal asthma symptoms[b] **Numerator** = Patients who were evaluated during at least one office visit during the reporting year for the frequency (numeric) of daytime and nocturnal asthma symptoms[b] **Denominator** = All patients aged 5-40 years with asthma
		Per Patient: Whether or not patient was evaluated during at least one office visit during the reporting year for the frequency (numeric) of daytime and nocturnal asthma symptoms[b] *Per Patient Population:* Percentage of patients who were evaluated during at least one office visit during the reporting year for the frequency (numeric) of daytime and nocturnal asthma symptoms[b]
Pharmacologic Therapy *Denominator Exclusion:* Documentation of patient reason(s)[c] for not prescribing either the preferred long-term control medication (inhaled corticosteroid) or an acceptable alternative treatment	A stepwise approach to therapy is recommended to maintain long-term control:[d,e,f] **Step 1: Mild Intermittent Asthma** No daily medication needed **Step 2: Mild Persistent Asthma** *Preferred treatment:* Low-dose inhaled corticosteroids (ICS) *Alternative treatment:* Cromolyn, leukotriene modifier, nedocromil, OR sustained-release theophylline	Percentage of patients with mild, moderate, or severe *persistent* asthma who were prescribed *either* the preferred long-term control medication (inhaled corticosteroid)* or an acceptable alternative treatment **Numerator** = Patients who were prescribed *either* the preferred long-term control medication (inhaled corticosteroid) or an acceptable alternative treatment **Denominator** = All patients aged 5-40 years with mild, moderate, or severe *persistent* asthma
	Step 3: Moderate Persistent Asthma *Preferred treatment:* Low-medium dose ICS + long-acting inhaled beta$_2$-agonists (LABA)* *Alternative treatment:* Increase medium-dose ICS OR low-medium dose ICS and either leukotriene modifier or theophylline (If needed, may increase ICS within medium-dose range in either treatment) **Step 4: Severe Persistent Asthma** *Preferred treatment:* High-dose ICS + LABA* AND, if needed, corticosteroid tablets or syrup long term Studies comparing ICS to cromolyn, nedocromil, theophylline, or leukotriene receptor antagonists are limited, but available evidence shows that none of these long-term control medications appear to be as effective as ICS in improving asthma outcomes. For quick relief for all patients, a short-acting bronchodilator is recommended as needed for symptoms.[d,f] (NAEPP EPR-2 recommendations are based on strong evidence from clinical trials and the opinion of the Expert Panel)	*Per Patient:* Whether or not patient with mild, moderate, or severe *persistent* asthma was prescribed *either* the preferred long-term control medication (inhaled corticosteroid) or an acceptable alternative treatment *Per Patient Population:* Percentage of all patients with mild, moderate, or severe *persistent* asthma who were prescribed *either* the preferred long-term control medication (inhaled corticosteroid) or an acceptable alternative treatment Percentage of patients with mild, moderate, or severe *persistent* asthma who were prescribed *either* the preferred long-term control medication (inhaled corticosteroid) or an acceptable alternative treatment, with denominator exclusion applied Distribution of long-term control therapy by category of medication, severity classification, and age range
	* In patients with moderate or severe persistent asthma, strong evidence indicates that use of LABA *in combination with* ICS leads to improvements in lung function and symptoms, and reduced supplemental bronchodilator use. LABA is not recommended for use as monotherapy.	

a   Refers to all patients aged 5-40 years with diagnosed asthma.

b   To be counted in calculations of this measure, symptom frequency must be numerically quantified. Measure may also be met by physician documentation or patient completion of an asthma assessment tool/survey/questionnaire. Assessment tool may include the QualityMetric[12] Asthma Control Test™; NAEPP Asthma Symptoms and Peak Flow Diary.[13]

c   Patient reasons for not prescribing either the preferred long-term control medication (inhaled corticosteroid) or an acceptable alternative treatment: economic, social, and/or religious, etc.

d   See table of treatment recommendations on reverse side of Prospective Data Collection Flowsheet for recommended dosages and other information.

e   If optimal control of asthma is not achieved and sustained at any step of care, several actions may be considered, including: assessment of patient adherence and technique in using medications correctly; step up to the next higher step of care; consultation with an asthma specialist.[16]

f   Although quick-relief inhaled medications are not considered an acceptable alternative for long-term control of asthma, this information is being collected to further inform the Work Group.

FIGURE 8.4. Physician's Consortium recommendations for quality improvement monitoring. (Copyright 2005 by American Medical Association. All rights reserved.)

Physician Consortium for Performance Improvement
Asthma Core Physician Performance Measurement Set
Prospective Data Collection Flowsheet

Provider No. _____

Patient Name or Code _____   Birth Date _____ / _____ / _____   Gender M ❏ F ❏
(mm / dd / yyyy)

Monitoring — Asthma Vital Signs	Date of Initial Visit (mm / dd / yyyy):	Initial visit ❏ Yes ❏ No ___/___/___	___/___/___	___/___/___	___/___/___
	Patient completed an asthma assessment tool[a]	❏ Yes (if Yes, skip to Classification section)	❏ Yes (if Yes, skip to Classification section)	❏ Yes (if Yes, skip to Classification section)	❏ Yes (if Yes, skip to Classification section)
	Daytime asthma signs/symptoms (numeric frequency — over past 2-4 weeks, not just with acute attacks)	_____ (#) Per: (circle one) day week month	_____ (#) Per: (circle one) day week month	_____ (#) Per: (circle one) day week month	_____ (#) Per: (circle one) day week month
	Nocturnal asthma signs/symptoms (numeric frequency — over past 2-4 weeks, not just with acute attacks)	_____ (#) Per: (circle one) night week month	_____ (#) Per: (circle one) night week month	_____ (#) Per: (circle one) night week month	_____ (#) Per: (circle one) night week month
	Short-acting beta$_2$-agonists	# of puffs used/day: ____	# of puffs used/day: ____	# of puffs used/day: ____	# of puffs used/day: ____
	Frequency of acute attacks/exacerbations	_____ (#) Per: (circle one) day week month year	_____ (#) Per: (circle one) day week month year	_____ (#) Per: (circle one) day week month year	_____ (#) Per: (circle one) day week month year
Classification	**Classification of Asthma Severity[b,c] (check one)**	❏ Mild intermittent ❏ Mild persistent ❏ Moderate persistent ❏ Severe persistent			

Check all medication types prescribed (see table of treatment recommendations on reverse side)

Medications	**Quick-Relief Medications**				
	Short-acting beta$_2$-agonists				
	Anticholinergics				
	Long-Term-Control Medications	❏ Not prescribed (patient reasons*)	❏ Not prescribed (patient reasons*)	❏ Not prescribed (patient reasons*)	❏ Not prescribed (patient reasons*)
	Inhaled corticosteroids				
	Leukotriene modifiers				
	Cromolyn sodium				
	Nedocromil sodium				
	Sustained-release Methylxanthines				
	Long-acting beta$_2$-agonists				

*   Specify patient reasons (eg, economic, social, religious) for not prescribing therapy:

Other Medications					

a   Assessment tool may include the QualityMetric[12] Asthma Control Test™; NAEPP Asthma Symptoms and Peak Flow Diary.[13]

b   Classification should be based on clinical features before treatment.

c   If optimal control of asthma is not achieved and sustained at any step of care, several actions may be considered, including: assessment of patient adherence and technique in using medications correctly; step up to the next higher step of care; consultation with an asthma specialist.[19]

FIGURE 8.4. *Continued*

Classification of Asthma Severity (NAEPP EPR-2, p. 83-85; Update on selected topics, 2002) [10,11]
Clinical Feature Before Treatment[a]

	Symptoms[b]	Nighttime Symptoms	Lung Function	Recommended Treatment
Step 4: Severe Persistent[c]	Continual symptoms; Limited physical activity; Frequent exacerbations	Frequent	FEV_1 or PEF ≤60% predicted; PEF variability >30%	**Preferred treatment:** • High-dose inhaled corticosteroids **and** • Long-acting inhaled beta₂-agonists **And**, if needed, • Corticosteroid tablets or syrup long term (2 mg/kg/day; generally do not exceed 60 mg per day). (Make repeated attempts to reduce systemic corticosteroids and maintain control with high-dose inhaled corticosteroids.)
Step 3: Moderate Persistent[c]	Daily symptoms; Daily use of inhaled short-acting beta₂-agonist; Exacerbations affect activity; Exacerbations ≥2 times a week; may last days	>1 time a week	FEV_1 or PEF >60%-<80% predicted; PEF variability >30%	**Preferred treatment:** • Low-to-medium dose inhaled corticosteroids and long-acting inhaled beta₂-agonists **Alternative treatment** (listed alphabetically): • Increase inhaled corticosteroids within medium-dose range **or** • Low-to-medium dose inhaled corticosteroids and either leukotriene modifier or theophylline. If needed (particularly in patients with recurring severe exacerbations): **Preferred treatment:** • Increase inhaled corticosteroids within medium-dose range, and add long-acting inhaled beta₂-agonists **Alternative treatment** (listed alphabetically): • Increase inhaled corticosteroids in medium-dose range, and add either leukotriene modifier or theophylline
Step 2: Mild Persistent	Symptoms >2 times a week but <1 time a day; Exacerbations may affect activity	>2 times a month	FEV_1 or PEF ≥80% predicted; PEF variability 20-30%	**Preferred treatment:** • Low-dose inhaled corticosteroids **Alternative treatment** (listed alphabetically): cromolyn, leukotriene modifier, nedocromil, **or** sustained release theophylline to serum concentrations of 5-15 mcg/mL
Step 1: Mild Intermittent	Symptoms ≤2 times a week; Asymptomatic and normal PEF between exacerbations; Exacerbations brief (from a few hours to a few days); intensity may vary	≤2 times a month	FEV_1 or PEF ≥80% predicted; PEF variability <20%	No daily medication needed. Severe exacerbations may occur, separated by long periods of normal lung function and no symptoms. A course of systemic corticosteroids is recommended

Quick Relief for Patients in All Severity Classifications:
- Short-acting bronchodilator: 2-4 puffs short-acting inhaled beta₂-agonists as needed for symptoms.
- Intensity of treatment will depend on severity of exacerbation; up to 3 treatments at 20-minute intervals or a single nebulizer treatment as needed. Course of systemic corticosteroids may be needed.
- Use of short-acting inhaled beta₂-agonists on a daily basis, or increasing use, indicates the need to initiate or increase long-term control therapy.

Step down
Review treatment every 1 to 6 months; a gradual stepwise reduction in treatment may be possible.

Step up
If control is not maintained, consider step up. First review patient medication technique, adherence, and environmental control.

a The presence of one of the features of severity is sufficient to place a patient in that category. An individual should be assigned to the most severe grade in which any feature occurs. The characteristics noted in this figure are general and may overlap because asthma is highly variable. Furthermore, an individual's classification may change over time.

b Patients at any level of severity can have mild, moderate, or severe exacerbations. Some patients with intermittent asthma experience severe and life-threatening exacerbations separated by long periods of normal lung function and no symptoms.

c Referral to an asthma specialist is recommended if there are difficulties achieving or maintaining control of asthma or if the patient requires step 4 care. Referral may be considered if the patient requires step 3 care.

FIGURE 8.4. *Continued*

Asthma Assessment

Determine whether the goals of therapy are being met. Monitoring should be done in the six areas:

1. Signs and symptoms (daytime or nocturnal awakenings)
2. Pulmonary function (spirometry, peak flow testing)
3. Quality of life/functional status
4. History of asthma exacerbations
5. Pharmacotherapy: as-needed use of inhaled short-acting beta-agonist, adherence to regimen of long-term control medications
6. Patient–provider communication and satisfaction

Pharmacologic Therapy

Demonstrate evidence of a stepwise approach that is severity specific:

Step 1. Mild Intermittent Asthma—No daily medication needed. This clinical category will be deleted in the 2006 update of the NIH-NAEPP Guidelines for asthma management in recognition that 75% of asthma cases are Moderate-to-Severe Persistent.

Step 2. Mild Persistent Asthma—Preferred treatment: low-dose inhaled corticosteroids. Alternative treatment: leukotriene receptor antagonist, nedocromil, or sustained release theophylline.

Step 3. Moderate Persistent Asthma—Preferred treatment: low- to medium-dose inhaled corticosteroids and long-acting inhaled beta-2-agonist. Alternative treatment: Add either leukotriene receptor antagonist or theophylline to low- or medium-dose inhaled corticosteroids.

Step 4. Severe Persistent Asthma—Preferred treatment: high-dose inhaled corticosteroids and long-acting inhaled beta-2-agonists and, if needed, an oral corticosteroid. Table 8.8 compares equivalent potencies of various inhaled corticosteroid products.

Plan-Do-Study-Act

The most effective strategy to help a practice meet its targets for management is to use a registry in conjunction with Plan-Do-Study-Act (PDSA) interventions. Chapter 4 provides a detailed description of how to perform PDSA interventions for a chronic disease. The key questions you should ask in any PDSA activity are:

1. What are we trying to accomplish?
2. How will we know when we have reached our goal?
3. What interventions are likely to help us meet this goal?

It is best if the PDSA cycles are "rapid cycle," meaning that the entire process for intervention and review of data is over a short period of 2 to 3 weeks. The registry should be constructed so that important data are available to monitor the outcomes of PDSA interventions.

Expectations for full implementation of NIH-NAEPP and Physician's Consortium Guidelines, while laudable in the long run, cannot be accomplished overnight and often require years. It is imperative to begin immediately, however, to meet clinical performance measure goals and to pay for performance initiatives that will be instituted by Medicare and private health care insurance companies, to promote better quality of care by health care providers and better patient outcomes for a variety of chronic diseases, including asthma.

We employ the phrase, "pick every low-hanging fruit" as our guide to PDSA activities. Start with an assessment of one outcome of interest and look at interventions that can help you reach the goal:

1. Ensure that every patient with asthma in your practice has a continuity physician.

2. If you do not have a registry or an electronic medical record with the capacity to produce reports on asthma populations as described earlier in Monitoring, start a registry that is prospectively completed based on who comes in for asthma care. Reliance on ICD-9 codes (493.00-99) as a proxy is generally not recommended because of the large number of errors in ICD-9 coding. Although fraught with coding errors, it is nevertheless a good way to begin.

3. Develop a system of team-based care in your clinic. All chronic disease management is more effective when done as a team.

Members of your team can include nurses, RRTs, and pharmacists. Each member of the team can be responsible for a component of a comprehensive intervention. Team members who participate directly in patient care and education should be certified asthma educators (AE-C). Meet with your team and discuss the key clinical activities listed in Table 8.2 and build a rapid-cycle intervention around this. Step-by-step, multiple PDSA cycles will ultimately result in a practice that delivers high-quality care.

Alternative Therapies

Many patients use herbal remedies in an effort to control symptoms. It has been estimated that one third of patients use complementary and alternative medications. The most frequently used herbal remedies for patients with asthma are Echinacea, garlic, angelica, chamomile, ephedra (now banned), gingko, grape seed extract, licorice root, St. John's Wort, kava kava, peppermint oil, stinging nettle, and ginseng. Bielory [33] reviewed studies published from 1980 to 2003 and showed no proven beneficial effects of these medications. The study did express concerns for adverse side effects; usually in the form of a hypersensitivity reaction. The evidence supporting the use of these herbal remedies is lacking.

Acknowledgments. This chapter is dedicated to the memory of Eula Wiley, MSN, RN, C, dear friend and colleague. I am grateful to Professor Stanley M. Naguwa for mentoring a young fool and to Celeste Kivler and Claudia M. Vukovich who both brought new hope and vitality to the author. I am also grateful to Stephen W. Kutler who believed in the merit of new non-traditional ideas and brought one to life.

References

1. Centers for Disease Control and Prevention. Key clinical activities for quality asthma care: recommendations of the National Asthma Education and Prevention Program. MMWR 2003;52(No. RR-6):1–8.
2. Eisenberg SS. Building the case for asthma as a disease management program. Dis Manag 2004;7:202–215.
3. National Center for Health Statistics, Centers for Disease Control and Prevention. Asthma prevalence, health care use and mortality, 2002. http://www.cdc.gov/nchs/products/pub/pubd/hestats/asthma/asthma.htm. Accessed March 1, 2005.
4. Homa DM, et al. Asthma mortality in U.S. Hispanics of Mexican, Puerto Rican, and Cuban heritage, 1990–1995. Am J Respir Crit Care Med 2000; 161:504–509.
5. Bratton DL, et al. Impact of a multidisciplinary day program on disease and health care costs in children and adolescents with severe asthma: a two-year follow-up study. Pediatr Pulmonol 2001;31:177–189.
6. National Committee for Quality Assurance. Use of appropriate medications for people with asthma. The state of managed care quality, 2001. www.ncqa.org/somc2001/asthma/somc_2001_asthma.html.
7. National Center for Health Statistics, Centers for Disease Control and Prevention. Asthma prevalence and control among adults—United States 2001. MMWR 2003;52:357–360.
8. Kelly CS, et al. Outcomes evaluation of a comprehensive intervention program for asthmatic children enrolled in Medicaid. Pediatrics 2000;105: 1029–1035.
9. Rossiter LF, et al. The impact of disease management on outcomes and cost of care: a study of low-income asthma patients. Inquiry 2000;37:188–202.
10. Beckham S, et al. A community-based asthma management program: effects on resource utilization and quality of life. Hawaii Med J 2004;63: 121–126.
11. Twiggs JE, et al. Treating asthma by the guidelines: developing a medication management information system for use in primary care. Dis Manag 2004;7:244–260.
12. National Asthma Education and Prevention Program. Expert Panel Report 2: Guidelines for the Diagnosis and Management of Asthma. Bethesda, MD: National Institutes of Health, 1997. Publication No. 97-4051.
13. National Asthma Education and Prevention Program. Guidelines for the Diagnosis and Management of Asthma. Update on Selected Topics, 2002. Bethesda, MD: National Institutes of Health, 2002. Publication No. 02-5075.

14. Kivler C, et al. Cost savings parallel improved outcomes in severe asthma utilizing respiratory care practitioners. Am J Respir Crit Care Med 2003;167: A209.

15. Smith DH, et al. A national estimate of the economic costs of asthma. Am J Respir Crit Care Med 1997;156:787–793.

16. Fuhlbrigge AL, et al. The burden of asthma in the United States: level and distribution are dependent on interpretation of the national asthma education and prevention program guidelines. Am J Respir Crit Care Med 2002;166: 1044–1049.

17. Drazen JM, et al. Adherence to prescribed treatment for asthma. Am J Respir Crit Care Med 2000;161:A402.

18. Abramson MJ, et al. Are asthma medications and management related to deaths from asthma? Am J Respir Crit Care Med 2000;163:12–18.

19. Liu TA, et al. Culturally competent policies and other predictors of asthma care quality for Medicaid-insured children. Pediatrics 2004;114:e102–e110.

20. Wilson SR, et al. A controlled trial of two forms of self-management education for adults with asthma. Am J Med 1993;94:564–576.

21. Gallefoss F, Bakke PS. Cost-effectiveness of self-management in asthmatics: a 1-yr follow-up randomized, controlled trial. Eur Respir J 2001;17:206–213.

22. Krishna S, et al. Internet-enabled interactive multimedia asthma education program: a randomized trial. Pediatrics 2003;111:503–510.

23. Tinkelman D, Schwartz A. School-based asthma disease management. J Asthma 2004;41:455–462.

24. Piette JD, Heisler M, Wagner TH. Cost-related medication underuse. Arch Intern Med 2004;164:1749–1755.

25. Szefler SJ, et al. Significant variability in response to inhaled corticosteroids for persistent asthma. J Allergy Clin Immunol 2002;109:410–418.

26. Israel E, Chinchilli VM, Ford JG, et al. Use of regularly scheduled albuterol treatment in asthma: genotype-stratified, randomized, placebo-controlled cross-over trial. Lancet 2004;364:1505–1512.

27. McGraw DW, et al. Antithetic regulation by beta-adrenergic receptors of Gq receptor signaling via phospholipase C underlies the airway beta-agonist paradox. J Clin Invest 2003;112:619–626.

28. Shore SA, Drazen JM. Beta-agonists and asthma: too much of a good thing? J Clin Invest 2003;112:495–497.

29. Thomas PS, et al. Pseudo-steroid resistant asthma. Thorax 1999;54:352–356.

30. Buhl R. Omalizumab (Xolair) improves quality of life in adult patients with allergic asthma: a review. Respir Med 2003;97:123–129.

31. Tiotropium (Spiriva) for COPD. Med Lett 2004;46:1183.

32. Barnes PJ. New drugs for asthma. Natl Rev Drug Discov 2004;3:831–844.

33. Bielory L. Complementary and alternative interventions in asthma, allergy, and immunology. Ann Allergy Asthma Immunol 2004;93:S45–S54.

9
Heart Failure

WILLIAM LEWIS AND JIM NUOVO

Summary

Management

1. When performing the initial evaluation of a patient diagnosed with heart failure (HF), you should assess the following:
   a. The severity of the symptoms of impaired cardiac function (e.g., dyspnea on exertion, paroxysmal nocturnal dyspnea, orthopnea, fatigue, and leg edema)
   b. Evidence for risk factors strongly associated with HF: ischemic heart disease, hypertension, diabetes, valvular heart disease
   c. Evidence for risk factors also associated with HF: hyperlipidemia, excessive alcohol use, tobacco use, cocaine and amphetamine use
   d. Evidence for iatrogenic contributing factors associated with HF: use of nonsteroidal anti-inflammatory drugs and thiazolidinediones, chemotherapy and/or radiation therapy
   e. Comorbid conditions, particularly depression
2. Your intake history should assess the following:
   a. Patient's understanding of HF and its health effects
   b. Patient's perception of barriers to lifestyle modification
   c. Impact of HF on patient's quality of life
3. Initial testing should include the following:
   a. Laboratory tests to assess for comorbid conditions that may impact medical treatment: complete blood count, renal panel, liver function tests, blood glucose level, lipid panel, thyroid-stimulating hormone, and urinalysis
   b. Tests to assess cardiac function, for example, a two-dimensional echocardiogram for ejection fraction and evidence of valvular disease, and a 12-lead electrocardiogram (ECG) to assess for prior ischemic events, dysrhythmias, and evidence of heart block
   c. A chest x-ray to assess for evidence of fluid overload

4. Self-management support can be of substantial value in an effective HF management program. Techniques you can use to support self-management include the following:

   a. Ask you patients about their readiness to change; only 20% of patients are ready to make significant lifestyle changes at the time of initial evaluation. This can be accomplished by asking, "How likely are you to pursue changing your diet at this point?" or "To help you understand more about heart failure, what type of information would be most helpful to you at this time: a pamphlet, a Web site, a class?"

   b. Help your patients set goals. It is best if these goals are patient-generated, specific, short-term, achievable action plans, such as, "This week I will walk around the block before lunch on Monday, Tuesday, and Thursday."

   c. Ask your patients how confident they are that they can make changes to achieve these goals. This can be done in the following way: "On a 10-point scale, how confident are you that you can start a walking program three times a week?" Patients who score their confidence level as less than 7 are unlikely to be successful for that goal. If this occurs, the goal should be changed to one that is more likely to be achieved.

   d. Document patient-generated goals in the chart, and monitor for success in achieving the goals or note the barriers encountered.

   e. Have your office staff assist in reinforcing health behaviors, self-management goals, and emergency action plans. For example, have the office staff remind the patient that it is important to get a scale check weight every day.

5. Provide educational resources that are culturally sensitive and tailored to a patient's specific needs and goals. Resources available include:

   a. The American Heart Association

   b. The Heart Failure Society of America

6. Encourage your patients to learn the principles of healthy eating.

7. Reinforce the value of an exercise program. A progressive walking program offers the best chance for long-term success.

8. Reinforce the value of monitoring daily weight and reporting significant changes.

9. Depression is a common comorbid condition with all chronic diseases. Failure to recognize and treat depression often results in poor outcomes.

10. The evidence to support the use of angiotensin-converting enzyme (ACE) inhibitors and beta-adrenergic blocking agents (beta-blockers) is strong. In general, the approach is to start low and go slow to avoid adverse side effects. For patients unable to tolerate ACE inhibitors, use an angiotensin receptor blocker (ARB) in its place. Functional class II to IV patients should be considered for a beta-blocker unless

there is a contraindication. Although uncommon, the symptoms of HF may worsen acutely; however, within 2 to 3 months the positive impact of beta-blockers should be noticeable. Aldosterone agonists have an important effect on morbidity and mortality in functional class III and IV patients; however, it is unclear whether they should be considered first line. Digoxin also tends to be reserved for patients who fail to respond to an ACE inhibitor, a diuretic, and a beta-blocker.

11. Recent evidence suggests that the beneficial effects of ACE inhibitors may not apply to African Americans; the addition of the combination of hydralazine and nitrates to ACE inhibitor therapy may be more effective.

12. Areas of concern for medication regimens include the following:

   a. Patients unable to tolerate an ACE because of angioedema or cough; if mild, the cough may subside after 2 to 3 months.

   b. Acute worsening of HF in patients placed on a beta-blocker; mild worsening of symptoms should be anticipated acutely and adjustments made in the dosages of ACE inhibitors and/or diuretics.

   c. Use of an aldosterone agonist by patients with impaired renal function or relatively high serum potassium; gynecomastia is uncommon with spironolactone, but, if it occurs, eplerenone can be substituted.

   d. The costs of medical therapy are often prohibitive for patients, resulting in pill splitting or nonadherence. Many patients do not feel that their physician can help with this problem.

Monitoring

1. Many providers fall short in meeting well-published consensus goals for management and monitoring of HF and its complications. To improve the quality of care, you should consider the following:

   a. Developing a registry that includes the names of all patients with HF, their associated relevant outcomes, and their medication lists, weights, blood pressures, low-density lipoprotein cholesterol levels, electrolyte panels, renal function tests, ECGs, and echocardiograms.

   b. If you do not have a registry, use monthly billing reports of patients with an ICD-9 diagnosis of 428.0 as a proxy.

2. The most effective intervention for a practice is to use templates for each office visit and to develop a system by which ongoing performance can be assessed for a particular patient and for the practice. Although this can be facilitated with an electronic medical record, it can also be done with a standard paper checklist that includes an office visit template and flow sheet.

3. Support self-management goals by including these in the medical record. Patient-generated goals should be documented in the record; ongoing assessments can be made regarding successes and barriers.

4. Give all your patients with HF an action plan. The action plan should contain information that indicates when control is optimal and when interventions need to be made. An example of an action plan for HF can be found at www.improvingchroniccare.org. This can be used to support self-management goals.
5. Specific targets for optimal management include the following:
   a. Daily measurement of weights
   b. Use of an ACE inhibitor for all patients unless contraindicated
   c. Use of an ARB for patients unable to tolerate an ACE inhibitor
   d. Use of a beta-blocker: carvedilol, metoprolol succinate (Toprol XL), or bisoprolol (not currently FDA approved for HF)
   e. A two-dimensional echocardiogram to document systolic dysfunction and assess for valvular disease
6. Use the registry to develop reports for the office, for example, you can monitor how well the practice is doing in achieving the recommended targets of control and monitoring tests by determining the percentage of patients with HF who have an action plan.
7. Perform rapid-cycle Plan-Do-Study-Act interventions to help improve practice performance. They are the most effective means of improving outcomes in a practice. They are best when they are directed to one specific problem and involve participation from the practice team—provider and staff. For example, medical assistants can be trained to ask all patients with HF whether they have a scale at home and if measure their weight daily. The performance of the practice, the number of patients with a scale at home, can be measured before and after an intervention.

Burden as a Chronic Disease

Fast Facts

• Heart failure is the most prevalent and expensive chronic disease in the United States.
• The elderly bear a disproportionate burden of HF; most patients with HF are over age 65 years.
• More Medicare dollars are spent for the diagnosis and treatment of HF than for any other diagnosis.
• Readmission rates are as high as 50% within 6 months of discharge. The average admission for HF costs between $7,174 and $10,000.

Background

Heart failure is the most prevalent and expensive chronic disease in the United States. A substantial percentage of total health care costs come from the management of HF and its associated complications. More Medicare dollars are spent for the diagnosis and treatment of HF than for any other diagnosis [1].

Prevalence

Heart failure is the only cardiovascular disorder that is increasing in frequency, the result of an aging population, reductions in the death rate for those with ischemic heart disease, and greater longevity for those who develop HF [2]. Advances in the treatment of ischemic heart disease have contributed to the increasing number of patients with HF. About 22% of men and 46% of women who have had a myocardial infarction (MI) develop HF within 6 years.

The numbers of patients affected by this condition are substantial, as are the associated morbidity and mortality. Some facts that highlight the extent of this "epidemic" are presented in Table 9.1. Given the numbers affected, the burden on the elderly, the burden on the health care system, and the toll on patients and their families, we must make all reasonable efforts to investigate ways to prevent HF and to develop new methods of delivering effective care.

TABLE 9.1. The impact of heart failure in the United States.

- Numbers affected
  - ▲ Over 5 million patients in the United States have heart failure.
  - ▲ Each year, an additional 500,000 are diagnosed.
  - ▲ By 2007, 10 million people are expected to have HF.
- Burden on the elderly
  - ▲ The elderly bear much of the burden of this chronic disease.
  - ▲ Most HF occurs after age 65 years; 6% to 10% of the population over age 65 have HF.
- Burden on the health care system
  - ▲ Heart failure accounts for 15 million office visits, each patient averaging three outpatient visits a year.
  - ▲ Symptoms of HF are the leading cause of hospitalization.
  - ▲ National hospitalization data indicate that over the past 30 years HF discharge rates have tripled.
- Morbidity and mortality
  - ▲ Heart failure is the primary or secondary cause of death for approximately 300,000 per year in the United States.
  - ▲ Heart failure is lethal. In 1993, it was found that once HF is clinically detected, men have an average survival rate of only 1.7 years and women, 3.2 years.
  - ▲ From 1979 to 2000, HF deaths increased by 148%.
  - ▲ Sudden death is the most common cause of mortality; it occurs six to nine times more often in HF patients than in the general population.

Costs

Several cost-of-illness studies related to HF have been performed over the last few years. Not surprisingly, the findings all indicate that HF imposes a large economic burden on society. In the United States, the economic cost of HF in 1999 was estimated to be $56 billion per year. Of these costs, 57% are for hospitalizations, 15% for nursing home care, 10% for home health care, 10% for medications, and 8% for health professional services. It has been projected that HF will account for 3% to 5% of the health care budget [3]. Heart failure is the most common Medicare diagnosis-related group, and more Medicare dollars are spent for the diagnosis and treatment of HF than for any other diagnosis.

Heart failure accounts for 15 million office visits each year, with each patient averaging three outpatient visits per year. At least 1 in 5 patients seen in the outpatient setting is admitted to the hospital for exacerbation of their symptoms. Symptoms of HF are the leading cause of hospitalization worldwide in persons older than 65 years. In the United States, HF accounts for 6.5 million hospital days each year. Readmission rates are as high as 50% within 6 months of discharge. The average admission for heart failure costs between $7,174 and $10,000 [4]. The personal burden of this disease is substantial. Forty to sixty percent of patients with HF die within 5 years of their diagnosis. Sudden death occurs at a rate six to nine times that of the general population. Patients with HF are likely to have multiple comorbid conditions (e.g., diabetes, hypertension, osteoarthritis, chronic pain syndromes, and depression) that affect their quality of life.

Impact of Disease Management Programs

Summary

- Multiple studies on the care provided to patients with HF have shown poor adherence to well-known markers for quality of care. For example, in a study of Medicare patients, only 75% of patients with HF who are candidates for an ACE inhibitor are given one.
- Elderly patients with HF are at an increased risk for early rehospitalization.
- Disease management programs have been consistently shown to have a positive impact on costs, utilization, patient outcomes, patient satisfaction, and provider satisfaction.
- Programs that focus on enhancing patient's self-care activities reduce HF hospitalizations and all-cause hospitalizations by two-thirds. Strategies that use telephone contact and advised patients to see their primary care provider in the event of deterioration similarly reduce HF hospitalizations and all-cause hospitalizations.

- Behavioral factors, such as social isolation and nonadherence to medications and diet, frequently contribute to early readmissions, suggesting that many such admissions could be prevented.
- Disease management efforts will be most useful when there is a marked disparity between the best-case management for this disease and the management that is being applied.

Background

One of the challenges in caring for patients with any chronic condition, including HF, has been to provide those services that are recognized as having an impact on outcomes. Multiple studies on the care provided to patients with HF have shown poor adherence to well-known markers for quality of care [5]. For example, in a study of Medicare patients, only 75% of patients with HF who are candidates for an ACE inhibitor are given one. The elderly are uniquely susceptible to the adverse outcomes of HF. Elderly patients with HF are at an increased risk for early rehospitalization, with rates of readmission ranging up to 50% within 6 months of discharge. Moreover, behavioral factors, such as social isolation and noncompliance with medications and diet, frequently contribute to early readmissions, suggesting that many such readmissions could be prevented. For example, Tsuchihashi and associates [6] found that socioenvironmental variables (e.g., strained financial resources and social isolation) were strong predictors for hospital readmission and length of stay for patients with HF. Disease management programs have been consistently shown to have a positive impact on costs, utilization, patient outcomes, patient satisfaction, and provider satisfaction. Some examples of these interventions include the following:

1. McAlister and associates [5] reviewed 29 trials involving 5,039 patients. Programs that focused on enhancing patients' self-care activities reduced HF hospitalizations and all-cause hospitalizations by two-thirds. Strategies that used telephone contact and advised patients to see their primary care provider in the event of deterioration similarly reduced HF hospitalizations and all-cause hospitalizations. In the 15 of 18 trials that evaluated cost, multidisciplinary strategies were cost saving [5].

2. Rich and associates [7] performed a prospective, randomized trial of a nurse-directed, multidisciplinary intervention on the rates of readmission within 90 days of discharge. The intervention consisted of comprehensive education for the patient and family, a prescribed diet, social-service consultation, a review of medications, and intensive follow-up. They found that the intervention had significant positive effects on quality of life, utilization, and costs. The number of readmissions for HF was reduced by 56.2%, and the overall cost of care was $460 less per patient in the intervention group (over a 3-month observation period).

3. Berg and associates [8] investigated the impact of a telephonic disease management program for patients with HF. The study included 533 elderly patients. The intervention was a structured, protocol-driven, telephone nursing intervention designed to provide patient education, counseling, and monitoring services. Over a 1-year period there was a substantial decrease in utilization in the following areas: 23% fewer hospitalizations, 26% fewer inpatient bed days, 22% fewer emergency department visits, 44% fewer HF hospitalizations, 70% fewer 30-day readmissions, and 45% fewer skilled nursing facility bed days. Claims costs were $1,792 per person lower in the intervention group.

4. HealthPartners, a program that uses best practice guidelines and systematic team-based care for HF patients, has been able to reduce life-threatening exacerbations by over 60%. A Kaiser Permanente program in Ohio, using a similar intervention, reduced HF death rates to less than half of the state average [9].

5. The Organized Program to Initiate Lifesaving Treatment in Hospitalized Patients with Heart Failure (OPTIMIZE-HF) is a national collaborative program designed to improve medical care education of hospitalized patients with HF and to accelerate initiation of guideline-recommended therapies by administering them prior to discharge. This program uses a registry focused from the time of hospital admission to a 60-day follow-up period. Included with the registry is a care improvement strategy with a hospital toolkit and structured educational initiatives. The target of this program has been to include 500 participating hospitals caring for over 50,000 patients with HF. The outcome of this intervention is pending [10].

Many of the studies demonstrating cost savings are performed over a relatively short period of time, generally a few months. Given the fact that HF is a progressive disease for which there is no curative treatment, it is unclear whether disease management programs can impact costs and utilization over the long term. Galbreath and associates [11] studied the impact of a disease management program in a large, community-based population over a longer interval than most studies—18 months. They randomized 1,069 patients with systolic or diastolic HF using a telephone disease management program. All HF patients received a bathroom scale, an electronic blood pressure monitor, and finger pulse oximeter. Disease managers used a proprietary MULTIFIT protocol under which patient care was directed in accordance to treatment guidelines from the American College of Cardiology/American Heart Association. Initially call frequency was weekly, with a transition to monthly for the duration of the intervention. Patient education included instruction on a cardiac-prudent diet, medication compliance, exercise, and reaction to symptoms consistent with HF exacerbation. Patients had access to a 24-hour toll-free advice line. An extensive review of the records was done to assess a large number of outcomes. Their findings were remarkable for a significant survival benefit and improvement in New York Heart Association (NYHA) class; however, there were no clear differences in costs or health care utilization between the intervention and control groups. There was also no clear improvement in functional capacity as measured by a 6-minute walk test.

This study is significant in that it may be that disease management efforts will be most useful when there is a marked disparity between the best-case management for a disease and the management that is being applied. For example, in this study, 77% of the patients were taking an ACE inhibitor or an ARB, a significantly higher percentage than in studies of other populations. Therefore, the margin for improvement is smaller, and the value added by a disease management program is more difficult to demonstrate. The message from this study is that we should try to assess what level of care is currently being provided to our own population of patients who have HF. If the overall management of the practice population is consistent with national consensus guidelines, it is likely that the most effective disease management intervention will be targeted to those patients with the worst functional class. If the care currently being provided is substantially below these guidelines, then a comprehensive disease management program is more likely to benefit all HF patients [11].

Screening for Heart Failure

Summary

- The reliability of the symptoms given by our patients and the physical examination findings we tend to focus on for the detection of HF, particularly for mild disease, are problematic.
- The underlying mechanisms that explain most of the clinical findings of HF include an inotropic abnormality resulting in diminished systolic emptying (systolic dysfunction) and a compliance abnormality in which the ability of the ventricles to accept blood is impaired (diastolic dysfunction).
- Most patients with HF have systolic dysfunction. The primary cause is coronary artery disease.
- As many as 40% of patients with HF have diastolic dysfunction as defined by a normal left ventricular ejection fraction with clinical signs of HF. Patients with diastolic dysfunction are more likely to be women and more likely to be over 65 years of age.
- There is a close relationship between diabetes mellitus and HF. The relationship appears to be caused by a combination of ischemia from vascular disease along with a diabetes-related cardiomyopathy.
- There are no consensus screening recommendations for the early detection of HF in the general population. However, there is a growing body

of evidence that early detection and treatment of patients with asymptomatic left ventricular hypertrophy (LVH) may have a positive impact on the natural history of this disease.

- Electrocardiography has the capacity to detect some, but not all, patients with LVH. Accuracy of the ECG in part depends on the criteria used for defining LVH.
- A two-dimensional ECG coupled with Doppler flow studies is the primary method of detecting HF.
- Although there is some variation in the criteria used to detect systolic dysfunction, most research studies use the criteria of an ejection fraction <40%; however, an ejection fraction of <50% is abnormal, but the guidelines to treat are less clear cut. It is important to remember that a normal ejection fraction does not rule out diastolic dysfunction.
- Rapid measurement of brain natriuretic peptide (BNP) has become a common tool used in emergency departments, particularly in the evaluation of patients with dyspnea. It can accurately distinguish dyspnea caused by HF from dyspnea due to other causes. A challenge has been determining the ideal cut-off criteria for an abnormal test.
- The effectiveness of echocardiographic screening for LVH can be increased if providers target high-risk subgroups. These subgroups include:
  - ▲ Patients with a prior MI with anterolateral Q waves detected on ECG
  - ▲ Hypertensive patients with LVH detected on ECG
  - ▲ Patients with diabetes and LVH detected on ECG

Documenting Heart Failure

Although the diagnosis of HF is often established on clinical grounds, the reliability of symptoms and physical examination findings (particularly for mild disease) is problematic. Stevenson and Perloff [12] highlighted the problems in reliability of clinical examination findings in patients with HF. Rales, edema, and elevated mean jugular pressures were only 58% sensitive. They were absent in 18 of 43 patients with HF. Clinical criteria developed in the Framingham Study [13] are listed in Table 9.2. Given these criteria, the challenge for most of us is to recognize the early signs of HF in those patients who have only "minor criteria" signs or symptoms, and to differentiate these HF signs and symptoms from those of other diseases that present in a similar manner.

The following study highlights the challenges in making a clinical diagnosis of HF. Maisel and associates [14] assessed the value of BNP versus clinical assessment in the diagnosis of HF. The results of their study showed the following odds ratios in determining the presence of HF: rales, 2.24; cephalization of vessels on chest x-ray, 10.69; bilateral leg edema, 2.88; jugular venous distention, 1.87; and significantly elevated BNP, 29.60.

TABLE 9.2. Clinical criteria for heart failure.

- Major criteria
  ▲ Paroxysmal nocturnal dyspnea
  ▲ Neck vein distention
  ▲ Rales
  ▲ Cardiomegaly on chest x-ray
  ▲ Pulmonary edema on chest x-ray
  ▲ S3 gallop
  ▲ Positive hepatojugular reflux
- Minor criteria
  ▲ Bilateral leg edema
  ▲ Nocturnal cough
  ▲ Dyspnea on exertion
  ▲ Hepatomegaly
  ▲ Pleural effusion
  ▲ Tachycardia (>120 beats/min)
  ▲ Weight loss of more than 10 pounds over 5 days in response to treatment

Note: Definitive criteria for HF = 2 major or 1 major and 2 minor criteria.
Source: Data from McKee et al. [13].

The underlying mechanisms that explain most of the clinical findings of HF include an inotropic abnormality resulting in diminished systolic emptying (systolic dysfunction) and a compliance abnormality in which the ability of the ventricles to accept blood is impaired (diastolic dysfunction). Most patients with HF have systolic dysfunction. Approximately, two-thirds of patients with HF have systolic dysfunction, and the remaining one-third have diastolic dysfunction. The primary cause of systolic dysfunction is coronary artery disease. Aggressive treatment of ischemic heart disease has resulted in fewer patients who die from an MI, leaving more who survive with compromised ventricular function and eventual HF. The risks for HF are not dissimilar to the risk factors for all cardiovascular disease. There is also a close relationship between diabetes mellitus and HF. The relationship appears to be caused by a combination of ischemia from vascular disease along with a diabetes-related cardiomyopathy. A single risk factor may be sufficient to cause HF; however, a combination of factors substantially increases the risk. The risk factors associated with HF are presented in Table 9.3. Knowing these risk factors should help target efforts toward prevention and treatment of HF. In particular, we should work to ensure that risk factors for ischemic heart disease are adequately addressed in our patients, we should work to effectively control hypertension, we should work to optimally help manage our patients who have diabetes, we should address the epidemic of obesity, and we should identify those high-risk patients who have asymptomatic LVH.

A national survey of 13,000 men and women provided more precise estimates of the risks for HF: coronary artery disease, relative risk = 8.1; diabetes, relative risk = 1.9; smoking, relative risk = 1.6; valvular heart

TABLE 9.3. Risk factors for heart failure.

- Factors strongly associated with HF
  ▲ Ischemic heart disease
  ▲ Hypertension
  ▲ Diabetes mellitus
  ▲ Obesity
  ▲ ECG showing left ventricular hypertrophy
  ▲ Valvular disease
- Factors less consistently associated with HF
  ▲ Excessive alcohol use
  ▲ Cocaine or amphetamine use
  ▲ Tobacco use
  ▲ Hyperlipidemia
  ▲ Sleep apnea
  ▲ Sedentary lifestyle
  ▲ Impaired pulmonary function tests
- Iatrogenic factors contributing to HF
  ▲ Nonsteroidal anti-inflammatory drugs (NSAIDs)
  ▲ Thiazolidinediones (e.g., pioglitazone [Actos] and rosiglitazone [Avandia])
  ▲ Chemotherapy or mantle radiation
- Other factors
  ▲ Ethnicity: African Americans are more likely to develop HF, and the onset of symptoms tends to be in younger age groups; HF symptoms occur on average 10 years of age younger than whites. African-American patients tend to have more hospitalizations and readmissions, and their prognosis is generally worse.

disease, relative risk = 1.5; hypertension, relative risk = 1.4; and obesity, relative risk = 1.4.

Heart failure may occur with normal left ventricular systolic function, known as diastolic dysfunction. Patients with diastolic dysfunction are more likely to be women and more likely to be over age 65 years. Various studies suggest that as many as 40% of patients with HF have diastolic dysfunction as defined by a normal ejection fraction. There has been substantial variability in the reported prevalences of diastolic dysfunction because of the differing opinions on diagnostic criteria. A recent study by Kitsman and associates [15] was designed to clarify some of the questions around diastolic dysfunction: is it a "real disease," and what are the characteristic features that distinguish it from systolic dysfunction? They assessed 147 patients at least 60 years old. Of these, 59 had diastolic dysfunction showing clinically evident HF with an ejection fraction of at least 50% and having no evidence of coronary artery disease, valvular heart disease, or pulmonary disease. Their findings indicate that patients identified with diastolic dysfunction had similar, although not as severe, pathophysiologic characteristics compared with patients with typical systolic HF, including severely reduced exercise capacity, neuroendocrine activation, and impaired quality of life. This included an increased left ventricular mass and elevated BNP levels (diastolic HF 56 pg/mL versus systolic HF 154 pg/mL) [15]. Heart failure associated with diastolic dysfunction is also associated with more edema, whereas impaired systolic function is more often associated with an S3 gallop and other signs of ventricular dilatation. The most common conditions associated with diastolic dysfunction are aging, hypertension, diabetes mellitus, LVH, coronary artery disease, and infiltrative cardiomyopathies. Patients tend to be overweight, older, and have renal dysfunction.

Screening for Heart Failure

There are no consensus screening recommendations for the early detection of HF in the general population. However, there is a growing body of evidence that early detection and treatment of patients with asymptomatic LVH may have a positive impact on the natural history of this disease. Patients with asymptomatic LVH have a high rate of progression to overt HF. This appears to be true even for patients who have not had an MI. Vasan and associates [16] studied 4,774 patients with hypertension and LVH over an 11-year period. None of these patients had had a prior MI. The risk for HF in this group was 1.47.

Among patients with HF, antecedent evidence of LVH is present in approximately 20% as detected by ECG and in 70% as detected by echocardiogram. An important question has been whether early detection and treatment of asymptomatic LVH would have a positive effect on outcomes, thereby reducing the risk of HF. Devereux and associates [17] performed such a study, determining whether there was a prognostic significance in treating LVH in patients with hypertension. They performed a prospective cohort study on the effects of a Losartan Intervention for Endpoint Reduction in Hypertension (LIFE) randomized trial from 1995 to 2001. Nine hundred forty-one patients with hypertension and LVH were identified. Each had an echocardiogram and was evaluated annually for 5 years. A reduction in hypertrophy (LV mass index) was strongly associated with improved cardiovascular outcomes [17]. Another study by Okin and associates [18] looked at regression of ECG-detected LVH during antihypertensive treatment in a randomized trial of 9,193 patients with hypertension also in the LIFE study. Less severe LVH during antihypertensive therapy was associated with lower likelihoods of cardiovascular mortality [18]. In the Studies of Left Ventricular Dysfunction (SOLVD) trial, the incidence of death or symptomatic HF in high-risk patients treated with an ACE inhibitor was reduced from 39% to 30% over a 3-year study period [19].

Detection of Left Ventricular Hypertrophy

Electrocardiogram

Electrocardiography has the capacity to detect some, but not all, patients with LVH. Accuracy of the ECG in part depends on the criteria used for defining LVH. Common criteria are listed in Table 9.4 [20].

TABLE 9.4. Common criteria used to detect left ventricular hypertrophy.

- Sokolow-Lyon indices
  ▲ If the sum of the S wave in V1 and R wave in V5 or V6 is >35 mm and/or
  ▲ The R wave in aVL is >11 mm
- Cornell voltage criteria
  ▲ For men: If the sum of the S wave in V3 and R wave in aVL is >28 mm
  ▲ For women: If the sum of the S wave in V3 and R wave in aVL is >20 mm

Source: Data from Mirvis [20].

Conservative estimates of the sensitivity and specificity in the detection of moderate to severe LVH are sensitivity, 30% to 60%, and specificity, 80% to 90%. Sensitivity and specificity are improved in the presence of LVH with a strain pattern.

Two-Dimensional Echocardiogram

A two-dimensional echocardiogram coupled with Doppler flow studies is the primary method for detecting HF. The test measures the left ventricular ejection fraction and evaluates structural and valvular abnormalities that may affect cardiac function. There is some variation in the criteria used to detect systolic dysfunction. Most studies use an ejection fraction <40%; however, an ejection fraction <50% is abnormal. It is important to remember that a normal ejection fraction does not rule out diastolic dysfunction. As discussed above, some patients will have diastolic dysfunction alone. Doppler flow measurements of diastolic filling need to be interpreted in the context of the individual patient. An elderly patient with no clinical signs of HF may be labeled as having diastolic dysfunction because of an "overinterpretation" of echocardiographic indices of diastolic function.

Brain Natriuretic Peptides

Atrial natriuretic (ANP) and brain natriuretic peptides (BNP) are hormones that are released from myocardial cells in response to volume expansion and wall stress. Both hormones have diuretic effects, enhancing sodium excretion and lowering blood pressure. Plasma levels of both hormones are increased in patients with asymptomatic and symptomatic HF and are increased in patients with systolic or diastolic dysfunction. Rapid measurement of BNP has become a common tool used in emergency departments, particularly in the evaluation of patients with dyspnea. It can accurately distinguish dyspnea caused by HF from dyspnea due to other causes. A challenge has been in determining the cut-off criteria for an abnormal test. Maisel and associates [14] conducted a prospective study of

TABLE 9.5. Concerns on the use of brain natriuretic peptide (BNP).

- BNP is not sensitive enough to use as a screening tool for the presence of asymptomatic left ventricular hypertrophy.
- Most dyspneic patients with HF have values above 400 pg/mL.
- Pulmonary embolism and pulmonary hypertension may elevate BNP levels.
- Patients may present with more than one cause of dyspnea; a high BNP does not rule out other causes of dyspnea (e.g., pneumonia, anemia, dysrhythmia).

Source: Data from de Lemos et al. [21].

1,586 patients who came into an emergency room with acute dyspnea and whose BNP was measured. The BNP value was more accurate than any historical or physical examination findings, or laboratory values, in identifying HF as the cause of dyspnea. The diagnostic accuracy of BNP was 83.4% at a cut-off of 100 pg/mL. The negative predictive value of BNP under 50 pg/mL was 96%. A BNP of 50 was 79% accurate; a BNP of 80 and above was 83% accurate [14]. Measurement of BNP should not be used as a substitute for clinical judgment in caring for patients with HF. Some concerns for BNP as a diagnostic tool are presented in Table 9.5 [21]. The message from the data in Table 9.5 is to be cautious about overreliance on this test.

To summarize, detection of all patients with asymptomatic LVH would require periodic echocardiographic evaluation of large numbers of patients with coronary artery disease, diabetes, hypertension, and valvular disease. The effectiveness of echocardiographic screening for LVH can be increased if providers target high-risk subgroups [22]. These subgroups include:

1. Patients with a prior MI with anterolateral Q waves detected on ECG
2. Hypertensive patients with LVH detected on ECG
3. Patients with diabetes and LVH detected on ECG

Initial Evaluation

Summary

- The American College of Cardiology and the American Heart Association (ACC/AHA) have established guidelines for the evaluation of patients with different "stages" of HF.
- For those determined to be at high risk for developing HF (patients with hypertension, ischemic heart disease, and diabetes):
  - ▲ Treat reversible risk factors (control hypertension, hyperlipidemia, diabetes, and obesity; and advise patients to avoid use of tobacco and excessive amounts of alcohol). For example, a decrease in blood pressure can reduce the risk of HF substantially. A decrease in systolic blood pressure of 5 mm Hg has been shown to cut the risk of HF by 25%; a reduction of 10 mm Hg has been shown to cut the risk by 50%.

- ▲ Unless contraindicated, prescribe an ACE inhibitor.
- ▲ Periodically evaluate the patient for signs and symptoms of overt HF.
- For those patients who have developed structural heart disease (e.g., LVH, asymptomatic valvular disease, prior MI) and show no signs of over HF:
  - ▲ Perform the same interventions for those at high risk.
  - ▲ Again, unless contraindicated, prescribe an ACE inhibitor.
  - ▲ Unless contraindicated, prescribe a beta-blocker.
  - ▲ Perform regular evaluations for signs and symptoms of HF.
- Once the diagnosis of HF is made, your evaluation should include the following:
  - ▲ Determine the underlying cause, and assess for factors that may be reversible and that can aggravate the symptoms.
  - ▲ Assess for commonly associated comorbid conditions.
  - ▲ Assess the impact of HF on the patient's quality of life, including functional limitations.
  - ▲ Gauge the patient's understanding and awareness of the implications of HF for his or her health and the barriers that may impact effective management of the condition.
- Establishing a category for the severity of symptoms can help guide you toward the appropriate level of management. There are two commonly used classification systems: the NYHA and the ACC/AHA stages of HF. The NYHA system assigns patients to one of four classes, depending on the degree of effort required to elicit symptoms:
  - ▲ Class IV (Severe HF)—symptoms of HF at rest
  - ▲ Class III (Moderate HF)—symptoms on less than ordinary exertion
  - ▲ Class II (Mild HF)—symptoms on ordinary exertion
  - ▲ Class I (Mild HF)—symptoms only at levels that would limit normal individuals
- It is important to recognize that there is often a discordance between functional impairment (as identified by the stages of HF) and severity of systolic dysfunction (as identified by ejection fraction). Patients with a very low ejection fraction may be asymptomatic, whereas patient with preserved left ventricular systolic function may have severe disability. This phenomenon is not well understood.
- The ACC/AHA system of stages of HF also provides specific management guidance for each stage.

Patients at High Risk for Developing Heart Failure: "Pre-Heart Failure"

As described earlier, it appears reasonable to attempt to identify those patients at high risk for developing HF, as it is likely that early intervention will impact the long-term effects of the disease. Once identified, what

TABLE 9.6. Recommendations for patients at high risk for developing heart failure (ACC/AHA stage A).

- Strong evidence to support action
  - Control hypertension
  - Treat lipid disorders; at least target LDL cholesterol to <100 mg/dL
  - Avoid tobacco, excessive alcohol, and illicit substances
  - Use an ACE inhibitor if coronary artery disease, diabetes, or hypertension with associated cardiovascular risk factors is present
  - Periodic evaluation for signs and symptoms of HF
- Evidence to support action
  - Noninvasive evaluation of left ventricular function for patients with a strong family history of cardiomyopathy
- No clear evidence to support action
  - Reduction of dietary salt beyond what is prudent; 2 g sodium diet
  - Routine testing to detect left ventricular dysfunction in patients without signs or symptoms of HF or evidence of structural disease
  - Routine use of nutritional supplements

Source: Data from Hunt et al. [23].

action should you take with these patients? The ACC/AHA has recommended the label "pre-heart failure" for this group. A summary of the ACC/AHA consensus guidelines is provided in Table 9.6 [23]. The strongest evidence for action is to do the following for these high-risk patients (e.g., those with hypertension, coronary artery disease, and diabetes):

1. Treat reversible risk factors (control hypertension, hyperlipidemia, diabetes, and obesity, and advise patients to avoid use of tobacco and excessive amounts of alcohol).
2. Unless contraindicated, prescribe an ACE inhibitor.
3. Periodically evaluate the patient for signs and symptoms of overt HF.

Table 9.7 summarizes the recommendations for those patients who have developed structural heart disease (e.g., LVH, asymptomatic valvular

TABLE 9.7. Recommendations for patients with asymptomatic left ventricular (LV) dysfunction (ACC/AHA stage B).

- Strong evidence to support action
  - ACE inhibitor for patients with a history of myocardial infarction despite a normal ejection fraction
  - ACE inhibitor for patients with a reduced ejection fraction for any cause
  - Beta-blockade for patients with a myocardial infarction regardless of ejection fraction
  - Regular evaluation for signs and symptoms of HF
- No evidence to support action
  - Reduction of dietary salt beyond what is prudent; 2 g sodium diet
  - Routine testing to detect LV dysfunction in patients without signs or symptoms of HF or evidence of structural disease
  - Routine use of nutritional supplements

Source: Data from Hunt et al. [1].

disease, prior MI) and show no signs or symptoms of HF [1]. The strongest recommendations are to use ACE inhibitors and beta-blockers in appropriate situations and to perform regular evaluations for signs and symptoms of HF.

Given findings from recent studies, we must all be aware of patients at high risk for developing HF and take appropriate action to modify their risk. The best studies include those identified as having pre-HF. Any method that can cause a decrease in blood pressure can reduce the risk of HF. A decrease in systolic blood pressure of 5 mm Hg has been shown to cut the risk of HF by 25%; a reduction of 10 mm Hg has been shown to cut the risk by 50%.

Patients Identified with Heart Failure

Once the diagnosis of HF is made, the following factors should be determined:

1. The underlying cause and other factors that may be reversible or that can aggravate the symptoms
2. Common associated comorbid conditions
3. The impact of HF on the quality of life of the patient, including functional limitations
4. The patient's understanding and awareness of the implications of HF to his or her health, and the barriers that may impact effective management of the condition

These four points are incorporated into Table 9.8 [1]. The history you obtain should be focused to identify cardiac and noncardiac disorders that might lead to the development of HF or accelerate its progression. This includes an assessment of risk factors for cardiovascular disease (hypertension, diabetes, lipid disorders, family history of any cardiovascular disease, use of tobacco, alcohol, or illicit drugs). Common noncardiac disorders that can aggravate HF include renal dysfunction, pulmonary disease, and thyroid disease. The physical examination should target complications associated with HF especially the patient's volume status. Again, it is important to recognize that the classic physical stigmata of this condition may not necessarily be present, particularly in the mild stages; however, it still is reasonable to assess for jugular venous distention, heart rate, rhythm, presence of a murmur, evidence of pulmonary congestion, hepatojugular reflux, hepatomegaly, and peripheral edema. Even if some components are "normal" at the time of the initial evaluation, you can use them as a comparison for subsequent evaluations. All patients should have an initial 12-lead ECG, a chest x-ray, and a two-dimensional echocardiogram with Doppler flow studies to assess left ventricular systolic function and presence of valvular disease.

TABLE 9.8. Initial evaluation for patients with newly diagnosed heart failure.

- History: A thorough history to identify cardiac and noncardiac disorders that might lead to the development of HF or accelerate its progression
- Common considerations
  - ▲ Risk factors for HF: History of hypertension, coronary artery disease, diabetes, history of valvular disease, chemotherapy or mantle radiation, use of tobacco, excessive use of alcohol, and use of illicit drugs
  - ▲ Comorbid conditions: Chronic obstructive pulmonary disease, peripheral vascular disease, chronic renal insufficiency, anemia, depression, and thyroid disease
- Review of symptoms: Common considerations
  - ▲ Symptoms associated with HF: paroxysmal noctural dyspnea, orthopnea, bilateral leg edema, nocturnal cough, dyspnea on exertion, fatigue, weight gain
  - ▲ Symptoms associated with accompanying cardiovascular disease: exertional chest pain, palpitations
  - ▲ Symptoms that interfere with patient's ability to perform routine and desired activities of daily living
- Medication list: Medications that may aggravate cardiac function: NSAIDs, thiazolidinediones
- Habits
  - ▲ Diet
  - ▲ Exercise
  - ▲ Tobacco use
  - ▲ Alcohol, cocaine, amphetamine use
- Physical examination
  - ▲ Blood pressure
  - ▲ Pulse
  - ▲ Weight/BMI
  - ▲ Jugular veins
  - ▲ Cardiac examination
  - ▲ Lung examination
  - ▲ Hepatojugular reflux: An early sign of venous constriction that may be present before increased venous pressure is demonstrated by other means. Place the patient on a bed with a movable back rest. Lower the thorax until the head of the blood column is just visible in the jugular veins above the clavicle. Ask the patient to breath normally. Then place the hand in the right upper quadrant of the abdomen and press firmly upward under the costal margin. If venous constriction is present, displacement of this small amount of blood from the liver will cause a rise in the head of the blood column in the neck.
  - ▲ Peripheral edema
- Laboratory evaluation*: Diagnose precipitating, and sometimes reversible, causes or complications of HF: Complete blood count, urinalysis, serum electrolytes, calcium, magnesium, blood urea nitrogen, serum creatinine, blood glucose, liver function tests, and thyroid-stimulating hormone
- Additional tests[†]
  - ▲ 12-lead ECG
  - ▲ Chest x-ray
  - ▲ Two-dimensional echocardiogram with Doppler flow studies

*Measurement of BNP not currently recommended in the initial evaluation of patients with HF.
[†]Radionuclide ventriculography can provide highly accurate measurements of global and regional function and assessment of ventricular enlargement, but is unable to directly assess valvular abnormalities or cardiac hypertrophy. Therefore, echocardiography is the preferred test.
Source: Data from Hunt et al. [1].

Impact on Quality of Life

The evaluation of all patients should include an assessment of the impact on quality of life. There are a number of different methods to do this assessment. The Minnesota Quality of Life Measurement Tool has been a standard research tool in many different studies. An abbreviated version of this tool is given in Table 9.9 [24].

Classifying the Severity of Heart Failure

An important aspect of the initial evaluation is to determine the severity of impairment. Common symptoms and examination findings for different levels of impairment in patients with HF are listed in Table 9.10. Again, use caution in this assessment, as comorbid conditions may also be contributing to the patient's symptoms. The most commonly associated comorbid conditions include hypertension, diabetes, ischemic heart disease, chronic obstructive pulmonary disease, chronic renal insufficiency, peripheral vascular disease, cerebrovascular disease, obesity, and depression.

The importance of establishing a category for the severity of symptoms is that it can help guide you toward the appropriate level of management. There are two commonly used classification systems: the NYHA and the ACC/AHA stages of HF. They are presented in Tables 9.11 and 9.12. The NYHA system (Table 9.11) assigns patients to 1 of 4 classes depending on the degree of effort required to elicit symptoms: symptoms of HF at rest (class IV, Severe), on less than ordinary exertion (class III, Moderate), on

TABLE 9.9. Abbreviated version of the Minnesota Living with Heart Failure Questionnaire.

During the last month did your heart failure prevent you from living as you wanted by:

(No)	(Very little)				(Very much)
0	1	2	3	4	5

1. Causing swelling in your ankles, legs, etc.?
2. Making you sit or lie down to rest during the day?
3. Making your walking about or climbing stairs difficult?
4. Making your working around the house or yard difficult?
5. Making your going places away from home difficult?
6. Making your sleeping well at night difficult?
7. Making doing things with your family or friends difficult?
8. Making your recreational pastimes (hobbies) difficult?
9. Making your sexual activities difficult?
10. Making you tired or low on energy?
11. Making you short of breath?
12. Making you feel like a burden to your family or friends?
13. Making you feel a loss of self-control?
14. Making you feel depressed?

Source: Data from Rector and Cohn [24].

TABLE 9.10. Common symptoms and examination findings for different levels of impairment in patients with heart failure.

- Mild impairment
  - ▲ Symptoms: Easy fatigue, deteriorating exercise capacity, nocturia, and exertional shortness of breath
  - ▲ Examination findings: Basilar rales, S3 gallop, and enlarged point of maximal impulse
- Moderate impairment
  - ▲ Symptoms: Noctural cough, orthopnea, paroxysmal noctural dyspnea, wheezing (especially in those with no history of asthma), anorexia, and tachypnea at rest
  - ▲ Examination findings: Edema, prominent rales over bases, cool extremities due to vasoconstriction, hepatomegaly, hepatojugular reflux, S3 gallop, right pleural effusion, and cardiomegaly on physical examination or on chest x-ray
- Severe impairment
  - ▲ Symptoms: Ascites, cerebral dysfunction
  - ▲ Examination findings: Altered mental status, cyanosis, hypotension, anasarca, and frothy pink sputum

ordinary exertion (class II, Mild), or only at levels that would limit normal individuals (class I, Mild). It is important to recognize that there is often a discordance between functional impairment (as identified by the stages of HF) and severity of systolic dysfunction (as identified by ejection fraction). Patients with a very low ejection fraction may be asymptomatic, whereas patient with preserved left ventricular systolic function may have a severe disability. This phenomenon is not well understood. Advanced heart failure (NYHA class III or IV) affects a quarter of the people with HF and accounts for the majority of morbidity and mortality in HF.

TABLE 9.11. NYHA classification of heart failure.

Class	Patient symptoms
Class I (Mild)	No limitation of physical activity. Ordinary physical activity does not cause undue fatigue, palpitation, or dyspnea (shortness of breath).
Class II (Mild)	Slight limitation of physical activity. Comfortable at rest, but ordinary physical activity results in fatigue, palpitation, or dyspnea.
Class III (Moderate)	Marked limitation of physical activity. Comfortable at rest, but less than ordinary activity causes fatigue, palpitation, or dyspnea.
Class IV (Severe)	Unable to carry out any physical activity without discomfort. Symptoms of cardiac insufficiency at rest. If any physical activity is undertaken, discomfort is increased.

Note: To determine the best course of therapy, physicians often assess the stage of heart failure according to the New York Heart Association (NYHA) functional classification system. This system relates symptoms to everyday activities and to the patient's quality of life.
Source: Adapted from Hunt et al. [1], by permission of J Am Coll Cardiol.

TABLE 9.12. ACC/AHA stages of heart failure.

Stage	Descriptions	Examples
A	Patients at high risk of developing HF because of the presence of conditions that are strongly associated with the development of HF. Such patients have no identified structural or functional abnormalities of the pericardium, myocardium, or cardiac valves and have never shown signs or symptoms of HF	Systemic hypertension; coronary artery disease; diabetes mellitus; history of cardiotoxic drug therapy or alcohol abuse; personal history of rheumatic fever; family history of cardiomyopathy
B	Patients who have developed structural heart disease that is strongly associated with the development of HF, but who have never shown signs or symptoms of HF	Left ventricular hypertrophy or fibrosis; left ventricular dilatation or hypocontractility; asymptomatic valvular heart disease; previous myocardial infarction
C	Patients who have current or prior symptoms of HF associated with underlying structural heart disease	Dyspnea or fatigue due to left ventricular systolic dysfunction; asymptomatic patients who are undergoing treatment for prior symptoms of HF
D	Patients with advanced structural heart disease and marked symptoms of HF at rest despite maximal medical therapy, and who require specialized interventions	Patients who are frequently hospitalized for HF and cannot be safely discharged from the hospital; patients in the hospital awaiting heart transplantation; patients at home receiving continuous intravenous support for symptom relief, or being supported with a mechanical circulatory assist device; patients in a hospice setting for the management of heart failure

Source: Adapted from Hunt et al. [1], by permission of J Am Coll Cardiol.

The ACC/AHA stages of HF classification system (Table 9.12) emphasizes the importance of identifying high-risk patients and taking steps to avoid progression to overt HF. There are also recommendations for actions that are stage specific. Tables 9.6 and 9.7 describe the guidelines for stages A and B. Tables 9.13 and 9.14 present the recommendations for stages C and D. For both stages C and D, the general recommendations are the same as for stages A and B. For stages C and D, implementation of a disease management program will demonstrate the most immediate results by establishing a registry that can be used to monitor the progress of the patient and the population of patients in a practice; by ensuring proper laboratory testing and interventions for abnormal results; by ensuring effective use of medications to alleviate symptoms; and by establishing a program to enhance self-management.

TABLE 9.13. ACC/AHA guidelines for patients with left ventricular dysfunction with current or prior symptoms (stage C).

- General measures: The same as presented for stages A and B. In addition:
  ▲ Moderate sodium restriction
  ▲ Daily measurement of weight
  ▲ Immunization with influenza and pneumococcal vaccines
  ▲ Encourage prudent physical activity to avoid deconditioning
  ▲ Encourage close attention to symptoms and follow-up
  ▲ Encourage patient education and training in self-management
- Medications recommended: Most patients with symptomatic left ventricular dysfunction should be managed with a combination of four drugs: an ACE inhibitor, a diuretic, a beta-blocker, and (usually) digitalis
- Interventions to be considered for selected patients: The following agents have been considered useful for selected patients and are undergoing continued trials to determine the exact role in the treatment of HF: aldosterone antagonists, angiotensin receptor blockers, hydralazine and isosorbide dinitrate, and exercise training.

Source: Data from Hunt et al. [1].

Other Methods of Assessing Function: The Six-Minute Walk Test

The 6-minute walk test (6MWT) has been recommended as a more objective way to assess functional impairment in patients with HF. Patients are instructed to walk at their own pace while attempting to cover as much distance as possible during the allotted time. They are encouraged to give their best effort during the test. Two chairs are placed 50 feet apart, and the patient walks back and forth, stopping to rest when needed. The total distance covered is then determined. The 6MWT is considered a valid and reliable tool, and correlates well with outcomes such as need for hospitalization and mortality. Patients covering less than 300 feet have higher rates of hospitalization and death than those able to cover 450 feet [25].

Finally, because self-management has been shown to be an effective intervention in all chronic conditions, it is always important to gauge

TABLE 9.14. ACC/AHA guidelines for the management of heart failure in patients with refractory end-stage heart failure (stage D).

- General measures: Despite recommendations presented in Tables 9.6, 9.7, and 9.13, some patients fail to respond and develop severe symptoms at rest, and require repeated hospitalizations.
- Before a patient is considered to have refractory HF, it is important to confirm the diagnosis, assess for factors that may be contributing to the condition, and ensure that all medical therapies have been effectively used.
- Meticulous management of fluids can be an effective strategy for symptom control.
- Alternative surgical and mechanical approaches for the treatment of end-stage HF are under development.

Source: Data from Hunt et al. [1].

patients' understanding of the disease, their concerns associated with the diagnosis, and their willingness to make necessary lifestyle changes in order to optimize their health. Methods to support self-management and to provide patients with educational resources are discussed later.

Ongoing Evaluation

Once the nature and cause of HF have been defined, you should focus on the ongoing clinical assessment of each patient [26]. This ongoing review of clinical status is important to selecting and monitoring treatment. It should include an assessment of functional capacity, volume status, laboratory evaluation, and prognosis.

Management

Fast Facts

- To help reduce the burden of HF for those in ACC/AHA stages A and B (pre-HF), we should improve our efforts to:
  - ▲ Control hypertension
  - ▲ Lower serum lipid levels
  - ▲ Assist patients who are ready to quit smoking
  - ▲ Prescribe an ACE inhibitor, unless contraindicated, for patients with hypertension, diabetes, and coronary artery disease
  - ▲ Assess for LVH in high-risk groups: patients with hypertension, diabetes, and coronary artery disease
  - ▲ For those with LVH, ensure that they are prescribed an ACE inhibitor and a beta-blocker (unless contraindicated) and are monitored for signs and symptoms of developing HF
- To have the greatest short-term impact on the burden of HF for those in stages C and D, we should improve our efforts to help our patients:
  - ▲ Adhere to modest dietary sodium restriction
  - ▲ Monitor daily weights
  - ▲ Engage in prudent physical activity
  - ▲ Pay attention to the signs and symptoms of worsening HF
- For those identified as having end-stage HF, we should ensure that:
  - ▲ We have confirmed the diagnosis of HF
  - ▲ We have adequately addressed comorbid conditions that may be aggravating the symptoms
  - ▲ We pay meticulous attention to intake of fluids and volume status
  - ▲ We address end-of-life issues with the patients and their families
- Effective treatment of HF requires enhancing each patient's self-management skills.

- Perhaps the most critical component of this intervention is to appreciate the importance of "self-efficacy," the confidence to carry out a behavior necessary to reach a desired goal. On a 10-point scale, patients who rate their level of confidence under 7 are unlikely to be successful for that goal.
- Assessment of a patient's readiness to change is an important part of chronic disease management; approximately 20% of patients are ready for change at the time of initial evaluation. Failing to assess the patient's readiness often results in ineffective management, especially provider frustration, which often ends with the patient being labeled as "noncompliant."
- Important barriers to promoting self-management include ambiguous and unclear symptoms as indicators of illness, vague timeline features associated with symptom worsening, and inaccurate perceived causes of symptoms. Heart failure is one of the most difficult disease processes to objectively define signs and symptoms of early exacerbation. Newly diagnosed HF patients report the greatest difficulty identifying symptoms associated with their disease, but even long-term HF patients have trouble.
- A delay in action in a response to symptoms often results in a hospital visit for most HF patients. Coordinating patient education, particularly in supporting self-care, improves outcomes such as length of hospital stay, readmission frequency, and medication adherence. Some examples of effective interventions you can take in your practice include the following:
  - ▲ Assess what patients and caregivers perceive as causative factors for decompensation.
  - ▲ Use verbal and written instructions that prompt patients about their disease and the actions required to maintain a stable condition.
  - ▲ Patients with HF must be instructed to:
    - ♦ Identify and monitor personal signs of an early exacerbation
    - ♦ Monitor weight daily
    - ♦ Maintain a low-sodium diet
  - ▲ Provide an emergency action plan to all patients.
- Socioeconomic barriers are recognized as contributing to poor outcomes in patients with HF. Patients with low literacy skills are particularly at risk for frequent hospitalizations and high utilization of care, aggravated by having less knowledge about self-care. For the patients in your practice who are doing poorly, you should work to identify and help those who have this barrier as a contributing factor for their symptoms of HF.
- A key feature to self-management education is the patient-generated short-term action plan. The action plan must be patient generated, realistic, and have a reasonably high self-efficacy (the level of confidence that the goal can be achieved).

- The following techniques should help promote self-management for your patients:
  - ▲ Elicit patient-generated goals for each visit, for example, "What goal would you like to focus on in managing your heart failure?"
  - ▲ Assess self-efficacy for each goal. Provide patients with a 10-point response scale with the following lead question: "How confident are you that you can achieve this goal?" A patient's self-efficacy rating of less than 7 is a strong indicator that the patient will be unlikely to achieve that particular goal.
  - ▲ Provide a means to document patient-generated goals and to monitor success in achieving the goals or barriers encountered. Recognize achievement in meeting self-generated goals.
  - ▲ Work with office staff to reinforce health behavior and self-management goals, for example, reinforcing monitoring and control of hypertension when blood pressure is being taken and prompting patients to discuss self-generated goals with the physician.

Management of High-Risk Patients

As described, the ACC/AHA has categorized HF into four stages. This classification includes recommendations for treatment. These are presented in Tables 9.6, 9.7, 9.13, and 9.14. The estimated numbers of patients in each group are stage A, 60 million; stage B, 32 million; stage C, 6 million; and stage D, 200,000.

These numbers suggest that we can make a substantial impact in reducing the overall burden of HF in the population by targeting those patients in stages A and B. Specifically, we should improve our efforts to:

1. Control hypertension
2. Lower serum lipid levels
3. Assist patients who are ready to quit smoking
4. Prescribe an ACE inhibitor, unless contraindicated, for patients with hypertension, diabetes, and coronary artery disease
5. Assess for LVH in high-risk groups: patients with hypertension, diabetes, and coronary artery disease
6. For those with LVH, ensure that they are prescribed an ACE inhibitor and a beta-blocker (unless contraindicated) and are monitored for signs and symptoms of developing HF

For those patients who already have overt HF, we are likely to demonstrate short-term benefits, such as lowering costs and high-resource utilization, by addressing those in stages C and D. Specifically, we should improve our efforts to help our patients:

1. Adhere to modest dietary sodium restriction
2. Monitor daily weights

3. Engage in prudent physical activity
4. Pay attention to the signs and symptoms of worsening HF

We should pay particular attention to those identified as having end-stage HF by ensuring that:

1. We have confirmed the diagnosis of HF
2. We have adequately addressed comorbid conditions that may be aggravating the symptoms
3. We pay meticulous attention to intake of fluids and volume status
4. We address end-of-life issues with the patients and their families

Self-Management Support and Assessing Readiness to Change

The evidence strongly suggests that the key to effective disease management of any chronic condition, including HF, is to set an environment that promotes self-management. Self-management education includes information/instruction, counseling, and behavioral intervention. Although this chapter focuses on self-management training in the office setting, it is important to recognize that effective settings also include work sites, churches, senior centers, community centers, home, and extended-care facilities. The two critical components that can enhance a patient's efforts in self-management are:

1. Appreciating the importance of self-efficacy and the confidence to carry out a behavior necessary to reach a desired goal
2. Assessing the patient's readiness to change

Assessment of a patient's readiness to change for a given recommendation has been associated with greater efforts with self-care and improved control and lifestyle modification. Approximately, 20% of patients at the time of initial diagnosis are ready to accept and act on necessary lifestyle changes. Failing to assess the patient's readiness often results in ineffective management, especially provider frustration, which often ends up with the patient being labeled as noncompliant. An example of this is sending patients to an education class on dietary change and lifestyle modification when they are not ready to make these changes. Assessment of readiness to change can be accomplished by asking questions such as "How likely are you to pursue changing your diet at this point?" and "To help you understand more about HF, which of the following information would be helpful to you at this time: a pamphlet, a Web site, a class?" More information on assessment of readiness to change can be found in the works listed in Table 7.7 in Chapter 7 and in Chapter 2.

Studies on the Effectiveness of Self-Management Support

A number of studies have assessed the impact of self-management support. Although the methods used to support self-management varied, most show a positive impact on quality of life, patient satisfaction, utilization of services, and outcomes. Riegel and associates [27] have published research on the testing of a survey tool that can be used to assess a patient's abilities in self-care. The tool is presented in Table 9.15. The information from this survey can be helpful with patients who have frequent exacerbations of their HF symptoms and have moderate to severe intensity of symptoms. It is important to provide this survey to your patients in a "no fault" manner; emphasize that you are trying to help them identify areas that may help them achieve better control of their symptoms.

Self-management support for patients with chronic disease is a relatively new concept. There have been different methods used in organizations to help promote self-management. The impact of these interventions has been variable; some interventions have been found to be effective while other interventions are not. Findings from studies that target self-management enhancement are as follows.

Predictors of Self-Care

Chriss and associates [28] used the self-care index presented in Table 9.15 to determine the profile of patients who were most likely to be successful with self-care. They found that older, male patients who had fewer comorbid illnesses were most likely to be successful with self-care.

Methods of Promoting Self-Management

Use of a Pharmacy-Based Support Intervention

Murray and associates [29] are performing a trial with patients with HF who will receive 9 months of pharmacy support. The pharmacist provides written and verbal education for each patient along with icon-based labeling of medication containers. The pharmacist identifies patient barriers to medications, coaches them on overcoming these barriers, and coordinates medication use with their primary care provider. They also provided ongoing monitoring.

Web-Based Communication

Ross and associates [30] assessed the impact of a Web-based communication tool for patients: the SPPARO (System Providing Access to Records Online) Program. One hundred seven patients were included in the trial. At 1 year the intervention group was no better in terms of confidence in managing symptoms; however, their adherence to the treatment regimen

TABLE 9.15. Self-care of heart failure index.

1. How often do you do the following?
   (Answers are NEVER, RARELY, SOMETIMES, FREQUENTLY, ALWAYS)
   Weigh yourself daily
   Eat a low-salt diet
   Take part in regular physical activity
   Keep your weight down
   Get a flu shot every year

2. Many patients have symptoms because of their heart failure. Trouble breathing and ankle swelling are common symptoms. In the past 3 months, have you had trouble with breathing or ankle swelling?
   (Answers are YES or NO)

3. The last time you had trouble with breathing or ankle swelling, how quickly did you recognize it as a symptom of heart failure?
   (Answers are I DID NOT RECOGNIZE IT, NOT QUICKLY, SOMEWHAT QUICKLY, QUICKLY, VERY QUICKLY)

4. Listed below are remedies that people with heart failure use. When you have trouble with breathing or ankle swelling, how likely are you to try one of these remedies?
   (Answers are NOT LIKELY, SOMEWHAT LIKELY, VERY LIKELY)
   Reduce salt intake
   Reduce fluid intake
   Take an extra water pill
   Call you doctor or nurse for guidance

5. If you tried any of these remedies the last time you had trouble with ankle swelling or fluid, how sure were you that the remedy helped?
   (Answers are I DIDN'T TRY ANYTHING, NOT SURE, SOMEWHAT SURE, VERY SURE)

6. How confident are you that you can evaluate the importance of your symptoms?
   (Answers are NOT CONFIDENT, SOMEWHAT CONFIDENT, VERY CONFIDENT, EXTREMELY CONFIDENT)

7. Generally, how confident are you that you can recognize changes in your health if they occur?
   (Same answer choices as last question)

8. Generally, how confident are you that you can do something that will relieve your symptoms?
   (Same answer choices as last question)

9. How confident are you that you can evaluate the effectiveness of whatever you do to relieve your symptoms?
   (Same answer choices as last question)

Source: Data from Riegel et al. [27].

was greater. The intervention group also experienced no effect on health status, and they had more emergency room visits.

Peer Support

Peer support has been used for a variety of patient populations. Riegel and Carlson [31] studied the effect of training nine persons with HF to mentor other HF patients. This study targeted those patients admitted for a decompensated exacerbation. At the end of 3 months, there were no differences in HF readmissions, lengths of stay, or costs. Small group meetings lead by a peer support did not work in this setting.

Home Health Intervention

Feldman and associates [32] studied the impact of a home health intervention. They looked at 371 Medicare patients with HF served by 205 home health nurses. The intervention consisted of an evidence-based protocol, patient self-care guide, and training to improve nurses' teaching and support skills. The intervention was associated with a marginally significant reduction in the volume of skilled nursing visits and a reduction in the number of visits provided. There was no change in physician or emergency room use. Expected outcome improvements did not occur.

Patient Training

Holman and Lorig [33] have done extensive work on self-management training for patients. They summarized the responsibilities of the patient in the presence of chronic disease as follows:

* Using medications properly
* Changing behaviors to improve symptoms or slow disease progression
* Adjusting to social and economic consequences
* Interpreting and reporting symptoms accurately

Their research also describes what patients with chronic conditions want, but are not typically getting, from their health are providers:

* Information concerning the diagnosis, its implications, and its treatments and their consequences
* Understanding of the potential impact on their future
* Continuity of care and ready access to it
* Coordination of care, particularly with specialists
* Infrastructure improvements: flexible scheduling, wait times, billing
* Ways to cope with symptoms, such as pain, fatigue, disability, and loss of independence, and ways to adjust to disease consequences, such as uncertainty, fear and depression, anger, loneliness, sleep disorders, memory loss, exercise needs, nocturia, sexual dysfunction, and stress

Barriers to Self-Care

Frantz [34] has described significant barriers to promoting self-care among patients. The most notable were ambiguous and unclear symptoms as indicators of illness; vague timeline features associated with symptom worsening, and inaccurate perceived causes of symptoms. Heart failure is one of the most difficult disease processes to objectively define the signs and symptoms of early exacerbation. Newly diagnosed HF patients report the greatest difficulty identifying symptoms associated with their disease, but even long-term HF patients can have trouble. Heart failure symptoms most frequently reported by patients were shortness of breath, fatigue, difficulty breathing while sleeping, palpitations, and sudden weight gain. Early signs of HF exacerbation included bloating, loss of appetite, increased fatigue, and lack of concentration. Patients usually attributed these symptoms to "overdoing it," "not sleeping well," or "getting old."

DeGeest and associates [35] found that vague or ambiguous symptoms delayed care and thwarted ongoing self-monitoring behavior. A delay in action in a response to symptoms resulted in a hospital visit for most HF patients. Jaarmsa and associates [36] found that, despite intensive education and support in the hospital, HF patients had limited knowledge of the disease process as well as limited decision-making skills. In their home care study of patients with HF, Miranda and associates [37] found that coordinating patient education, particularly in supporting self-care, improved outcomes such as length of hospital stay, readmission frequency, and medication adherence.

Some examples of effective interventions that you can make in your practice include the following:

1. Assess what patients and caregivers perceive as causative factors for decompensation.
2. Use verbal and written instructions that prompt patients about their disease and the actions required to maintain a stable condition.
3. Patients with HF must be instructed to:
   a. Identify and monitor personal signs of an early exacerbation
   b. Monitor weight daily
   c. Maintain a low-sodium diet
4. An emergency action plan should be provided to all patients (Table 9.16).

Socioeconomic barriers are recognized as contributing to poor outcomes in patients with HF. Patients with low literacy skills are particularly at risk for frequent hospitalizations and high utilization of care, aggravated by having less knowledge about self-care. DeWalt and associates [38] tested a disease management intervention for patients with low literacy skills (mean skills at the fifth grade level). The survey they used is presented in Table 9.17. Their intervention included a 1-hour educational session and scheduled supportive phone calls that were tapered over 6 weeks. Although the mean knowledge score did not change after the intervention (mean = 67%), the proportion of patients weighing themselves daily increased from 32% at baseline to 100% at 12 weeks. There was an overall improvement in one class based on the NYHA Classification System.

TABLE 9.16. Emergency action plan.

Green zone: all clear	Green zone means
Your goal weight:	
No shortness of breath	Your symptoms are under control
No swelling	Continue taking your medications as ordered
No weight gain	Continue daily weights
No chest pain	Follow low-salt diet
No decrease in your ability to maintain your activity level	Keep all physician appointments
Yellow zone: caution	**Yellow zone means**
If you have any of the following signs and symptoms	Your symptoms may indicate that you need an adjustment of your medications
Weight gain of 3 or more pounds	Call your physician, nurse coordinator, or home health nurse
Increased cough	Name:
Increased swelling	Number:
Increase in shortness of breath with activity	Instructions:
Increase in the number of pillows activity needed	
Anything else unusual that bothers you	
Call your physician if you are going into the yellow zone	
Red zone: medical alert	**Red zone means**
Unrelieved shortness of breath: shortness of breath at rest	Any of these indicates that you need to be evaluated by a physician right away
Unrelieved chest pain	
Wheezing or chest tightness at rest	
Need to sit in a chair to sleep	

Source: Courtesy of www.improvingchroniccare.org.

TABLE 9.17. Heart failure knowledge questionnaire for patients with low literacy skills.

1. Heart failure means that:
   a. Your heart is beating out of rhythm
   b. Your heart might stop beating sometime soon
   c. Your heart is not pumping blood as well as it should
   d. You are having a heart attack
   e. Don't know
2. Which of the following symptoms can come from your heart failure?
   a. A headache
   b. Yellowing of the skin
   c. Shortness of breath when you lay down flat
   d. Vomiting blood
   e. Don't know

TABLE 9.17. *Continued*

3. Which of the following are signs that you are dehydrated (lost too much water)?
   a. Dizziness
   b. Shortness of breath
   c. Chest pain
   d. Peeing a lot
   e. Don't know
4. I'm going to read a list of problems, and I want you to tell me if each one is a sign your heart failure is getting worse?
   a. Is shortness of breath a sign that your heart failure is getting worse
      Yes; No; Don't know
   b. Is swelling of the legs or ankles a sign your heart failure is getting worse?
      Yes; No; Don't know
   c. Is waking up a night short of breath a sign your heart failure is getting worse?
      Yes; No; Don't know
   d. Is gaining weight a sign your heart failure is getting worse?
      Yes; No; Don't know
5. If you use a lot of salt it will:
   a. Make your heart failure worse
   b. Make your heart failure better
   c. Won't affect your heart failure
   d. Don't know
6. What should you do when you feel more short of breath and your weight has increased by 6 pounds?
   a. Stop taking your fluid pill
   b. Call your doctor
   c. Go on a diet
   d. Weigh yourself tomorrow to see if you gained more
   e. Don't know
7. What should you do when your legs swell up more than normal?
   a. Take an extra dose of your fluid pill
   b. Walk more
   c. Eat more salt
   d. Eat more protein
   e. Don't know
8. Compared with someone without heart failure, a person with heart failure should drink:
   a. More fluids than usual
   b. About the same amount of fluids
   c. Less fluids than usual
   d. Don't know
9. People with heart failure should weigh themselves
   a. Every day
   b. Once a week
   c. Once a month
   d. Only when they feel bad
   e. Don't know

Provider Support for Self-Management

Self-management promotion represents a paradigm shift for most patients, providers, and practices. The key element to the paradigm shift is a patient-centered approach, with the provider functioning as a health coach. This is an important shift, as many physicians feel helpless or ineffective in providing counseling for health promotion. Of physicians surveyed in 1991, less than 10% thought that they could be successful in modifying patients' behaviors.

Developing a Short-Term Action Plan

A key feature to self-management is the patient-generated short-term action plan. As described by Bodenheimer and associates [39], this is "similar to a New Year's resolution, but of shorter duration, such as 1 to 2 weeks." It is also more specific, for example, "This week I will walk around the block before lunch on Monday, Tuesday, and Thursday." The action plan must be patient-generated, realistic, and have reasonably high self-efficacy.

Providers should query the likelihood that a patient will be able to achieve the short-term action plan. This can be done by asking the following question: "On a scale of 1 to 10, how sure are you that you can accomplish this goal?" If the answer is 7 or greater, the action plan is likely to be accomplished. If the answer is below 7, it would be reasonable to reassess the plan and help make it more realistic.

Based on our experience, we believe the following techniques will help promote self-management:

1. Elicit patient-generated goals for each visit, for example, "What goal would you like to focus on in managing your HF?"

2. Assess self-efficacy for each goal. Provide patients with a 10-point response scale with the following lead question: "How confident are you that you can achieve this goal?" A patient's self-efficacy rating of less than 7 is a strong indicator that the patient will be unlikely to achieve that particular goal.

3. Provide a means to document patient-generated goals and to monitor success in achieving these goals or the barriers encountered. Recognize achievement in meeting self-generated goals.

4. Work with office staff to reinforce health behavior and self-management goals, for example, reinforcing the importance of monitoring and control of hypertension when the blood pressure is being taken and prompting the patient to discuss self-generated goals with the physician.

Helping Patients Set Their Goals

How should the providers emphasize the patient's role? It begins with a simple message: "HF is a serious condition. There are things you can do to live better with HF and things that the medical team can do to assist you. We are going to work together on this." In setting goals it is important for you to assist your patients to set realistic goals, understand and use an action plan, assess the barriers to achieving goals, make appropriate changes, and recognize achievement of objectives. You can support this in the following way:

1. Promote goal setting. It is better to pursue one goal at a time, a goal that focuses on a behavior and not on an outcome, that is patient-generated, and that is achievable.
2. Ensure that the system allows you to keep track of the goals so that during follow-up visits you will remember to inquire about how the patient did.
3. Be nonjudgmental/nonfatalistic about failures.
4. Remember to recognize success.

Education to Support Self-Management

Education is clearly important in promoting self-management. Key areas of understanding include monitoring symptoms of HF, nutrition therapy, weight control, exercise, stress reduction.

Monitoring Symptoms

An important goal of medical therapy of patients with HF is to improve how patients feel and function during daily activities. Numerous physiologic end points such as exercise tolerance tests have been used as surrogate measures of therapeutic benefit. Rector and Cohn's previously described Minnesota Living with Heart Failure Questionnaire [24] (see Table 9.9) may be used to monitor symptoms over time. The 6MWT (also described earlier) can be used as well to provide a measurable method of monitoring symptoms over time.

Nutrition Therapy

Helping patients follow a heart-healthy diet with appropriate restrictions on dietary sodium and total fluid intake is an important adjunct to managing patients with HF. Some patients experience acute decompensation caused by excessive consumption of foods or fluids that they thought were healthy (e.g., tomato juice or oysters), not realizing that they are significant sources of sodium. To obtain proper information on the necessary dietary changes, it is important for you to guide your patients to resources such as dietitians, nurse educators, and online and in-print materials (books and pamphlets). For printed materials, excellent resources are available from the American Heart Association (www.amhrt.org).

Changing a lifelong pattern of eating is a substantial challenge for patients. Prior to referral to educational resources, providers should do the following:

1. Assess the patient's readiness to change. If the patient is not yet ready to make dietary changes, it is better, initially, to provide the patient with printed or online educational resources.
2. Assist the patient in establishing reasonable nutritional goals.
3. Assess the patient's self-efficacy (the confidence to make changes).

Nutritional goals described by the AHA include the following:

1. Provide regular meal planning advice and guidelines. Balance food intake with drug therapy and exercise.
2. Maintain reasonable weight by monitoring calorie consumption (10% to 20% of calories from protein; less than 10% of calories from saturated fat; less than 10% of calories from polyunsaturated fat; 60% to 70% of calories from monounsaturated fat and carbohydrates; and less than 300 mg of cholesterol per day).

Exercise

Sixty percent of Americans do not engage in any form of moderate activity, and 30% do not exercise at all. Many patients with HF have comorbid conditions that add barriers to engaging in exercise. Physical deconditioning can accelerate the symptoms of HF. Is it wise to recommend an exercise program to those patients with HF? What are the benefits to a patient in starting such a program? A study by Hambrecht and associates [40] looked at the effects of exercise training on patients with left ventricular dysfunction. They performed a randomized trial of 73 men all with systolic dysfunction (mean ejection fraction = 27%). Patients underwent a training program in the hospital involving the use of a bicycle ergometer. They started with 10 minutes of exercise 4 to 6 times a day for 2 weeks followed by 6 months of exercise. The exercise involved the use of an in-home bicycle ergometer for 20 minutes per day at a level of 70% of peak oxygen uptake. They received instruction on monitoring the heart rate necessary to achieve this level of activity. At the end of the study, patients in the exercise group experienced significant improvement in their stroke volume and in their NYHA class. ACTION HF is an ongoing randomized trial assessing the effects of an exercise program on mortality. Information on this trial can be obtained through on the Web at www.hfaction.org. Of course, all patients starting an exercise program should undergo testing to ensure that they do not have clinically significant ischemia.

There are many barriers to patients with HF engaging in an exercise program. Corvera-Tindel and associates [41] studied the predictors of noncompliance to participation in exercise training. Exercise training was a 12-week home walking exercise program, averaging 30 minutes per day.

Thirty-nine HF patients participated. Only 35% of the patients actively complied with the requirements for this program. Patients with comorbid illness and who had HF for longer periods of time were more likely to drop out of the activity.

For patients who are motivated and have satisfactory confidence in participating in exercise activities, a pedometer can help patients set reasonable goals and receive daily feedback. Asakuma and associates [42] found that use of a pedometer gave reasonable, noninvasive estimates of function and quality of life. It is important to encourage patients to:

1. Pick an exercise that they enjoy
2. Start slowly, increasing length, frequency, and intensity gradually
3. Set reasonable goals for their exercise program

Educate patients with HF that exertional chest pain or a significant change in exertional shortness of breath warrants consideration for underlying ischemia.

Behavioral Concerns

Patients with HF have a twofold increased rate of depression. Depression is associated with suboptimal control and increased rates of end-organ complications. Murberg and Furze [43] studied the connection between depression and poor outcomes in 119 patients with HF. They found that symptoms of depression were a significant predictor of mortality. Despite this knowledge, fewer than 25% of patients with HF and depression receive treatment for this condition. Given the rate of depression in this population and the impact on quality of life and control of the disease, all patients with HF should undergo periodic screening for signs of depression.

Education Resources

There are a number of resources available to assist patients in dealing with common barriers, including symptom management, fatigue management, relaxation, and managing emotions, nutrition, exercise, and medications. They are listed in Table 9.18. In addition, the Centers for Disease Control and Prevention (CDC) includes patient information on HF treatment at their Web site (see http://cdc.gov/cvh/library/fs_heart_failure.htm). Another resource for patients with access to the Internet is the Heart Failure Society of America (www.abouthf.org). This site includes 11 different education modules for patients and their families. Topics include how to follow a low-sodium diet; self-care: following your treatment plans and dealing with your symptoms; exercise and activity; how to evaluate claims of heart failure treatments and cures; and advanced directives.

TABLE 9.18. Resources for information about heart failure.

1. Lists of phone and Internet resources for patients and physicians:
American Heart Association
7272 Greenville Avenue
Dallas, TX 75231-4596
(800)242-8721

Agency for Healthcare Policy and Research
P.O. Box 8547
Silver Spring, MD 20907
(800)358-9295

"Living with Heart Disease: Is it Heart Failure?"
National Heart, Lung and Blood Institute Information Center
P.O. Box 30105
Bethesda, MD 20824-0105

2. Internet resources:
www.abouthf.org: Patient education site from the Heart Failure Society of America
www.amhrt.org: The American Heart Association's site with multiple links about HF for
patients and health care professionals
www.mayoclinic.com: Patient education materials, including advice on coping skills, self-
care, prevention, and treatment
www.nhlb.nih.gov/health/public/heart/other/hrtfail/htm: The official site of the National
Heart, Lung and Blood Institute, with articles for patients and providers
http://www.heartcenter.ccf.org:8080: The Cleveland Clinic Heart Center
http://www.amhrt.org: American Heart Association

3. Other patient resources:
http://www.amhrt.org: American Heart Association—Home, Health and Family
www.abouthf.org: A website from the Heart Failure Society of America that includes a
video designed to explain heart failure, it symptoms, and treatment options

Medications

Summary

- The evidence is overwhelming that ACE inhibitors can reduce mortality,
  hospitalizations, and symptoms, and increase exercise capacity in patient
  with HF.
- Despite the drug's known efficacy, the number of patients found to be
  taking an ACE inhibitor is less than optimal.
- The evidence for the efficacy of ARBs in HF is less persuasive, and for
  the present this class of medication should be prescribed only when an
  ACE inhibitor cannot be tolerated.
- Beta-blockers are indicated for stages II through IV HF secondary to
  systolic dysfunction if the patient is free from cardiogenic shock, acute
  pulmonary edema, or evidence of gross fluid retention.

- Beta-blocker therapy should be strongly considered when a patient is stabilized in the hospital rather than waiting for 2 weeks after discharge.
- Beta-blockers exert their effect by retarding or reversing the progression of ventricular dysfunction and HF and by decreasing the risk of sudden death. The effect occurs over a period of months, and the effect on sudden death may be by a reduction in arrhythmias.
- Long-term beta-blockade reduces myocardial hypertrophy and filling pressures, and increases ejection fraction, a process called *ventricular remodeling.*
- Carvedilol, bisoprolol, and metoprolol succinate have undergone the most rigorous studies. There is no conclusive evidence for a difference between these beta-blockers in their benefits, but one study showed generic metoprolol tartrate to be inferior to carvedilol.
- When prescribing beta-blockers, the general principle should be "start low and go slow." Treatment should be started at low dose and titrated upward at 2- to 4-week intervals to target dose or a resting heart rate of 60, depending on the clinical response.
- Use caution when prescribing beta-blockers for patients with severe COPD, for those taking a calcium channel blocker, for those with relative hypotension, and for those taking digoxin.
- It may take 2 to 3 months to see the benefits of beta-blocker therapy.
- Spironolactone should be restricted to patients with severe or progressive HF caused by systolic dysfunction whose serum creatinine level is less than or equal to 2.0mg/dL and serum potassium level is less than 5.0mEq/L at baseline.
- Discontinue potassium supplementation when starting spironolactone, and question the patients about the use of potassium-containing salt substitutes and high-potassium foods such as orange juice or bananas.
- Serum potassium level should be monitored at the end of 1 week of treatment and periodically for the first 2 to 3 months. If serum potassium levels increase to 5.5mEq/L or greater, reduce the dosage to 12.5mg daily or 25mg every other day.
- Discontinue spironolactone for any patient whose serum potassium level is 6.0mEq/L or higher.
- Spironolactone is indicated for edema and can be a useful addition to Lasix for patients with all classes of HF and can obviate the need for potassium supplementation.
- Digoxin remains a therapeutic option for the outpatient management of those with chronic symptomatic HF caused by systolic dysfunction.
- Current consensus guidelines recommend digoxin for patients with NHYA class II to IV HF if symptoms persist despite therapy with an ACE inhibitor, diuretics, and a beta-blocker.
- When you prescribe digoxin, you should consider the following:

▲ Digoxin is not indicated as the primary treatment for the stabilization of patients with acutely decompensated HF.

▲ Digoxin should not be administered to patients who have significant sinoatrial or atrioventricular block unless the block has been treated with a permanent pacemaker. It should be used with caution with drugs, such as amiodarone or a beta-blocker, known to affect the sinus or atrioventricular node.

▲ The dose should be 0.125 to 0.25 mg each day for most patients. Those over 70 years of age, with impaired renal function, or a low lean body mass should take the lower dose.

▲ Loading of digoxin is not necessary.

▲ Serial assessments of serum levels is not necessary for most patients.

▲ There appears to be little relationship between levels and therapeutic effect; therefore, target serum levels are between 0.5 and 1.0 ng/mL.

▲ Digoxin toxicity is commonly associated with levels >2 ng/mL but may occur at lower levels in patients with hypokalemia or hypomagnesemia.

▲ For patients with HF and atrial fibrillation with rapid ventricular response, the administration of high doses of digoxin (>0.25 mg each day) for rate control is not recommended. Additional rate control can be achieved with a beta-blocker or amiodarone.

• Medication costs can pose a substantial barrier for your patients with HF. In a recent study by AHRQ, about two-thirds of chronically ill adults do not tell their physicians when they have to cut back on their medications because of the cost. Of those who did not tell their physician, 58% said they did not believe their physician could help them with the cost problem. Patients who did talk to their physician said their medications were not changed to less expensive alternatives, and few reported getting any assistance, such as information about programs that help pay drug costs or where to buy cheaper drugs.

The medications used in HF are directed toward the key physiologic changes that result in cardiac decompensation: pump failure and neurohormonal changes. The most common medications used are ACE inhibitors, ARBs, diuretics, beta-blockers, aldosterone antagonists, and digoxin. Table 9.19 summarizes the key features of each of these agents, including initial and maximum dosages, common adverse reactions, and costs.

Angiotensin-Converting Enzyme Inhibitors

Perhaps the most important advance in the treatment of HF was the introduction of diuretics and ACE inhibitors. The combination of these two agents is the foundation of HF therapy. There is an ongoing debate over the mechanisms by which ACE inhibitors bring about their beneficial effects. The combination of effects on the kidneys, on modulators such as

TABLE 9.19. Medications for the treatment of heart failure.

Medications	Initial dose/maximum dose	Adverse reactions/cautions
Loop diuretics		Hypersensitivity to sulfonylureas, renal or hepatic impairment,
Demadex/torsemide	5 mg QD/200 mg QD	hypokalemia, metabolic alkalosis
Lasix/furosemide	20 mg QD/600 mg QD	
Bumex/bumetanide	0.5 mg QD/10 mg QD	
Aldosterone antagonists		
Aldactone/ spironolactone	25 mg QD/50 mg QD	Hyperkalemia; requires ongoing monitoring. Discontinue if serum potassium level is >6.0 mEq/L. Lower dosage to 12.5 mg QD or 25 QOD if serum potassium level is between 5.5 and 6.0 mEq/L
Inspra/eplerenone	50 mg QD/50 mg BID	Hyperkalemia requires ongoing monitoring. Do not give to patients with creatinine clearances below 50 mL/min
ACE inhibitors		
Accupril/quinapril	10 mg QD/80 mg/day	Angioedema, hypotension, renal failure, hyperkalemia, cough
Altace/ramipril	2.5 mg QD/20 mg/day	
Captoten/captopril	12.5 mg TID/450 mg/day	Caution for patients with renal
Lotensin/benazepril	10 mg QD/80 mg/day	failure
Prinivil/lisinopril	10 mg QD/80 mg/day	
Vasotec/enalapril	5 mg QD/40 mg/day	
Zestril/lisinopril	10 mg QD/80 mg/day	
Angiotensin receptor blockers*		
Atacand/candesartan	4 mg QD/32 mg QD	Fatigue, diarrhea, dizziness, hypotension, angioedema, and hyperkalemia/Caution for patients with hepatic or renal impairment or patients who are volume depleted. Avoid potassium-containing salt substitutes
Avapro/irbesartan	75 mg QD/300 mg QD	
Cozaar/losartan	2.5 mg QD/100 mg QD	
Diovan/valsartan	40 mg BID/160 mg BID	
Beta-blockers		
Coreg/carvedilol	3.125 QD/25 mg BID	Hypotension, severe bradycardia, initial worsening of heart failure, fatigue, depression, bronchospasm
	50 mg BID for patients >85 kg	

TABLE 9.19. *Continued*

Medications	Initial dose/maximum dose	Adverse reactions/cautions
Toprol XL/metoprolol succinate	12.5 mg QD/200 mg/day	
Zebeta/bisoprolol Digoxin	1.25 mg QD/10 mg/day	
Lanoxin/digoxin	0.125 mg QD/0.25 mg QD	Atrioventricular block, bradycardia, ventricular arrhythmias, dizziness, nausea. Caution for the elderly and for those with impaired renal function

*Only diovan has FDA approval and that is for ACE-intolerant patients. Candesartan may get approval soon based on CHARM.

bradykinin and catecholamines, and on the heart muscle, is likely to be responsible for the improved outcomes. The evidence is overwhelming that ACE inhibitors can reduce mortality, hospitalizations, and symptoms and increase exercise capacity in patient with HF [1]. There are some subsets of patients, such as the very old and those with a normal ejection fraction, for whom uncertainty still exists. Despite its known efficacy, the number of patients found to be taking an ACE inhibitor is less than optimal. For those prescribed an ACE inhibitor, approximately 15% to 30% of patients discontinue the medication because of its side effects. The most common side effect causing discontinuation is cough. For some, the cough is mild and resolves in 2 to 3 months. For others, the severity of cough is not tolerable and requires switching to an ARB. Other problematic side effects include angioedema, hyperkalemia, and renal impairment. Most guidelines recommend starting low and titrating the dose upward [44]. If further studies provide more support for the idea that ACE inhibitors prevent ischemic episodes and delay the onset of HF, then a new indication for ACE inhibitors will be the prevention of HF.

Angiotensin Receptor Blockers

The evidence for the efficacy of ARBs in HF is less persuasive, and for the present this class of medication should be prescribed only when an ACE inhibitor cannot be tolerated. Caution should be used for patients with liver disease and for those with renal impairment. Problematic side effects include angioedema, hyperkalemia, excessive hypotension, dizziness, fatigue, and diarrhea. Within 1 week substantial benefits are generally seen; however, it may take 3 to 6 weeks to see maximal effects. Some have advocated the combined use of ACE inhibitors and ARBs for patients with HF. The theory is that ACE inhibitors alone only partially block the adverse effects of the renin–angiotensin–aldosterone system. At present, there are insufficient data to support the combined use of ACE inhibitors and ARBs [45].

Beta-Blockers

Beta-blockers were avoided for decades because their pharmacologic profile did not fit the understanding of the pathophysiology of the disease. Activation of the sympathetic nervous system was thought to be an important compensatory mechanism in HF, giving inotropic support to the heart and therefore maintaining blood pressure. It was assumed that blocking a "protective mechanism" would aggravate the symptoms of HF. Almost 30 years ago the first observations about the positive effects of beta-blockade were made. A reduction in heart rate remains an important predictor of the benefit from beta-blockade; however, neurohormonal modulation and reduced sympathetic stimulation may also contribute. Left ventricular ejection fraction increases within 3 to 6 months after the start of therapy. Multiple randomized trials involving more than 15,000 patients have demonstrated a cumulative relative reduction of 30% to 40% in both morbidity and mortality. The observed benefits translate into the prevention of 3 to 4 deaths for every 100 patients treated for mild to moderate HF over a 1-year period [46]. Beta-blockers exert their effects by retarding or reversing the progression of ventricular dysfunction and HF and by decreasing the risk of sudden death. The effect occurs over a period of months, and the effect on sudden death may be by a reduction in arrhythmias. Long-term beta-blockade reduces myocardial hypertrophy and filling pressures and increases ejection fraction, a process called *ventricular remodeling*. Reduction in heart rate is likely to play a major role in the benefits of beta-blockade. It is unclear whether it is necessary to block only the beta-1-receptor or whether nonselective agents might prove superior. Carvedilol, bisoprolol, and metoprolol succinate have undergone the most rigorous studies. There is no conclusive evidence for a difference between these beta-blockers in their benefits. However, the COMET trial demonstrated superiority of carvedilol over generic metoprolol tartrate in the dosages used.

Beta-blockers are indicated for stages II to IV HF secondary to systolic dysfunction if the patient is free from cardiogenic shock, acute pulmonary edema, or evidence of gross fluid retention. It is important to remember that beta-blockers are not effective for the short-term rescue of patients with worsening HF. However, treatment should be initiated soon after achieving a moderate degree of stability.

Concerns for the use of beta-blockers include the following:

1. Many patients with HF have COPD, but, unless the patient has severe obstructive impairment, such patients usually tolerate beta-blockers. More selective beta-blockers (bisoprolol, metoprolol succinate) can be used by patients with sensitivity to beta-2-blockade.

2. Concomitant use with calcium channel blockers should be done with caution. There may be an additive effect of blocking on the atrioventricular node, resulting in severe bradycardia. Calcium channel blockers are associated with increased mortality in HF, with the exception of amlodipine and felodipine, which have been demonstrated to be mortality neutral.

3. A low arterial pressure indicates that additional care needs to be taken with the introduction of a beta-blocker because of the risk of syncope. Hypotension is most frequently a problem related to the initiation of therapy. As ventricular function improves, a process that may take 2 to 3 months, these symptoms usually improve.

4. Diabetes was considered to be a contraindication to beta-blockers in the past because of the masking symptoms of hypoglycemia. Most studies confirm that diabetics obtain marked benefits with the use of a beta-blocker.

5. Beta-blockers usually have little impact on claudication or overall walking distance in patients with peripheral vascular disease. They can be used safely.

6. Hemodynamic decompensation can be aggravated; therefore, beta-blockers are not recommended for patients with little reserve as indicated by obvious fluid retention or symptoms of HF at rest.

If there are no contraindications, treatment should be started as soon as possible after a diagnosis of HF secondary to systolic dysfunction. Patients with severe HF should have therapy started in the hospital prior to discharge, provided fluid retention has been controlled and they do not require intravenous therapy with a vasodilator or positive inotropic agent.

Starting Beta-Blockers

The general principle is "start low and go slow." Treatment should be started at low dose and titrated upward at 2- to 4-week intervals to a target dose or resting heart rate of 60, depending on the clinical response. For example:

Bisoprolol: First dose 1.25 mg each day; target dose 10 mg each day
Carvdiol: First dose 3.12 5 mg each day; target dose 25 mg BID
Metoprolol: First dose 50 mg BID; target dose 200 mg each
Toprol XL: First dose 25 mg each day; target dose 200 mg each day

Asymptomatic bradycardia should be managed by reassurance alone, always recognizing that excessive bradycardia could cause increased fatigue or breathlessness. If bradycardia is symptomatic, the need for other medications that affect heart rate should be considered. If the withdrawal of medication is not an option, then the dose of beta-blocker should be reduced to relieve symptoms. Patients who cannot tolerate a beta-blocker because of bradycardia should be considered for a pacemaker.

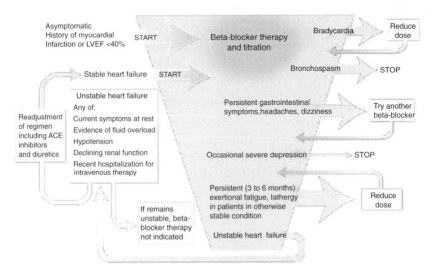

FIGURE 9.1. Funnel diagram on the use of beta-blockers in stable HF. (From Stevenson [47].)

Management of Worsening Heart Failure During Beta-Blockade

Increased fluid retention should be assessed by weighing the patient daily. Patients should be instructed to increase the doses of diuretic, temporarily. For patients with a mild exacerbation of symptoms, treatment consists of reassurance, control of fluid retention with diuretics, and waiting for the effects of beta-blockers to appear [46].

In summary, beta-blockers are an important adjunct in the treatment of HF and can have a significant impact on morbidity and mortality. Their use requires paying attention to the appropriate indications, careful titration, and monitoring of symptoms. Stevenson [47] created a "funnel diagram" (Figure 9.1) to assist physicians who prescribe beta-blockers for their HF patients.

Aldosterone Antagonists

Aldosterone is a major prognostic determinant in HF. Emerging data suggest that ACE inhibitors and ARBs are insufficient to suppress aldosterone. The Randomized Aldactone Evaluation (RALES) study provided proof that aldosterone is important for patients with HF. Based on the results of this trial, the use of spironolactone should be restricted to patients with severe or progressive HF caused by systolic dysfunction in whom serum creatinine level is less than or equal to 2.0 mg/dL and serum potassium less than 5.0 mEq/L at baseline. Prior to initiating therapy, potassium supplementation should be discontinued or significantly decreased. Patients should be questioned regarding the use of potassium-containing salt substitutes and the use of high-potassium foods such as orange juice or bananas. Spironolactone should be started at 25 mg a day. Serum potassium should be monitored at the end of 1 week of treatment and periodically for the first 2 to 3 months. If serum potassium levels increase to 5.5 mEq/L or greater, you should reduce the dose to 12.5 mg daily or 25 mg every other day. You should discontinue spironolactone for any patient whose serum potassium level is 6.0 mEq/L or higher [48]. The importance of careful monitoring of serum potassium levels is highlighted in a study by Juurlink and associates [49] as a follow-up to the RALES study. They found that the publication of the RALES results was associated with abrupt increases in the rate of prescriptions for spironolactone and in associated hyperkalemia-associated morbidity and mortality.

Digoxin

Digoxin remains an important therapeutic option for the outpatient management of patients with chronic symptomatic HF caused by systolic dysfunction. Randomized controlled trials have confirmed its efficacy in improving ejection fraction and exercise capacity. The Digitalis Investigation Group [50] confirmed its efficacy and long-term use. Current consensus guidelines recommend it for patients with NHYA class II through IV HF if symptoms persist despite therapy with an ACE inhibitor, diuretics, and a beta-blocker. The benefits are evident regardless of the underlying rhythm (normal sinus rhythm versus atrial fibrillation), the etiology of HF, or concomitant therapy. Unlike other agents with a positive inotropic action, digoxin does not increase all-cause mortality and has a substantial benefit in reducing HF hospitalizations. According to the Heart Failure Society of America, concerns about the use of digoxin are the following:

1. Digoxin is not indicated as the primary treatment for the stabilization of patients with acutely decompensated HF.

2. Digoxin should not be administered to patients who have significant sinoatrial or atrioventricular block unless the block has been treated with a permanent pacemaker. It should be used with caution with drugs known to affect the sinus or atrioventricular node, such as amiodarone or a beta-blocker.

3. The dose should be 0.125 to 0.25 mg each day for most patients. Those over 70 years of age, with impaired renal function, or a low lean body mass should use the lower dosage.

4. Loading of digoxin is not necessary.

5. Serial assessments of serum levels are not necessary for most patients. The appropriate therapeutic range of digoxin for HF patients continues to be debated.

6. There appears to be little relationship between levels and therapeutic effects. Current data suggest that up to 80% of the maximum inotropic effect of digoxin is obtained when the serum concentration is within the range of 1.0 to 1.5 ng/mL at the 24-hour trough point. Other studies suggest that maximal clinical benefit is achieved with a therapeutic range of 0.5 to 1.5 ng/mL.

7. Digoxin toxicity is commonly associated with levels >2 ng/mL but may occur at lower levels in patients with hypokalemia or hypomagnesemia.

8. For patients with HF and atrial fibrillation with rapid ventricular response, the administration of high doses of digoxin (>0.25 mg each day) for rate control is not recommended. Additional rate control can be achieved with beta-blocker or amiodarone [51].

Isosorbide Dinitrate and Hydralazine

A recent study published in the New England Journal of Medicine assessed the efficacy of a fixed combination of isosorbide dinitrate and hydralazine. The study included 1,050 African Americans who had moderate to severe HF. A total dose of 120 mg of isosorbide and 225 mg of hydralazine was given to these patients in addition to standard therapy (ACE inhibitor, beta-blocker, diuretic, digoxin, and spironolactone). The group receiving isosorbide and hydralazine had significantly lower mortality (6.2% for the treatment group versus 10.2% not treated with the combination). The treatment group also had improved outcomes with respect to quality of life measures and rates of hospitalization. The rate of side effects was quite high in the treatment group, with 30% complaining of dizziness and 48% complaining of headache [52]. It is certainly reasonable to consider this combination for selected patients who fail to respond to the "standard" medical interventions. The guidelines regarding the use of aldosterone antagonists have been upgraded from "should be considered" to "recommended" for patients classified as NYHA class IV, who have reasonable renal function, a serum potassium level less than 5 mmol/L, and a creatinine level less than 2 mg/dL.

Cost-Effective Considerations

Given that most of your patients with HF will be on multidrug regimens and many will have limited financial means, the costs of medications will play a role in their ability to adhere to their medical treatment. The Agency for Healthcare Research and Quality (AHRQ) released the results of a study on medication usage by patients with chronic illnesses. About two-thirds of chronically ill adults do not tell their physicians when they have to cut back on their medications because of the cost. The AHRQ surveyed more than 4,000 adults who were taking medications for diabetes, HF, and other conditions. More than 600 patients said they had stopped taking some medication in the past year because of the cost, and two-thirds of this group said they did not tell their physicians in advance. Of those who did not tell their physicians, 58% said they did not believe their physician could help them with the cost problem. Patients who did talk to their physicians said their medications were not changed to less expensive alternatives, and few reported getting any assistance, such as information about programs that help pay drug costs or where to buy cheaper drugs [53]. Many patients have taken action by purchasing their medications through pharmacies in Canada. Other resources are NeedyMeds.com and BenefitsCheckUp.org.

Monitoring

Summary

- Many practices fall short in meeting well-published goals for the management of HF and its complications.
- The evidence demonstrating the importance of setting up an effective monitoring system is seen in the:
  - ▲ High rates of readmission of patients for exacerbation of HF
  - ▲ Failure to ensure that patients with HF receive appropriate medical therapy (only 75% of patients with HF who are candidates for an ACE inhibitor are given a prescription)
- Only 70% of Medicare patients with HF have an ejection fraction measured (for more information and updates, see www.ama-assn.org/go/quality).
- The underutilization of appropriate medications and other evidence-based, guideline-recommended therapies represents a major clinical practice and public health issue.
- One method to improve documentation is to use a template for each office visit and a flow sheet to monitor outcomes to assess quality of care.

Background

Many practices fall short in meeting well-published goals for the management of HF and its complications. Concerns for the quality of care delivered to patients with chronic conditions, including HF, come from a number of organizations, including the Institute of Medicine, the National Committee on Quality Assurance, the Centers for Medicare & Medicaid Services, AHRQ, the ACC/AHA, and the Physician Consortium for Performance Improvement. Each of these organizations has presented data to demonstrate how we fall short in multiple areas in caring for patients with chronic disease, including ongoing monitoring of individual patients and the practice population. Evidence demonstrating the importance of setting up an effective monitoring system includes the following:

1. High rates of readmission of patients for exacerbation of HF
2. Failure to ensure that patients with HF receive appropriate medical therapy (only 75% of patients with HF who are candidates for an ACE inhibitor are given a prescription)
3. Only 70% of Medicare patients with HF have an ejection fraction measured (for further information and updates, see www.ama-assn. org/go/quality)

The underutilization of appropriate medications and other evidence-based, guideline-recommended therapies represents a major clinical practice and public health issue [54]. Disease management programs have consistently shown improvements in process outcomes, patient satisfaction, utilization of resources, and costs. Although there are multiple components in setting up an effective disease management program, as described in the Chronic Care Model (www.improvingchroniccare.org), a key feature is the ability to adequately document the outcomes of interest, to maintain this information in the form of a registry, to retrieve relevant data, to analyze these data in the form of reports, and to implement practice changes that are aimed at improving outcomes for all patients.

Documentation

One method to improve documentation is to use a template for each office visit and a flow sheet to monitor outcomes that can assess quality of care. The means to achieve this level of documentation can be as sophisticated as an electronic medical record or as simple as a paper checklist. An HF-specific office visit template and flow sheet should be available at the time of each visit. An example of a template is presented in Figure 9.2. We believe it is very important to reinforce the principle of patient self-management, and therefore the flow sheet should include a summary of each patient's generated goals. It is also important to document that each patient has received an action plan (Table 9.16).

Measures to Improve Quality of Care

There are a number of methods to help improve the quality of care. These can be used in both inpatient and outpatient settings.

Inpatient Programs

Fonarow and associates [55] recommended an in-hospital intervention for those patients admitted for HF. They found that an intervention prior to

Date					
Current Heart Failure Medications					
β-Blocker agent/dosage					
ACE Inhibitor agent/dosage					
Digoxin dosage					
Spironolactone dosage					
Loop diuretic agent/dosage					
Thiazide diuretic agent/dosage					
Other cardiovascular agents(s)/dosage(s)					
New or increased adverse effects (Specify)					
Current Patient Data					
NYHA class (I-IV)					
Symptoms, eg, orthopnea (Specify if increased or decreased)					
Blood pressure					
Pulse					
Weight					
Physical findings, eg, edema (Specify if increased or decreased)					
Plan					
Medication or dosage changes					
Other					

FIGURE 9.2. Office template for patients with HF. (By permission of MH Farrell, et al., JAMA 287:890, 2002.)

discharge, along with a patient education program, had a positive effect on long-term patient compliance and clinical outcomes. Phillips and associates [56] performed a meta-analysis of comprehensive discharge planning programs designed to reduce readmission rates and improve outcomes, such as survival and quality of care. They reviewed 18 studies from 8 countries involving 3,304 patients observed for an average of 8 months. The interventions included medication review and counseling, education on diet, exercise, and stress, social work assessment, and telephone and home health follow-up. They found that readmission rates, survival, and quality of life were improved, without increasing costs.

American College of Cardiology, American Heart Association, and Physician Consortium for Performance Improvement Heart Failure Core Physician Performance Measurement Set
Prospective Data Collection Flowsheet

Allergies
_____
_____

Provider No. _____   Patient Name or Code _____   Birth Date ___ / ___ / _____   Gender M ❑ F ❑
(mm / dd / yyyy)

Initial Laboratory Tests Performed: (select all that apply)			
❑ CBC	❑ BUN	❑ Blood glucose	❑ Other
❑ Serum electrolytes	❑ Serum creatinine	❑ Thyroid stimulating hormone	
❑ Left ventricular function assessed: ___/___/____		❑ Left ventricular systolic dysfunction (left ventricular ejection fraction < 40% or moderately or severely depressed left ventricular systolic function)	
Results:			

Clinical Assessment

Date of Visit (mm / dd / yyyy)	____/____/____	____/____/____	____/____/____	____/____/____
Weight (lb/kg)	❑Unable to weigh	❑Unable to weigh	❑Unable to weigh	❑Unable to weigh
Heart Rate				
Blood Pressure	L R sitting supine standing	L R sitting supine standing	L R sitting supine standing	L R sitting supine standing
Assessment of Clinical Symptoms of Volume Overload (Excess)	Dyspnea Y or N Fatigue Y or N Orthopnea Y or N	Dyspnea Y or N Fatigue Y or N Orthopnea Y or N	Dyspnea Y or N Fatigue Y or N Orthopnea Y or N	Dyspnea Y or N Fatigue Y or N Orthopnea Y or N
Level of Activity	❑ Standardized scale or assessment tool used[a]	❑ Standardized scale or assessment tool used[a]	❑ Standardized scale or assessment tool used[a]	❑ Standardized scale or assessment tool used[a]
Assessment of Clinical Signs of Volume Overload (Excess)	Peripheral edema Y or N Rales Y or N Hepatomegaly Y or N Ascites Y or N Assessment of jugular venous pressure Y or N S3 or S4 gallop Y or N Other: _____	Peripheral edema Y or N Rales Y or N Hepatomegaly Y or N Ascites Y or N Assessment of jugular venous pressure Y or N S3 or S4 gallop Y or N Other: _____	Peripheral edema Y or N Rales Y or N Hepatomegaly Y or N Ascites Y or N Assessment of jugular venous pressure Y or N S3 or S4 gallop Y or N Other: _____	Peripheral edema Y or N Rales Y or N Hepatomegaly Y or N Ascites Y or N Assessment of jugular venous pressure Y or N S3 or S4 gallop Y or N Other: _____

Education

Patient Education	❑ Patient education provided[b]	❑ Patient education provided[b]	❑ Patient education provided[b]	❑ Patient education provided[b]

a   Standardized scale or assessment tools may include the New York Heart Association Functional Classification of Congestive Heart Failure (level of activity only), Kansas City Cardiomyopathy Questionnaire; Minnesota Living with Heart Failure Questionnaire; or Chronic Heart Failure Questionnaire (Guyatt).

b   Patient education should include one or more of the following: weight monitoring; diet (sodium restriction); symptom management; physical activity; smoking cessation; medication instruction; minimizing or avoiding use of NSAIDs; referral for visiting nurse or specific educational or management programs; or prognosis/end-of-life issues.

© 2005 American Medical Association. All Rights Reserved.

FIGURE 9.3. American College of Cardiology, American Heart Association, and Physician Consortium for Performance Improvement Heart Failure Physician Performance Measurement Set. (Copyright 2003 American Medical Association. By permission.)

The ACC/AHA and the Physician Consortium for Performance Improvement provide evidence-based clinical performance measures, including a data collection flow sheet (Figure 9.3) that can be used for quality improvement activities. The consortium is a physician-led initiative that includes experts from 50 national medical specialty societies, state medical societies, AHRQ, and the Centers for Medicare and Medicaid Services. Updates on practice guidelines are available at www.ama-assn. org/go/quality. Current clinical recommendations are as follows:

**American College of Cardiology, American Heart Association, and
Physician Consortium for Performance Improvement
Heart Failure Core Physician Performance Measurement Set
Prospective Data Collection Flowsheet**

Provider No. _____   Patient Name or Code _____

Adverse Drug Reactions

	Date of Visit (mm / dd / yyyy)	____ / ____ / ____	____ / ____ / ____	____ / ____ / ____	____ / ____ / ____
Medication Management	**Beta-Blocker Therapy**	❑ Prescribed ❑ Not prescribed (medical reasons*) ❑ Not prescribed (patient reasons*)	❑ Prescribed ❑ Not prescribed (medical reasons*) ❑ Not prescribed (patient reasons*)	❑ Prescribed ❑ Not prescribed (medical reasons*) ❑ Not prescribed (patient reasons*)	❑ Prescribed ❑ Not prescribed (medical reasons*) ❑ Not prescribed (patient reasons*)
	ACE Inhibitor or ARB Therapy	❑ Prescribed ❑ Not prescribed (medical reasons*) ❑ Not prescribed (patient reasons*)	❑ Prescribed ❑ Not prescribed (medical reasons*) ❑ Not prescribed (patient reasons*)	❑ Prescribed ❑ Not prescribed (medical reasons*) ❑ Not prescribed (patient reasons*)	❑ Prescribed ❑ Not prescribed (medical reasons*) ❑ Not prescribed (patient reasons*)
	Warfarin Therapy ❑ Chronic or paroxysmal atrial fibrillation	❑ Prescribed ❑ Not prescribed (medical reasons*) ❑ Not prescribed (patient reasons*)	❑ Prescribed ❑ Not prescribed (medical reasons*) ❑ Not prescribed (patient reasons*)	❑ Prescribed ❑ Not prescribed (medical reasons*) ❑ Not prescribed (patient reasons*)	❑ Prescribed ❑ Not prescribed (medical reasons*) ❑ Not prescribed (patient reasons*)

*Specify medical (eg, allergy, contraindication) or patient (eg, economic, social, religious) reasons for not prescribing therapy:

Other Medications

AP21:05-0629:PDF:8/05

FIGURE 9.3. *Continued*

- Laboratory tests: Initial management should include CBC; urinalysis; measurement of serum electrolytes, calcium, magnesium, blood urea nitrogen, creatinine, and glucose levels; liver function tests; and thyroid-stimulating hormone. Serial monitoring of electrolytes and renal function should be done.
- Left ventricular function assessment. For patients with HF, an assessment of left ventricular systolic function with two-dimensional echo-cardiography or radionuclide ventriculography is recommended. For

patients with a change in clinical status or clinical event with significant effects on cardiac function, repeated measurement of ejection fraction is recommended.

- Weight measurement: A thorough physical examination is recommended to identify cardiac and noncardiac disorders that may accelerate the progression of HF. This physical examination may include initial and ongoing assessments of the patient's volume status.
- Blood pressure: A thorough physical examination is recommended to identify cardiac and noncardiac disorders that may accelerate the progression of HF.
- Assessment of clinical symptoms of volume overload: A thorough history is recommended to identify cardiac and noncardiac disorders that may accelerate the progression of HF. The history may include initial and ongoing assessments of volume status.
- Assessment of activity level: A thorough history is recommended to identify cardiac and noncardiac disorders that may accelerate the progression of HF. This history may include initial and ongoing assessment of the patient's activity level.
- Examination of the heart: A thorough physical examination is recommended to identify cardiac and noncardiac disorders that may accelerate the progression of HF.
- Patient education: Patient education and close supervision are recommended for patients with HF, to reduce the likelihood of noncompliance and lead to the detection of changes in body weight or clinical status early enough for effective treatment to be instituted. Avoidance of patient behaviors that may increase the risk of HF (e.g., smoking, alcohol, and illicit drug use) should be encouraged.
- Beta-blocker therapy: Beta-blocker therapy is recommended for all patients with asymptomatic LVH, a recent MI, and symptomatic left ventricular systolic disease.
- ACE inhibitors: Therapy with ACE inhibitor is recommended for all patients with stage B disease, HF patients with a recent MI, and symptomatic left ventricular systolic disease.
- Warfarin therapy for patients with atrial fibrillation: Anticoagulant use is recommended for patients with HF and concomitant diseases, paroxysmal or chronic atrial fibrillation, or a previous thromboembolic event.

The most effective strategy to help a practice meet these targets for management is the use of a registry in conjunction with Plan-Do-Study-Act (PDSA) interventions. Chapter 4 provides a summary of how to perform PDSA interventions with a specific chronic disease. The key questions to ask in any PDSA performance improvement activity are:

1. What are we trying to accomplish?
2. How will we know when we have reached our goal?
3. What interventions are likely to help us meet this goal?

It is best if the PDSA cycles are "rapid cycle" (meaning the entire process of intervention and review of data is over a short period, e.g., a few weeks). The registry should be constructed so that important data are available to monitor the outcomes of PDSA interventions.

Other suggestions for interventions based on our experience include the following:

1. Ensure that every person with HF in your practice has a continuity physician. Start a registry, if one has not been used, and include documentation of the primary care provider. If you cannot start a registry, use monthly billing reports of patients with a 428.XX diagnosis as a proxy.

2. Develop systems of team-based care with standing orders. Think of HF as a disease that requires a team for management. Members of the team can include nurses, clinic assistants, receptionists, educators, nutritionists, and pharmacists. Each member of the team can be responsible for a component of a comprehensive intervention. Standing orders can be adopted from evidence-based guidelines through ACC/AHA, Consortium for Performance Improvement Evidence-Based Guidelines.

3. Measure performance at the level of the office practice. This can include summarizing performance data on the entire practice as well as generating a list of patients who need a specific service. For example, a "report card" can assess the percentage of patients receiving a beta-blocker who meet guideline criteria for this intervention.

As noted, the literature supports the use of disease management programs in an effort to improve these process outcomes. For providers and groups with no experience in setting up a disease management program, the Improving Chronic Illness Care Foundation provides the opportunity to participate through a "learning collaborative." This can be accessed at www.improvingchronicillnesscare.org. There are also organizations that help providers assess their practice performance against consensus standards.

The Organized Program to Initiate Lifesaving Treatment in Hospitalized Patients with Heart Failure (OPTIMIZE-HF) is a national collaborative designed to improve medical care and education of hospitalized heart failure patients and to accelerate initiation of evidence-based heart failure guideline-recommended therapies by administering them prior to discharge [10].

Alternative Therapies

Summary

- Many patients use herbal remedies in an effort to control symptoms of their chronic problems.

- Challenges in dealing with herbal remedies include possible toxicity of herbal components, presence of adulterants, potential interactions with prescription medications, and variable quality of preparations.
- The most frequently used herbal remedies by those with HF include coenzyme Q-10, creatine, hawthorn, L-arginine, L-carnitine, propionyl-L-carnitine, taurine, terminalia, vitamin E, and ginseng panax. These drugs have not undergone adequate evaluation for potential interactions with ACE inhibitors, diuretics, beta-blockers, spironolactone, or digoxin.
- Given the widespread use of herbal remedies, it is advisable to ask all of your patients whether they are taking any of these preparations.
- The *Physician's Desk Reference* (PDR) provides a summary of the potential effects of most herbal treatments (www.pdr.net).

Usage

The total out-of-pocket expenditures for herbal medicines were $5.1 billion in 1997. The top 10 best-selling herbals are ginko biloba, echinacea, garlic, ginseng, soy, saw palmetto, St John's wort, valerian, cranberry, and black cohosh. Challenges in dealing with herbal remedies include possible toxicity of herbal components, presence of adulterants, potential interactions with prescription medications, and variable quality of preparations. The following are the most frequently used herbal remedies by those with HF: coenzyme Q-10, creatine, hawthorn, L-arginine, L-carnitine, propionyl-L-carnitine, taurine, terminalia, vitamin E, and ginseng panax. Although information from the Natural Medicine Comprehensive Database (www. naturaldatabase.com) suggests that most of these medications are possibly effective, except for vitamin E and Ginseng it is important to know that these drugs have not been evaluated for potential interactions with ACE inhibitors, diuretics, beta-blockers, spironolactone, or digoxin and that no well-conducted RCTs (randomized controlled trials) have been done. Given the widespread use of herbal remedies, it is advisable to ask all of your patients whether they are taking any of these preparations. The *Physician's Desk Reference* (PDR) includes summaries of the potential effects of most herbal treatments (www.pdr.net). It is also important to recognize that many patients who access the Internet for medical information will receive a broad spectrum of advice on the use of herbal remedies. For your patients who choose to use the Internet as a medical reference source, you should direct them to sites that provide quality information (Table 9.18).

Summary

Heart failure has become the most common and problematic cardiovascular disease. Many patients with HF have multiple comorbid conditions, including ischemic heart disease, diabetes, and chronic renal insufficiency.

The impacts on the quality of life for patients and their families are substantial. All patients with HF should have an evaluation to determine the underlying cause, and an assessment for comorbid conditions. You should always be alert for signs of depression. Failing to recognize depression can affect outcomes. All patients should receive appropriate education to enhance their understanding of HF and the lifestyle changes that can improve their quality of life. The available medications for patients with HF can have a substantial impact on symptoms and on morbidity and mortality. Optimal use of these medications requires careful dosage adjustments and the ability to monitor for adverse side effects. Disease management programs can help avoid needless use of emergency services and hospitalization. Included in these disease management activities are the use of an emergency action plan and self-management support.

References

1. Hunt SA, Baker DW, Chin MH, Cinquegrani MP, et al. ACC/AHA guidelines for the evaluation and management of chronic heart failure in the adult: executive summary. J Am Coll Cardiol 2001;38:2101–2113.
2. Massie BM, Shah NB. Evolving trends in the epidemiologic factors of heart failure: rationale for preventive strategies and comprehensive disease management. Am Heart J 1997;133:703–712.
3. Nohria A, Lewis E, Stevenson LW. Medical management of advanced heart failure. JAMA 2002;287;628–640.
4. O'Connell JB. The economic burden of heart failure. Clin Cardiol 2000;23: III6–III10.
5. McAlister FA, Stewart S, Ferrua S, McMurray JJJV. Multidisciplinary strategies for the management of heart failure patients at high risk for admission. J Am Coll Cardiol 2004;44:810–819.
6. Tsuchihashi M, et al. Medical and socioenvironmental predictors of hospital readmission in patients with congestive heart failure. Am Heart J 2001;142:703.
7. Rich MW, Beckham V, Wittenberg C, Leven CL, Freedland KE, Carney RM. A multidisciplinary intervention to prevent the readmission of elderly patients with congestive heart failure. N Engl J Med 1995;333:1190–1195.
8. Berg GD, Wadhwa S, Johnson AE. A matched-cohort study of health services utilization and financial outcomes for a heart failure disease-management program in elderly patients. J Am Geriatr Soc 2004;52:1655–1661.
9. Halvorson GC, Isham GJ. Epidemic of Care: A Call for Safer, Better, and More Accountable Health Care. San Francisco: Jossey-Bass, 2003.
10. Fonarow GC. Strategies to improve the use of evidence-based heart failure therapies: OPTIMIZE-HF. Rev Cardiovasc Med 2004;5(Suppl 1):S45–S54.
11. Galbreath AD, Krasuski RA, Smith B, Stajduhar KC, Kwan MD, Ellis R, Freeman GL. Long-term healthcare and cost outcomes of disease management in a large, randomized, community-based population with heart failure. Circulation 2004;110:1–9.
12. Stevenson LW, Perloff JK. The limited reliability of physical signs for estimating hemodynamics in chronic heart failure. JAMA 1989;261:884–888.

13. McKee PA, Castelli WP, et al. The natural history of congestive heart failure. The Framingham Study. N Engl J Med 1971;285:1441–1447.
14. Maisel AS, et al. Rapid measurement of b-type natriuretic peptide in the emergency diagnosis of heart failure. N Engl J Med 2002;347:161–167.
15. Kitzman DW, et al. Pathophysiological characterization of isolated diastolic heart failure in comparison to systolic heart failure. JAMA 2002;288:2144–2150.
16. Vasan RS, et al. Left ventricular dilatation and the risk of congestive heart failure in people without myocardial infarction. N Engl J Med 1997;336:1350–1355.
17. Devereux RB, et al. Prognostic significance of left ventricular mass change during treatment of hypertension. JAMA 2004;292:2350–2356.
18. Okin PM, et al. Regression of electrocardiographic left ventricular hypertrophy during antihypertensive treatment and the prediction of major cardiovascular events. JAMA 2004;292;2343–2349.
19. Hernandez AF, O'Connor CM. Lessons from the studies of left ventricular dysfunction (SOLVD). J Am Coll Cardiol 2003;42:709–711.
20. Mirvis DM. Electrocardiography: A Physiologic Approach. St. Louis: Mosby, 1993.
21. de Lemos JA, McGuire DK, Drazner MH. B-type natriuretic peptide in cardiovascular disease. Published online April 23, 2003, at http://image.thelancet.com/extras/02art2325web.pdf.
22. Kannel WB, D'Agostino RB, Silbershatz H, et al. Profile for estimating risk of heart failure. Arch Intern Med 1999;159:1197.
23. Hunt SA, et al. ACC/AHA guidelines for the evaluation and management of chronic heart failure in the adult: Executive summary. A report of the American College of Cardiology/American Heart Association Task Force on Practice Guidelines (Committee to Revise the 1995 Guidelines for the Evaluation and Management of Heart Failure). J Heart Lung Transplant 2002;21: 189–203.
24. Rector TS, Cohn JN. Assessment of patient outcome with the Minnesota Living with Heart Failure questionnaire: reliability and validity during a randomized, double-blind, placebo-controlled trial of pimobendan. Am Heart J 1992;124:1017–1025.
25. Demers C, et al. Reliability, validity, and responsiveness of the six-minute walk test in patients with heart failure. Am Heart J 2001;142:698–703.
26. ACC/AHA, and Physician Consortium for Performance Improvement Heart Failure Core Physician Performance Measurement Set: Prospective Data Collection Flowsheet, available at www.ama-assn.org/go/quality.
27. Riegel B, et al. Psychometric testing of the self-care of heart failure index. J Cardiac Failure 2004;10:350–360.
28. Chriss PM, Sheposh J, Riegel B. Predictors of successful heart failure self-care maintenance in the first three months after hospitalization. Heart Lung 2004;33:345–353.
29. Murray MD, et al. Methodology of an ongoing, randomized, controlled trial to improve drug use for elderly patients with chronic heart failure. Am J Geriatr Pharmacother 2004;2:53–65.
30. Ross SE, Moore LA, Earnest MA, Wittevrongel L, Lin CT. Providing a Web-based online medical record with electronic communication capabilities to

patients with congestive heart failure: randomized trial. J Med Internet Res 2004;6:e14.

31. Riegel B, Carlson B. Is individual peer support a promising intervention for persons with heart failure? J Cardiovasc Nurs 2004;19:174–183.

32. Feldman PH, et al. A randomized intervention to improve heart failure outcomes in community-based home health care. Home Health Care Serv Q 2004;23:1–23.

33. Holman H, Lorig K. Patient self-management: a key to effectiveness and efficiency in care of chronic disease. Public Health Rep 2004;119:239–243.

34. Frantz AK. Breaking down the barriers to heart failure patient self-care. Home Health Nurse 2004;22:109–115.

35. DeGeest S, et al. Complexity in caring for an ageing heart failure population: concomitant chronic conditions and age related impairments. Eur J Cardiovasc Nurse 2004;3:263–270.

36. Jaarmsa T, Halfens R, Tan F, Abu-Saad HH, Dracup K, Diederiks J. Self-care and quality of life in patients with advanced heart failure: the effect of a supportive educational intervention. Heart Lung 2000;29:319–330.

37. Miranda MB, et al. An evidence-based approach to improving care of patients with heart failure across the continuum. J Nurs Care Qual 2002;17:1–14.

38. DeWalt DA, et al. Development and pilot testing of a disease management program for low literacy patients with heart failure. Patient Educ Counseling 2004;55:78–86.

39. Bodenheimer T, Lorig K, Holman H, Grumbach K. Patient self-management of chronic disease in primary care. JAMA 2003;288:2469–2475.

40. Hambrecht R, et al. Effects of exercise training on left ventricular function and peripheral resistance in patients with chronic heart failure: a randomized trial. JAMA 2000;283:3095–3101.

41. Corvera-Tindel T, Doering LV, Gomez T, Dracup K. Predictors of non-compliance to exercise training in heart failure. J Cardiovasc Nurs 2004;19:269–277.

42. Asakuma S, Ohyani M, Iwasaki T. Use of pedometer counts in heart failure. Congest Heart Fail 2000;6:250–255.

43. Murberg TA, Furze G. Depressive symptoms and mortality in patients with congestive heart failure: a six-year follow-up study. Med Sci Monit 2004;10:CR643–CR648.

44. Poole-Wilson PA. ACE inhibitors and ARBs in chronic heart failure: the established, the expected, and the pragmatic. Med Clin North Am 2003;87:373–389.

45. Cruden NL, Newby DE. Angiotensin antagonism in patients with heart failure: ACE inhibitors, angiotensin receptor antagonists or both? Am J Cardiovasc Drugs 2004;4:345–353.

46. Cleland JGF. Beta-blockers for heart failure: why, which, when, and where. Med Clin North Am 2003;87:339–371.

47. Stevenson LW. Beta-blockers for stable heart failure. N Engl J Med 2002;346:1346–1347.

48. Rajagopalan S, Pitt B. Aldosterone as a target in congestive heart failure. Med Clin North Am 2003;87:441–457.

49. Juurlink DN, Mamdani MM, Lee DS, Kopp A, Austin PC, Laupacis A, Redelmeier DA. Rates of hyperkalemia after publication of the Randomized Aldactone Evaluation Study. N Engl J Med 2004;351:543–551.

50. Jones RC, Francis GS, Lauer MS. Predictors of mortality in patients with heart failure and preserved systolic function in the Digitalis Investigation Group trial. J Am Coll Cardiol 2004;44:1025–1029.

51. Dec GW. Digoxin remains useful in the management of chronic heart failure. Med Clin North Am 2003;87:317–337.

52. Taylor AL, et al. Combination of isosorbide dinitrate and hydralazine in blacks with heart failure. N Engl J Med 2004;351:2049–2057.

53. Piette, et al. Cost-related medication underuse: do patients with chronic illnesses tell their doctors? Arch Intern Med 2004;164:1749–1755.

54. Stafford RS, Radley DC. The underutilization of cardiac medications of proven benefit, 1990 to 2002. J Am Coll Cardiol 2003;41:56–61.

55. Fonarow CG, Gheorghiade M, Abraham WT. Importance of in-hospital initiation of evidence-based medical therapies for heart failure—a review. Am J Cardiol 2004;94:1155–1160.

56. Phillips CO, Wright SM, Kern DE, Singa RM, Shepperd S, Rubin HR. Comprehensive discharge planning with postdischarge support for older patients with congestive heart failure. A meta-analysis. JAMA 2004;291:1358–1367.

10
Osteoarthritis

Ernesto Zatarain

Chapter Summary

Management

1. Initial steps in the management of a patient recently diagnosed with osteoarthritis (OA) should include the following:
   a. Patient education
   b. Pain control
   c. Limiting disability
   d. Optimizing function
   e. Slowing or stopping disease progression
   f. Fostering self-management support
2. The history should include an assessment for the following:
   a. Comorbidities
   b. Clinical severity of the OA
   c. Site of OA involvement
   d. Individual preferences for treatment
   e. Cost of interventions
3. The core interventions should include the following:
   a. Educate the patient about the disease, using literature, opportunities for group classes, and self-management programs.
   b. Emphasize exercise; discuss with the patient that aerobic conditioning, stretching, and strengthening exercises are almost universally effective. It may be helpful to do this in consultation with a physical or occupational therapist.
   c. Manage local mechanical risk factors for disease progression, including malalignment, joint laxity, and previous joint damage.
   d. Educate the patient on how to implement joint protection principles.
   e. Consult with occupational therapist, hand therapist, and other allied professionals to evaluate for aids, devices, and adaptive methods for joint protection. These include proper use of long-handled appliances, utensils, elevated chairs, canes, and appropriate footwear,

      including shock-absorbing insoles or lateral wedge insoles, splints, and knee braces.

f. Provide nutritional counseling for weight loss if the patient is overweight.

g. Psychosocial factors need to be addressed, with extension of the education to the spouse or family. Occasional telephone contacts targeting identification of anxiety or depression have been proven to enhance compliance with treatment plans.

h. Introduce physical modalities to relieve discomfort, including heat or cold applications, or alternating both modalities, based on patient preferences.

i. Optimal management of OA frequently requires a combination of nonpharmacological and pharmacological interventions.

j. Acetaminophen is the drug of first choice for OA. It is the preferred long-term analgesic, recommended by the American College of Rheumatology, because of its safety and efficacy.

k. Nonsteroidal anti-inflammatory drugs (NSAIDs) at the lowest effective doses, and preferably used intermittently, should be added or substituted, for patients who respond poorly to acetaminophen. Special attention should be paid to risk factors for gastrointestinal (GI) complications as well as a risk for cardiovascular and renal side effects. Risk factors for GI toxicity include age over 65 years, history of previous peptic ulcer disease, history of upper GI bleeding, use of anticoagulants including aspirin, heavy alcohol use, and use of oral corticosteroids. For renal and cardiovascular toxicities, identified risk factors include history of hypertension, history of congestive heart failure, concomitant use of angiotensin-converting enzyme inhibitors, and other advanced medical conditions.

l. Topical creams such as capsaicin, prescribed at a concentration of 0.25% to 0.75%, can be used up to four times per day with the maximum benefit seen after 3 to 4 weeks of use. The evidence for sustained clinically significant benefit, beyond 2 weeks, from topical agents is limited, but their use appears safe.

m. Intra-articular steroid injections may be considered for patients with symptomatic exacerbation that is unresponsive to systemic analgesics, including NSAIDs.

n. Viscosupplementation of the knee with intra-articular injections of hyaluronan appears superior to placebo, with beneficial effects on pain, function, and patient global assessment according to a recent systematic review. The agents are expensive and require an office visit for their administration.

o. Glucosamine, which has been reported to have analgesic effects similar to those of acetaminophen, has not been shown conclusively to have any structural modification properties or to reduce the progression of joint space narrowing.

p. Other systemic analgesic agents, besides acetaminophen and NSAIDs, include tramadol and opioid agents. Although they are commonly prescribed, there is limited published clinical research about their usefulness in OA. Tramadol can be started at a dose of less than 50 mg/day, slowly increasing to a maximum of 100 mg four times a day. It is as effective as acetaminophen and 30 mg of codeine, but more expensive. It can be used in combination with an NSAID. Stronger narcotics may be of use for selected patients with difficult-to-control OA as rescue medications for severe pain or while other treatment modalities can be instituted.

q. For patients who fail to respond to medical treatment, including the nonpharmacological interventions, referral for specialized consultation and possible surgical intervention should be considered for refractory pain, increasing medication requirements, unacceptable impact on daily activities, or impaired sleeping. Consider the use of a sedating tricyclic antidepressant such as amitriptyline for those patients who experience sleeping problems because of their OA.

4. Always consider the possibility of comorbid depression, particularly in the patient who seems to be failing to respond to the "usual" treatment (see Chapter 12 for more details about depression).

5. During follow-up examinations, consider focusing a visit on any of the following areas:
   a. Joint protection methods
   b. Appropriate use of aids and devices when indicated
   c. Participation in exercise programs with emphasis on range of motion, strengthening, and aerobic conditioning
   d. Attempts to help the patient achieve an optimal body mass index
   e. Regular use of acetaminophen
   f. Evaluating for stress-related complications of OA (i.e., depression)

6. Further information for patients can be found at:
   a. www.niams.nih.gov/hi/topics/arthritis/oahandout.htm
   b. www.rheumatology.org
   c. www.arthritis.org

Burden as a Chronic Disease: Summary

1. Osteoarthritis is the most common form of arthritis and the most common form of disability in the United States.
   a. Over one-third of adults over 30 years of age have radiographic evidence of OA.
   b. Only a portion of patients with radiographic evidence of OA will develop symptoms.

2. Because of the aging of the population, the prevalence of OA is expected to increase. It is estimated that, over the next 20 years, the number of individuals affected by OA will increase from 43 million to

more than 60 million, with an annual cost that will reach nearly $100 billion by 2020.

3. It appears that lifelong exercise and fitness with good muscle tone may help prevent the development of OA.
   a. On the other hand, repetitive activities at work and intense competitive sport participation, especially in the presence of intrinsic joint vulnerabilities, may contribute to the development of symptomatic OA.
   b. Other vocational activities, such as lifting, kneeling, and squatting, increase the risk of knee OA, particularly if these activities are repeated over an extended period of time.
   c. Obesity is clearly associated with developing knee OA and, to a lesser degree, hip OA.

4. Our ability to implement preventive measures is limited at the present time. There are no agents currently available that can slow or stop the biochemical and structural changes that are associated with OA.

5. Several studies lend support for the efficacy of self-management interventions, primarily in relation to enhanced knowledge, compliance with exercise and disease self-management, self-efficacy, health care utilization, and pain. These programs have been adopted for diverse ethnic groups with similar successes and should be equally important to the pharmacological, occupational, and physical therapy interventions.

6. The initial assessment should include evaluation of the particular area of involvement and a discussion of treatment preferences. The issues that will determine which of the management options may help the individual patient include the following:
   a. Age
   b. Comorbidities
   c. Clinical severity of OA; impact on quality of life and ability to perform desired tasks
   d. Cost

7. Age will have a significant effect on the decision to use selected analgesic agents, particularly NSAIDs and opioid medications. The presence of comorbid conditions—cardiovascular, pulmonary, renal or neurologic, common in many elderly individuals—may limit or prevent the use of some of the drugs or the adherence to nonpharmacological interventions.

8. The investigation of the clinical severity should include the assessment of the impact of pain, the degree of disability or functional limitation, as well as the physician's and patient's global assessment of the activity of the disease.

9. A number of standardized, well-validated, self-reported instruments are available for use by patients with OA. These include:
   a. The Western Ontario and MacMaster Osteoarthritis Index (WOMAC)
   b. The Health Assessment Questionnaire (HAQ)

10. In clinical practice, however, restrictions in time and resources may limit the use of these instruments, and a practical classification of global assessment, pain, and functional impact can be quickly achieved. Table 10.1 (see later) presents my suggested method for a rapid, clinical assessment.

11. A short examination of the ability to arise unassisted from a chair, gait evaluation, and functional screening of the arms with ability to place hands behind the head, touch waist in back, and place hand in the contralateral hip will test the ability to stand, transfer, and maneuver for hygiene. Standing unassisted and touching tips of shoes will inform about standing and dressing lower extremities.

12. In most cases, pain is the main reason leading the individual with OA to see a physician.

13. Although a moderate amount of inflammation is part of the pathogenesis of OA, its suppression with NSAIDs has not been proved to relieve pain, change the natural course of the disease, or have an advantage over other analgesics for most patients.

14. Acetaminophen is the analgesic of first choice for the management of patients with OA. This position has been adopted by the American College of Rheumatology and the European Union League Against Rheumatism (EULAR). Often underestimated and underused, acetaminophen's efficacy is comparable with that of NSAIDs, including ibuprofen and diclofenac, and is frequently effective in substituting for the chronic use of an NSAID.

15. Nonsteroidal anti-inflammatory drugs are frequently used before acetaminophen, although the magnitude of reduction in pain scores is similar for most patients, with both types of analgesics.

    a. Nonsteroidal anti-inflammatory drugs differ in their capacity to penetrate the central nervous system and their ability to cause upper GI side effects. The renal side effects that may result in aggravation of hypertension, edema, or deterioration of renal function (elevated serum creatinine level) can occur with all NSAIDs.

    b. Nonsteroidal anti-inflammatory drugs can be used at less than maximum dosages with significant analgesic effects but with less risk of GI complications. An increase in dosage is not necessarily accompanied by an increase in efficacy.

    c. The need to avoid NSAIDs altogether, or to limit their use to the lowest effective dose and for a limited period of time, is particularly important for patients older than 65 years of age, with a prior history of peptic ulcer disease, comorbid conditions such as heart disease, renal insufficiency, and concurrent use of systemic corticosteroids, an anticoagulant, or aspirin.

    d. For those patients at risk for upper GI side effects, gastroprotective agents such as misoprostol, 200µg four times daily or a proton pump inhibitor, should be used.

16. Several COX-2–selective inhibitors have been withdrawn from the market due to concerns for adverse cardiovascular events.
17. Tramadol and opioid agents are often prescribed for patients with chronic pain unresponsive to other modalities. Their use should be tempered, however, by the fact that they are associated with tolerance, dependence, and addiction.
18. Glucosamine is widely proclaimed and used; however, it has rarely been tested in well-designed trials. There have been multiple studies with different preparations, many sponsored by the manufacturers. These studies tend to provide contradictory results. Systematic reviews of the pooled results from these studies revealed equivalence with placebo or a modest effect in pain and WOMAC function.
19. Intra-articular corticosteroid injections have been used for years for patients with OA.
    a. Several studies have attempted to identify predictive factors of response. Despite the long-term use of steroids, there are a surprisingly small number of studies looking at differences among the available steroid preparations, duration of effects, and optimal frequency of injections.
    b. In general, it is considered that the longer acting, more hydrophobic steroids are more effective (e.g., triamcinolone hexacetomide).
    c. The effect, in general, is short-lived, frequently 4 to 8 weeks.
    d. It has been suggested that after a year of injections given every 3 months, patients may have improvement in pain, severity of nocturnal pain, and range of motion.
20. Hyaluronan (HA) is a large glycosaminoglycan synthesized and secreted by type B cells of the synovial lining.
    a. Reports of their effectiveness have been contradictory over the years, but a recent systematic review concluded that it is an effective treatment for OA of the knee, the beneficial effects being in reducing pain on weight bearing, especially at 5 to 13 week postinjection.
    b. There are few randomized, head-to-head comparisons of the different available agents, and therefore no definitive conclusions can be reached about the relative value of the different products; part of their efficacy could be due to placebo effect.
    c. Given their cost, they should be considered an alternative for selected patients who have failed multiple other therapeutic modalities.
    d. There is no clear evidence that intra-articular viscosupplementation therapy slows progression of joint damage in humans with OA.
21. Some patients have the misconception that activity will aggravate OA, and they limit their physical activity. Multiple studies have demonstrated that improvements in range of motion, strengthening, and

aerobic exercises improve health and function in people with OA, particularly of lower extremities, and do not exacerbate joint pain or disease progression in the absence of joint instability or mechanical derangement.

22. The goals of the exercise program should be to reduce the impairment, improve function with reduction of pain, increase range of motion and strength, normalize gait, and improve performance of daily activities.

23. The prescription of exercise, frequently recommended by most practitioners, is difficult for patients to comply with if no specific information is provided for its implementation, adoption, and maintenance.

24. The challenge for patients with OA is to find and maintain a safe and effective exercise routine and to adopt it. In general, daily exercise that includes full active range of motion and periods of weight bearing and nonweight bearing should be used for joint health. If needed, initial gentle musculoskeletal flexibility improvement with stretching exercises, followed by progressive muscle strengthening, should prepare the patient for a graded program of aerobic exercise.

25. Involvement of an occupational therapist and education of the patient about techniques to reduce excessive loading on joints can further contribute to symptomatic alleviation and prevention of disease progression. Devices for assisting grip strength, elevated seats, shock-absorbing footwear, proper use of canes and other ambulation aids, items of daily use made of lighter materials, and advice on adaptive methods to get in and out of bed, bathtub, and cars are examples of interventions easily implemented and frequently overlooked.

26. The extensive work of Kate Lorig and Hal Holman in self-management support serves as a model for the treatment of chronic conditions, including arthritis.

   a. Self-management support should be considered an intervention on par with all of the previously mentioned techniques.

   b. Self-management tasks direct patients to learn how to:
      i. Take care of their illness
      ii. Carry out normal activities
      iii. Manage emotional changes

   c. For those patients who prefer online information, the Arthritis Self-Management (Self-Help) Program is available at http://patient-education.stanford.edu/programs/asmp.html. Topics in this self-help course include the following:
      i. Techniques to deal with problems such as pain, fatigue, frustration, and isolation
      ii. Appropriate exercise regimens
      iii. Use of medications
      iv. Communicating effectively with family, friends, and health professionals
      v. Healthy eating

  vi. Making informed treatment decisions
  vii. Disease-related problem-solving techniques
  viii. Getting a good night's sleep
 d. Patients involved in self-management activities tend to experience less pain, improved quality of life, and a lower need for office visits.

Introduction

Osteoarthritis (OA) is the most common form of arthritis and the most common form of disability in the United States. It is also the most common reason for total hip replacement and total knee replacement. More than one-third of adults older than 30 years have radiographic evidence of OA. Only a portion of patients with radiographic evidence of OA develop symptoms. However, because age is the most powerful risk factor, an increasing portion of the population will develop symptomatic osteoarthritis.

Osteoarthritis is the most common form of chronic musculoskeletal pain. Eighty percent of persons over the age of 55 years will have radiographic evidence of OA in the hands, knees, or hips. A smaller number will develop daily, activity-limiting symptoms; 10% to 15% of the elderly have this level of symptomatic hand, hip, or knee OA. These figures are from studies that define symptomatic disease as having pain most days of the month. If intermittent symptoms or occasional flares are allowed in the definition, then the prevalence increases, and a large proportion of the population more than 55 years old is symptomatic. Osteoarthritis is frequently associated with aging, to the point that some people believe it is an expected component of the aging process. Although not all elderly people will have symptomatic or radiographic manifestations of OA, important risk factors, in addition to age, include obesity, history of joint deformity and malalignment, female gender, presence of disability, history of previous joint injuries or damage (e.g., meniscectomy), muscle weakness or deconditioning, proprioception deficiencies, and joint laxity. It can also occur in younger individuals, leading to premature and prolonged disability, usually because of a combination of intrinsic joint vulnerabilities and certain occupations, sports, or comorbid conditions [1,2].

Because of the aging of the population, the prevalence of OA is expected to increase. The combination of an aging population, increased rates of obesity, and increasing joint damage with vocational and avocational activities suggests that the burden of OA will increase in this century. It is estimated that over the next 20 years the number of individuals affected by OA will increase from 43 million to more than 60 million, with an annual cost that will reach nearly $100 billion by 2020 [1–3]. Part of the cost of OA comes from joint replacements because OA is the cause of 80% of all total hip and knee replacements. The elements for primary prevention of OA include the identification of risk factors and activities that have been associated with the premature development or progression of OA. Some of these are not amenable to modification, like age, gender, and genetic susceptibility. Others are notoriously difficult to control (e.g., obesity, poor fitness, and joint laxity). Running and playing soccer and other sports when practiced in a recreational manner have not been associated with development of knee or hip OA unless there is a prior history of knee or hip injury, ligament damage, or internal derangement of the joint. Competitive running more than 20 miles per week, however, may be associated with an increased risk of knee OA. Overall, it appears that lifelong exercise and fitness with good muscle tone may help prevent the development of OA, while other repetitive activities at work and intense competitive sport participation, especially in the presence of intrinsic joint vulnerabilities, may contribute to the development of symptomatic OA [1–4]. Other vocational activities like lifting, kneeling, and squatting increase the risk of knee OA particularly if these activities are repeated over an extended period of time. Obesity is clearly associated with developing knee OA and, to a lesser degree, hip OA.

Secondary prevention, that is, introduction of interventions that prevent progression to the disease, is of great interest to researchers and the pharmaceutical industry. Our ability to implement preventive measures is limited at the present time. There are no agents currently available that can slow or stop the biochemical changes that are thought to be involved in the breakdown of the articular cartilage, or agents that affect the progression of changes in the underlying bone. Most of the time, interventions should focus on the management of symptoms, and minimizing pain and disability, while optimizing function and quality of life. At the primary level of care, the identification of risk factors already mentioned should be coupled with the recognition of the need for psychosocial management. Effective psychosocial management includes identification of comorbid stressors including depression, patient education on the management of OA, and active support of self-management. It is well established that patients' beliefs about disease and treatment can influence their response to illness and disease management. Patients can be effective and active agents of change in their treatment [5]. The self-management approach, as discussed elsewhere in this book, is based on the rationale that providing information about the disease and teaching skills in problem solving, communication, and disease management enhances the patient's ability to practice self-care. It has been found to be very helpful in chronic diseases in general and in arthritis in particular [6,7]. Several studies lend support for the efficacy of self-management interventions, primarily in relation to enhanced knowledge, compliance with exercise and disease self-management, self-efficacy, health care utilization, and pain [8,9]. These programs have been adopted for diverse ethnic groups with similar successes and should be equally important components of the treatment plan as are the pharmacological, occupational, and physical therapy interventions in the long-term management of these patients [8].

Initial Evaluation

Osteoarthritis results from disease processes that affect not only the articular cartilage but also the entire joint, including the subchondral bone, ligaments, joint capsule, synovial membrane, and periarticular muscles. At the end, the articular cartilage degenerates, with the formation of fissures, ulceration, and loss of the full thickness of the joint surface. The capsule undergoes fibrosis, the synovium shows a mild inflammatory infiltrate, and there is atrophy of the periarticular muscles. These different processes help explain, in part, why the presence of radiographic OA does not always correlate with the presence of symptoms. The origins and mechanisms of joint pain in patients with OA, therefore, seem to have a multifactorial etiology, including subchondral bone edema, microfractures, and the development of osteophytes, which stimulate the nerve endings in the periosteum. Affected joints show stretching of ligaments and joint capsule. Periarticular muscle weakness leads to diminished joint stability. Furthermore, a mild or moderate degree of inflammation can be found in the synovium. These events translate clinically into morning stiffness, usually lasting less than 30 minutes, pain, bony enlargement, effusions, and joint crepitation in late stages.

Because different treatment options are available to patients with OA, and given the different and overlapping pathophysiological processes, the interactions of allied health professionals, including physical therapists, occupational therapists, podiatrists, orthotists, psychologists, dietitians, rheumatologists, and orthopedic surgeons, play an important role in the care of the individual patient [5,10–16].

The initial assessment should include evaluation of the particular area of involvement and a discussion of treatment preferences. The issues that will determine which of the management options may help the individual patient include the following:

1. Age
2. Comorbidities
3. Clinical severity of OA: impact on quality of life and ability to perform desired tasks
4. Cost

As mentioned earlier, age will have a significant effect on the decision to use selected analgesic agents, particularly NSAIDs, and opioid medications. Similarly, the presence of comorbid conditions (cardiovascular, pulmonary, renal, or neurologic, common in many elderly individual) may limit or prevent the use of some of the drugs or the adherence to nonpharmacological interventions. The investigation of the clinical severity should include the assessment of the impact of pain, the degree of disability or functional limitation, and both the physician's and the patient's global

TABLE 10.1. Rapid assessment tool to gauge the impact of osteoarthritis.

Global rating: Are you better, same, worse?		
Pain:	Numerical rating scale (1–5, with 5 being "severe")	
	Have you had:	
	Pain at rest?	
	Pain with any weight bearing?	
	Pain at night?	
Function:	What is the most:	(a) difficult thing for you to do in an average day?
		(b) important thing for us to work on?
	What can you not do:	(a) that you were able to do?
		(b) that you need or would like to do?
	Are you able to sleep through the night?	

assessments of the activity of the disease. A number of standardized, well-validated self-reported instruments are available for patients with OA. These include:

1. The Western Ontario and MacMaster Osteoarthritis Index (WOMAC)
2. The Health Assessment Questionnaire (HAQ)

In clinical practice, however, restrictions in time and resources may limit the use of these instruments, and a practical classification of global assessment, pain, and functional impact can be quickly achieved. Table 10.1 illustrates my suggested method for a rapid, clinical assessment.

A short examination of the ability to arise unassisted from a chair, gait evaluation, and functional screening of the arms with ability to place hands behind the head, touch waist in back, and place hand on the contralateral hip will test the ability to stand, transfer, and maneuver for hygiene. Standing unassisted and touching tips of shoes will inform about standing and dressing lower extremities. Finally, attention to leg length inequality, areas of tenderness in periarticular structures (such as bursitis), muscle atrophy, joint contractures, and joint deformities amenable to stabilization or treatment could provide targets for improvement [17]. If the visit is very short, focus on the single function most difficult to achieve. The tests, in addition to inquiring about the preferences of the patient and awareness of the cost of the interventions, will determine which modalities to use.

Systemic Analgesics

In most cases, pain is the main reason an individual with OA sees a physician. It is frequently the main determinant of disability and quality of life. As discussed earlier, pain in OA seems to originate in different structures in and around a joint. Although a moderate amount of inflammation is part of the pathogenesis of OA, its suppression with NSAIDs has not been proved to relieve pain, change the natural course of the disease, or have an advantage over other analgesics for most patients.

Acetaminophen

Acetaminophen is a safe, readily available, inexpensive, well-tolerated, and effective analgesic. It is the analgesic of first choice for the management of OA. This position has been adopted by the American College of Rheumatology and the European Union League Against Rheumatism (EULAR) [10,11,18,19]. Acetaminophen has a central mechanism of action and can be used up to 4,000 mg/day. Often underestimated and underutilized, acetaminophen's efficacy is comparable to that of NSAIDs, including ibuprofen and diclofenac, and is frequently effective in substituting for the chronic use of an NSAID [20,21]. Although other analgesics have limitations because of age and renal, GI, or cardiovascular comorbidities frequently encountered in patients affected by OA, acetaminophen is generally well tolerated and can be combined with other analgesics in an effort to improve analgesia and minimize dose-dependent side effects of individual drugs.

There are conflicting reports about the need to monitor the International Normalized Ratio (INR) for patients using coumadin and acetaminophen. The risk appears negligible, but the clinician should advise patients about the potential risk and monitor the INR accordingly. Patients taking phenytoins may have a reduced analgesic effect. Overdoses of acetaminophen may result in acute hepatic failure and death. These risks have been reported in small series and case reports, mostly involving patients who took large doses of acetaminophen or used alcohol. It is prudent to advise limited use of analgesics for patients who use alcohol on a regular basis, limiting acetaminophen to 2 g/day. The reported association of acetaminophen and nephropathy needs to be interpreted with caution because some of these reports studied populations with significant confounding factors.

Nonsteroidal Anti-Inflammatory Drugs

Nonsteroidal anti-inflammatory drugs include agents that may exhibit both a peripheral and a central mechanism of action. They are frequently used before acetaminophen, although the magnitude of reduction in pain scores are similar in most patients with both types of analgesics [20–24]. Nonsteroidal anti-inflammatory drugs differ in their capacity to penetrate the central nervous system and in their ability to cause upper GI side effects. The renal side effects that can result in aggravation of hypertension, edema, or deterioration of renal function (elevated serum creatinine level) can occur with all NSAIDs. Their actions are mediated by inhibition of cyclooxygenase (COX) and decreased production of prostaglandins. They can inhibit both COX-1 and COX-2 (nonselective) or be more selective for

COX-2 and spare COX-1 enzymes. Inhibition of COX-1 is associated with GI dyspepsia, gastritis, bleeding and ulceration, and inhibition of platelet activation. COX-2 inhibitors, some recently removed from the market, may be useful for the subset of patients intolerant to nonselective NSAIDs and/or in need of gastroprotective agents. Some of the COX-2–selective agents are still available, but their use has greatly diminished in the elderly population because of concerns for an increased rate of cardiovascular events and cost. Furthermore, the evidence indicates that they have similar analgesic efficacy to the nonselective NSAIDs. Many of the nonselective NSAIDs can be used at less than maximum doses with significant analgesic effects but with less risk of GI complications. An increase in dosage is not necessarily accompanied by an increase in efficacy, and these drugs at full "anti-inflammatory" dosages are usually not more effective than acetaminophen and do not change the course of OA. The need to avoid NSAIDs altogether or limit their use to the lowest effective dose and for a limited period of time is particularly important for patients older than 65 years of age and those with a history of peptic ulcer disease, GI bleeding, comorbid conditions such as heart disease and renal insufficiency, or concurrent use of systemic corticosteroids, an anticoagulant, or aspirin [25]. For those patients at risk for upper GI side effects, gastroprotective agents such as misoprostol 200 µg four times daily or a proton pump inhibitor should be prescribed. Alternatively, a short course of a COX-2 inhibitor, for patients with no cardiovascular risk factors, or a nonacetylated salicylate may be prescribed. Among the nonselective NSAIDs, aspirin, indomethacin, piroxicam, and sulindac have been associated with a higher risk of upper GI toxicity compared with ibuprofen, naproxen, and nabumetone. The COX-2 selective agents are the safest from the GI perspective, but have other limitations as mentioned earlier. Because most NSAIDs, COX-2 selective and nonselective, seem to increase the risk for myocardial infarction to a greater or lesser degree, use of NSAIDs should be limited in patients with coronary risk factors [26,27].

Other Analgesics

Tramadol and opioid agents are often used by patients with chronic pain unresponsive to other modalities. Their use should be tempered, however, by the fact that they are associated with tolerance, dependence, and addiction. Misunderstanding of these conditions sometimes leads to underutilization of these drugs by patients with intense pain [28]. Nonetheless, they are probably more frequently used for short-term courses during periods of symptom exacerbation, or as a temporary treatment while other maneuvers are instituted. Opioids have the greatest analgesic efficacy and a well-known side effect profile, including constipation, drowsiness, and potential for abuse. Depending on route of administration and the particular agent, they can be used as single agents or in combination with other analgesics.

Tramadol is a short-acting analgesic with dual inhibition of opioid receptors and inhibition of serotonin and norepinephrine reuptake. It has analgesic efficacy somewhere between nonopioid and opioid analgesics. When used in a dose of 50 to 100 mg up to four times a day, it provides pain relief comparable to 325 mg of acetaminophen and 30 mg of codeine taken up to four times a day. The potential side effects of tramadol are similar to those of codeine, and its abuse and addiction potential is very low. However, its cost and the increased risk of seizures in some patients who use alcohol, or with the concomitant use of antidepressants should be considered. Tramadol and NSAIDs at low doses may work well in combination with acetaminophen.

Without doubt, function and quality of life can be improved substantially by adequate control of joint pain. However, because of the concern for the adverse effects of opioid analgesics, the management of pain should not begin and end with a prescription of an analgesic. Choice of management must take into account all the contributing factors that could modulate or magnify the disability and pain associated with OA [29].

Glucosamine

Widely proclaimed and used, and rarely tested in well-designed trials, nutritional supplements are readily accessible. There have been multiple studies with different preparations, many sponsored by the manufacturers. These studies tend to provide contradictory results. Systematic reviews of the pooled results from these studies revealed equivalence with placebo or a modest effect in pain and in WOMAC function. However, the results were not uniformly positive; suitable patients were not well defined and clinically important structural modification is unclear [30]. Glucosamine appears to be as safe as placebo. There are multiple preparations, but their manufacture and origin varies significantly. Cost can be a substantial barrier to the use of this agent.

Intra-Articular Injections

Osteoarthritis is predominantly a joint disease with no systemic manifestations. Frequently, the affected joints are easily accessible for examination and treatment. The use of intra-articular corticosteroids has been part of the therapeutic armamentarium for many years. They are thought to decrease joint inflammation by decreasing the production of the enzyme phospholipase A_2, resulting in the decreased production of prostaglandins and leukotrienes. Intra-articular corticosteroid use should be considered a temporary intervention. It can be used in single or multiple joints, particularly when they are not responsive to other therapeutic maneuvers [31]. Several studies have attempted to identify predictive factors of response.

Despite their use for many years, there are a surprisingly small number of studies looking at differences among the steroid preparations commercially available, duration of effects, and optimal frequency of injections [31]. In general, it is considered that the longer acting, more hydrophobic steroids are more effective, (e.g., triamcinolone hexacetomide). The effect in general is short-lived, frequently 4 to 8 weeks. It has been suggested that after a year of injections every 3 months, patients may have improvement in pain, severity of nocturnal pain, and range of motion compared with patients receiving saline injections. The adverse effects are generally minor. The risk of infection, the most serious complication, is very low, in the order of 1 in 5,000 to 1 in 50,000 injections. Other adverse effects include local reactions, subcutaneous atrophy, and tendon rupture, less commonly seen with more soluble agents (e.g., hydrocortisone, prednisolone, or methylprednisolone). Some patients experience temporary flushing and occasionally a postinjection flare.

Hyaluronan

Hyaluronan (HA) is a large glycosaminoglycan synthesized and secreted by type B cells of the synovial lining. Normal concentration in the synovial fluid is 2 to 4 mg/mL and is a viscous liquid (lubricant) at low shear rates, as in walking, and an elastic solid (shock absorber) at high shear rates, as in running. Hyaluronan preparations available for intra-articular injections have been purified from rooster comb and human umbilical cords or synthesized by bacteria. Reports of its effectiveness have been contradictory over the years, but a recent systematic review concluded that it is an effective treatment for OA of the knee, the beneficial effects including reduced pain on weight bearing especially at 5 to 13 weeks postinjection.

However, there are few randomized, head-to-head comparisons of the different agents, and therefore no definitive conclusions could be reached about their relative values; part of their efficacy could be from a placebo effect [32]. The side effects include a low risk of infection and hypersensitivity reactions with swelling and pain. Given their cost, they should be considered an alternative for selected patients who have failed multiple other therapeutic modalities. There is no clear evidence that intra-articular viscosupplementation therapy slows progression of joint damage in humans with OA.

Exercise

Physical disability in the aging population with OA may be the result of interactions of pain, lower extremity impairments, poor physical fitness, obesity, other comorbidities, and the severity of OA itself. The deconditioning and disability associated with OA predispose the individual to inactivity associated diseases and an increased risk of mechanical falls. Some patients have the misconception that activity will aggravate OA, and they limit their physical activity. Multiple studies have demonstrated that improve range of motion and strength, as well as aerobic exercises, improve health and function in people with OA, particularly efforts to for OA of the lower extremities. The goals of the exercise program should be to improve function, reduce pain, increase range of motion, increase strength, normalize gait, and improve performance of daily activities.

You must try to be as specific as possible with recommendations for exercise. The challenge for patients with OA is to find and maintain a safe and effective exercise routine and to adopt it. In general, daily exercise that includes full active range of motion and periods of weight bearing and nonweight bearing should be used for joint health. If needed, initial gentle musculoskeletal flexibility improvement with stretching exercises, followed by progressive muscle strengthening should prepare the patient for a graded program of aerobic exercise [12,13,15]. Close collaboration with occupational and physical therapists for one-on-one education and adaptation of the program to the patient's treatment preferences are needed. The exercise program should include advice and occasion to provide a positive lifestyle change with an increase in physical activity. Compliance and adherence to a program is the principal predictor for long-term outcome from exercise in patients with hip or knee OA. Strategies to improve or maintain adherence should be adopted. An example of this is the use of the action plan (see Chapter 2).

There is evidence that improvement in muscle strength, range of motion, and overall fitness may reduce the progression of knee and hip OA. During the acute stage, the goals are to decrease pain, and maintain range of motion and strength without aggravating the inflammation. Judicious use of rest, isometric exercises (maximum muscle tension but no muscle shortening or joint movement) and active range of motion exercises to prevent contractures are appropriate. During the chronic stages, the goals are to increase strength, range of motion, and function. Appropriate interventions are aquatic exercises, dynamic isotonic (involving shortening or lengthening of muscle and joint motion) exercises, and passive range of motion followed by progressive aerobic exercises. The physician is uniquely positioned to positively influence the patient's beliefs about exercise. There are few contraindications for exercise therapy. These include significant aortic stenosis, obstructive cardiomyopathy, and exercise-induced arrhythmias.

Assistive Devices and Joint Protection

Involvement of an occupational therapist and education of the patient on techniques to reduce excessive loading on joints can further contribute to symptomatic alleviation and prevention of disease progression. Devices for assisting grip strength, elevated seats, shock-absorbing footwear, proper use of canes and other ambulation aids, items of daily use made of lighter materials, and advice on adaptive methods to get into and out of bed, bathtub, and cars are examples of interventions easily implemented and frequently overlooked. Knee braces for varus deformity and hand splints for stabilization and decreased pain can also be very effective. These interventions help preserve functional independence, improve symptoms, decrease the use of medications, and result in enhanced self-efficacy.

Other, invasive, interventions include tidal irrigation of the knee and arthroscopic debridement and lavage. However, these have been shown to be no more effective than sham interventions [33].

Surgical Treatment

The impact of disease on lifestyle is the most important factor when considering a surgical approach. Poorly controlled pain, progressive medication requirements, functional decline, impaired rest, and partial success or failure of nonpharmacological interventions are all valid reasons to refer to a surgeon. The clinician should avoid an excessive delay and prolonged pain, disability and deconditioning before considering surgery, since the rate of complications is higher in weakened individuals. There are several well-established treatments to consider before performing a total joint replacement. Total joint arthroplasty is the most significant advance in the treatment of OA over the past 50 years, and surgical approaches continue to evolve toward better outcomes and less invasive techniques.

Self-Management Support

The extensive work of Kate Lorig, Hal Holman, and their associates [34] in self-management support serves as a model for the treatment of chronic conditions, including arthritis. Self-management support should be considered an intervention on par with all of the previously mentioned techniques. Self-management tasks help patients learn how to:

1. Take care of their illness
2. Carry out normal activities
3. Manage emotional changes

Their book provides education and materials that can be used for most patients with OA [34]. For those patients who prefer online information, the Arthritis Self-Management (Self-Help) Program is available at http://patienteducation.stanford.edu/programs/asmp.html. This self-help course includes the following topics:

1. Techniques to deal with problems such as pain, fatigue, frustration, and isolation
2. Appropriate exercise regimens
3. Use of medications
4. Communicating effectively with family, friends, and health professionals
5. Healthy eating
6. Making informed treatment decisions
7. Disease-related problem-solving skills
8. Getting a good night's sleep

Patients involved in self-management activities tend to experience less pain, have improved quality of life, and need fewer office visits.

References

1. Silman AJ, Hochberg MC. Epidemiology of the Rheumatic Diseases. Oxford, UK: Oxford University Press, 2001.
2. Felson D, Lawrence R, Dieppe P, Hirsch R, Helmick C, Jordon J, et al. Osteoarthritis: new insights. Part 1. The disease and its risk factors. Ann Intern Med 2000;133:635–646.
3. Elders MJ. The increasing impact of arthritis on public health. J Rheumatol 2000;27(Suppl 60):6–8.
4. Guccione AA, Felson DT, Anderson JJ, Anthony JM, Zhnag Y, Wilson PWF, et al. The effect of specific medical conditions on the functional limitations of elders in the Framingham Study. Am J Public Health 1994; 84:351–358.
5. Dieppe P, Brandt KD. What is important in treating osteoarthritis? Whom should we treat and how should we treat them? Rheum Dis Clin North Am 2003;29:687–716.
6. Bodenheimer T, Lorig K, Holman H, Grumbach K. Patient self-management of chronic disease in primary care. JAMA 2002;288:2469–2475.
7. Holman H, Lorig K. Patient self-management: a key to effectiveness and efficiency in care of chronic disease. Public Health Rep 2004;119:239–243.
8. Superio-Cabuslay E, Ward MM, Lorig KR. Patient education interventions in osteoarthritis and rheumatoid arthritis: a meta-analytic comparison with non-steroidal anti-inflammatory drug therapy. Arthritis Care Res 1996;9: 292–301.
9. Barlow J, Lorig K. Patient education. In Brandt KD, Doherty M, Lohmander LS (eds). Osteoarthritis. New York: Oxford University Press, 2003:321–326.
10. American College of Rheumatology Subcommittee on Osteoarthritis Guidelines. Recommendations for the medical management of osteoarthritis of the hip and knee: 2000 update. Arthritis Rheum 2000;43:1905–1915.
11. Jordan KM, Arden NK, Doherty M, et al. EULAR recommendations 2003: an evidence-based approach to the management of knee osteoarthritis: report of a task force of the Standing Committee for International Clinical Studies Including Therapeutic Trials (ESCISIT) Ann Rheum Dis 2003;62:1145–1155.

12. American Geriatrics Society Panel on Exercise and Osteoarthritis. Exercise prescription for older adults with osteoarthritis pain: consensus practice recommendations. J Am Geriatr Soc 2001;49:808–823.

13. Minor MA: Exercise for the patient with osteoarthritis. In Brandt KD, Doherty M, Lohmander LS (eds). Osteoarthritis. New York: Oxford University Press, 2003:299–305.

14. Felson DT, Lawrence RV, Hochberg MC, McAlindon T, Dieppe PA, Minor MA, et al. Osteoarthritis: new insights. Part 2. Treatment approaches. Ann Intern Med. 2000;133:726–737.

15. Roddy E, Zhang W, Doherty M, Arden NK, Barlow J, et al. Evidence-based recommendations for the role of exercise in the management of osteoarthritis of the hip and knee—the MOVE consensus. Rheumatology (Oxford) 2005;44:67–73.

16. Fransen M, McConnell S, Bell M. Exercise for osteoarthritis of the hip or knee. Cochrane Database Syst Rev 2003;3:CD004286.

17. Bischoff HA, Roos EM, Liang MH. Outcome assessment in osteoarthritis: a guide for research and clinical practice. In Brandt KD, Doherty M, Lohmander SL (eds). Osteoarthritis. New York: Oxford University Press, 2003:381–390.

18. Towheed TE, Judd MJ, Hochberg MC, Wells G. Acetaminophen for osteoarthritis. Cochrane Database Syst Rev 2003;2:CD004257.

19. Zhang W, Jones A, Doherty M. Does paracetamol (acetaminophen) reduce the pain of osteoarthritis? A meta-analysis of randomized controlled trials. Ann Rheum Dis 2004;63:91–97.

20. Brandt KD. Non-surgical treatment of osteoarthritis: a half century of "advances." Ann Rheum Dis 2004;63:117–122.

21. Pincus T, Koch GG, Sokka T, Lefkowith J, Wolfe F, Jordan JM, et al. A randomized, double-blind, cross-over clinical trial of diclofenac plus misoprostol versus acetaminophen in patients with osteoarthritis of the hip or knee. Arthritis Rheum 2001;44:1587–1598.

22. Scholes D, Stergachis A, Penna PM, Normand EH, Hansten PD. Non-steroidal anti-inflammatory drug discontinuation in patients with osteoarthritis. J Rheumatol 1995;22:708–712.

23. Eccles M, Freemantle N, Mason J for the North of England Non-steroidal Anti-Inflammatory Drug Guidelines Development Group. Summary guidelines for non-steroidal anti-inflammatory drugs versus basic analgesia in treating the pain of degenerative arthritis. BMJ 1998;317:526–530.

24. Wolfe MM, Lichtenstein DR, Singh G. Gastrointestinal Toxicity of non-steroidal anti-inflammatory drugs. N Eng J Med 1999;340:1888–1899.

25. Drazen JM. COX-2 inhibitors—A lesson in unexpected problems. N Eng J Med 2005;352:1131–1132.

26. Fries JF, Murtagh KN, Bennett M, Zatarain E, Lingala B, Bruce B. The rise and decline of non-steroidal anti-inflammatory drug-associated gastropathy in rheumatoid arthritis. Arthritis Rheum 2004;50:2433–2440.

27. Hippisley-Cox J, Coupland C. Risk of myocardial infarction in patients taking cyclo-oxygenase-2 inhibitors or conventional non-steroidal anti-inflammatory drugs: population based nested case-control analysis. BMJ 2005;330:1366–1369.

28. Greene B, Lim SS. The role of physical therapy in management of patients with osteoarthritis and rheumatoid arthritis. Bull Rheum Dis 1999;52:4.
29. Ballantyne JC, Mao J. Opioid therapy for chronic pain. N Engl J Med 2003;349:1943–1953.
30. Towheed TE, Maxwell L, Anastassiades TP, Shea B, Houpt J, et al. Glucosamine therapy for treating osteoarthritis. Cochrane Database Syst Rev 2005;2: CD002946.
31. Bellamy N, Campbell J, Robinson V, Gee T, Bourne R, Wells G. Intra-articular corticosteroid for treatment of osteoarthritis of the knee. Cochrane Database Syst Rev. 2005;2:CD005328.
32. Bellamy N, Campbell J, Robinson V, Gee T, Bourne R, Wells G. Viscosupplementation for the treatment of osteoarthritis of the knee. Cochrane Database Syst Rev 2005;2:CD005321.
33. Felson DT, Buckwalter J. Debridement and lavage for osteoarthritis of the knee. N Eng J Med 2002;347:132–133.
34. Lorig K, Holman H, Sobel D, Laurent D, Gonzalez V, Minor M. Living a Healthy Life with Chronic Conditions, 2nd ed. Boulder, CO: Bull Publishing Company, 2000.

11
Obesity

JIM NUOVO

Background: Burden as a Chronic Disease

1. Obesity is an epidemic in the United States. The third National Health and Nutrition Examination Survey (NHANES III) indicated that 22% of adults are obese (body mass index [BMI] >30 kg/m^2), and 34% are overweight (BMI 25 to 30 kg/m^2) [1].
2. The prevalence of obesity is increasing regardless of age, gender, ethnicity, or education [2].
3. Childhood obesity is also increasing, with reported rates varying between 25% and 37%.
4. Obesity is linked to many other comorbid conditions, including type 2 diabetes, coronary artery disease, heart failure, hyperlipidemia, hypertension, osteoarthritis, obstructive sleep apnea, and depression.

Costs

The costs of obesity are difficult to measure; however, perhaps 7% of the annual U.S. health care costs are related to obesity. About $50 billion is spent each year on methods to lose weight. In 1999, $321 million was spent on prescription medications to treat obesity.

Impact of Disease Management Programs

Disease management programs similar to those used for diabetes, asthma, and heart failure have not been reported in the treatment of obesity.

Initial Evaluation

Most cases of obesity are caused by nonmedical disorders, being sedentary, and consuming excess calories. Although they occur infrequently, medical conditions associated with weight gain (e.g., hypothyroidism and adverse effects of medications, particularly neuroleptic drugs) should be ruled out.

1. Calculate your patient's BMI (BMI = weight in kilograms/height in meters squared). A BMI chart is available on the Internet at www.nhlbi.nih.gov/health.
   a. A BMI of 25 to 29.9 kg/m^2 is overweight.
   b. A BMI of 30 kg/m^2 is obese.
   c. A BMI >40 kg/m^2 is the criterion to consider surgical interventions; use >35 kg/m^2 if comorbid conditions exist.
2. Assess all of your overweight and obese patients for central adiposity; patients with central adiposity are at increased risk for heart disease and diabetes and for some forms of cancer. Central adiposity can be assessed with waist circumference (measured at the level of the natural waist line or the narrowest part of the torso) and hip circumference (measured in the horizontal plane at the level of the maximal circumference, including the maximum extension of the buttocks posteriorly).
   A BMI of 25 to 35 kg/m^2 and a waist circumference >40 inches for men and >35 inches for women is considered high-risk for cardiovascular disease. A waist to hip ratio of >0.95 for men or >0.85 for women is another measure of central adiposity.
3. Screen all your overweight and obese patients for associated comorbid conditions:
   a. Hypertension
   b. Hyperlipidemia
   c. Type 2 diabetes
   d. Depression
   e. Obstructive sleep apnea (sleep apnea is more common in obese patients)
4. Consider a sleep study if your patient has clinical signs that suggest obstructive sleep apnea.
5. Laboratory tests to consider include:
   a. Fasting lipid panel
   b. Fasting glucose.
   c. Thyroid-stimulating hormone
6. Medications that increase weight should be avoided if possible. The most common problematic medications are the neuroleptic agents.

Management

1. Assess your patients' "readiness to change" with regard to diet and exercise (see Chapter 2).
2. Promote self-management techniques for all of your overweight and obese patients.
3. Help your patients set goals. It is best if these goals are patient-generated, specific, and short-term achievable action plans, for example, "This week I will walk around the block before lunch on Monday, Tuesday, and Thursday."
4. Promote self-generated goals that are reasonable and achievable. On a scale of 0 to 10 in which your patient is extremely confident in their ability to achieve the goal, a reasonable goal will have a self-rating of 7 or greater. If a patient's self-rating is 6 or less, that specific goal is not likely to be achieved; help your patient develop a more realistic goal.
5. Document patient-generated goals in the medical record, recognize achievements, and address barriers.
6. Provide appropriate educational materials to help patients understand the principles of healthy eating, the importance of exercise, and the methods to reduce stress. The National Heart, Lung, and Blood Institute maintains a culturally sensitive Web site that contains helpful information on a variety of health conditions, including obesity. It is available at www.nhlbi.nih.gov/health/index.htm.
7. Self-management training alone will be insufficient to provide long-term success in weight management [3].
8. Encourage your patients to learn the principles of healthy eating:
   a. Emphasize fruits, vegetables, and whole grains.
   b. Emphasize the need to limit portion sizes.
   c. Advise your patients to limit calories from liquids.
   d. For those patients who eat when they are not hungry, suggest that they look for other things to do: go for a walk, talk to a friend, chew sugarless gum.
9. There is no demonstrated advantage to any one of the most popular diets available. In a comparison trial of the Atkins, Ornish, Weight Watchers, and Zone diets for weight loss and heart disease risk reduction, no substantive difference in weight loss was found [4].

   Commercial weight loss programs provide treatment to millions of clients, but the efficacies of these programs have not been evaluated in a rigorous long-term trial. In a 2-year randomized comparison of a commercial weight loss program with a self-help program (consisting of two 20-minute counseling sessions with a nutritionist and provision of self-help resources), patients on the commercial weight loss program lost more weight (−4.3 kg vs. −1.3 kg) [5].

10. Target intakes for a weight loss program are 1,600 kcal/day for men and 1,300 kcal for women. This should result in a weight loss of 1 to 2 pounds per week. For patients wanting help with their meal plan, the National Heart, Lung, and Blood Institute's Web site includes an interactive menu planner.
11. Reinforce the value of an exercise program.
    a. Consider having sedentary patients take an exercise treadmill test before starting an exercise program, particularly if they have multiple cardiovascular risk factors.
    b. A progressive walking program offers the best chance for long-term success.
    c. A pedometer can serve as an excellent means to help patients set reasonable goals and receive daily feedback. Patients who wish to participate in a 10,000 steps program can get further information at www.shapeup.org.

Medications

1. Medications currently approved for weight loss fall into two broad categories: those that decrease food intake by reducing appetite or increasing satiety and those that decrease nutrient absorption.
    a. Appetite suppressants work by increasing the levels of anorexigenic neurotransmitters, namely, norepinephrine, serotonin, and dopamine.
    b. An example of a noradrenergic agent is phentermine (Adipex, Fastin, Ionamin).
    c. An example of a mixed noradrenergic and serotonergic agent is sibutramine (Meridia).
    d. Appetite suppressant contraindications include hypertension, cardiovascular disease, hyperthyroidism, agitated states, and history of drug abuse.
    e. Orlistat (Xenical) is a unique agent that decreases fat absorption through inhibiting lipase in the gastrointestinal tract. Diarrhea, abdominal cramping, and chronic malabsorption syndromes are recognized adverse side effects.
    f. Herbal remedies containing ephedra are now prohibited because of the drug's potential to cause serious adverse side effects.
2. Surgery for weight loss should be considered only for patients with a BMI $>40 kg/m^2$ (or $>35 kg/m^2$ if there are accompanying comorbid conditions).
3. An evidence-based algorithm for the treatment of obesity has been prepared by the National Institutes of Health (Figure 11.1) [6].

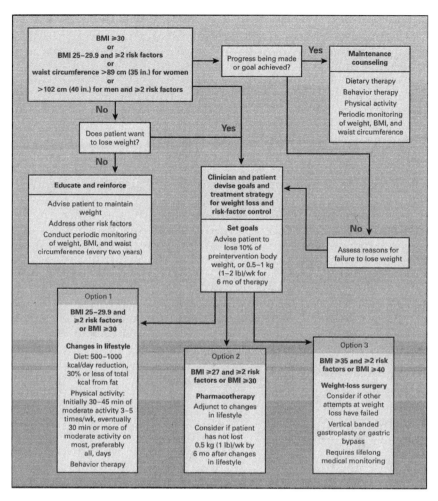

FIGURE 11.1. Evidence-based algorithm for the treatment of obesity. From Yanovski and Yanovski [6], by permission of N Engl J Med.

Monitoring

1. The first step in obesity treatment is to identify patients who are at increased risk for cardiovascular disease.
2. Abdominal adiposity may be the most sensitive marker of risk.
3. Patients identified as having an increased risk for cardiovascular disease need more regular monitoring and more rigorous management of other recognized risk factors, particularly hypertension, hyperlipidemia, and hyperglycemia.

4. Provide a means to monitor patient-generated goals in the medical record; recognize successes and address barriers in achieving these goals.

Alternative Therapy

1. Herbal remedies containing ephedra (ma huang) are now prohibited because of the potential for serious adverse side effects.
2. Inform your patients that some products listed as "ephedrine free" may actually contain other sources of similar substances, particularly herbals containing bitter orange or country mallow.
3. All ephedrine or ephedrine-like substances should be considered potentially dangerous.
   Inform your patients that many herbal weight loss remedies contain caffeine derivatives. These include guarana, cola nut, mate, and tea extract.

Summary

Obesity has become an epidemic health problem throughout the United States. Obesity is associated with many chronic health problems, including hypertension, heart failure, type 2 diabetes, osteoarthritis, obstructive sleep apnea, and depression. All overweight and obese patients should be evaluated for the presence of these comorbid conditions. Education and self-management support are important parts of a multidimensional approach to obesity. Medications for obesity are rarely effective in the long run.

References

1. National Heart, Lung, and Blood Institute. www.nhlbi.nih.gov/guidelines/obesity/ob_home.htm.
2. Mokdad AH, et al. The spread of the obesity epidemic in the United States, 1991–1998. JAMA 1999;282:1519–1522.
3. Latner JD. Self-help in the long term treatment of obesity. Obesity Rev 2001;2:87–97.
4. Dansinger ML, Gleason JA, Griffith JL, Selker HP, Schaefer E. Comparison of the Atkins, Ornish, Weight Watchers, and Zone diets for weight loss and heart disease risk reduction. A randomized trial. JAMA 2005;293:43–53.
5. Heshka S, et al. Weight loss with self-help compared with a structured commercial program: a randomized trial. JAMA 2003;289:1792–1798.
6. Yanovski SZ, Yanovski JA. Drug therapy: obesity. N Engl J Med 2002;346: 591–602.

12
Depression

Jim Nuovo

Background: Burden as a Chronic Disease

1. Depression is one of the most common chronic diseases you will see in your clinic. It affects approximately 20 million Americans.
2. The lifetime prevalence of depression in the general population is 16%.
3. Depression is more likely to occur in patients who have chronic medical problems. Your patients with diabetes, heart failure, osteoarthritis, and stroke have 1 ½ to 2 times the rate of depression.
4. Depression is a challenging disease to diagnose; symptoms of depression are often overlooked. For example, it is estimated that depression is identified in fewer than 50% of cardiac and diabetes patients, and only one-half of those identified receive treatment.
5. For many of your patients, somatic pain (e.g., headache, back pain, abdominal pain) will accompany the symptoms of depression; for 69% of patients with depression, the only complaint is pain.
6. In most patients, major depression is a relapsing illness. After the first episode, there is a 40% recurrence rate over the next 2 years; after two episodes, the risk of recurrence is 75%.

Costs

1. The economic costs for depression exceeded $81 billion in 2000.
2. The costs to employers are estimated to be about $3,000 per year for each employee.
3. Major depression is associated with 50% to 100% increases in medical costs. These costs are from increased utilization of emergency and primary care clinics, prescription medications, and laboratory tests and increased hospital days.
4. Patients with heart failure or diabetes and accompanying depression are significantly more costly to treat and tend to have poorer clinical outcomes [1,2].

Impact of Disease Management Programs

Depression often is unrecognized, and of those cases detected, only 30% to 50% receive adequate treatment. Disease management programs targeted to the treatment of depression have been shown to improve detection and outcomes. Primary care practices that implement depression quality improvement programs usually show improvements in measures of quality of care, in mental health outcomes, and in patient and provider satisfaction [3].

Many programs use telephone follow-up as a component to the disease management program. Examples of telephone interventions include the following:

1. Katon and associates [4] found that use of a phone follow-up protocol involving three telephone visits over a 1-year period, along with two office visits with a primary care doctor, improved detection of relapse and resulted in greater adherence to medical treatment.
2. Simon and associates [5] found that a program of systematic follow-up and care management by phone significantly improved clinical outcomes.
3. In separate studies, Tutty and associates [6] and Simon and associates [7] found that a telephone counseling and medication monitoring intervention was well-accepted and improved outcomes.

Studies that do not use a comprehensive program following the Chronic Care Model generally fail to show improvements in outcomes. Examples of these include the following:

1. Vergouwen and associates [8] found that educational interventions to enhance adherence failed to demonstrate a clear benefit to adherence or outcome. Most of these interventions were pharmacy based.
2. Capoccia and associates [9] performed a study in which patients with depression were randomized to usual care versus enhanced care with a pharmacist facilitating patient education and monitoring of adherence and adverse side effects. Frequent telephone contact did not result in increased adherence or improved outcomes.

The impact on overall costs remains unclear. The costs to run a depression management program compare favorably with other interventions when measured by quality of life-years; however, improving depression care does not appear to save money for health insurers or health care systems in the short term.

Few studies have been designed to assess the long-term impact of a depression management program. Most studies are designed to improve acute management and last 6 months or less. Rost and associates [10] assessed the impact of a long-term depression management program. Their intervention included guideline-directed pharmacotherapy or psychotherapy, the use of a nurse case manager, and regularly scheduled contacts to encourage treatment adherence. Their program resulted in significant improvements in the number of depression-free days (648 vs. 588) when compared with usual care. Health plan costs decreased significantly as a result of reduced overall health care utilization [10].

Initial Evaluation

All of your patients identified as having depression should have a history taken, a physical examination, and laboratory testing. This evaluation should be used in part to screen for medical conditions that may present with similar symptoms. At a minimum, laboratory tests should include a complete blood count and a thyroid-stimulating hormone assay (TSH). Other diagnostic tests should be guided by specific findings in the history or physical examination.

Use a standardized evaluation tool to assess the diagnosis of depression and its severity, as well as the response to treatment. The Patient Health Questionnaire (PHQ-9) is a commonly used instrument (Figure 12.1) [11]. Other assessment tools include the following:

1. The Beck Depression Inventory [12]
2. The General Health Questionnaire [13]
3. The Zung Self-Assessment Depression Scale [14]

Screen all of your patients with depression for common comorbid conditions. These include:

1. Anxiety disorders
2. Substance abuse
3. Other psychiatric diagnoses (particularly bipolar disorder)

Clues to the presence of an anxiety disorder are recurrent episodes of chest pain, hyperventilation, shortness of breath, epigastric distress, irritable bowel disease, headache, dizziness, paresthesias, panic attack, or frequent emergency room visits.

Alcohol and other drug problems can be screened for by asking a few questions that can be integrated into the interview, including the following:

1. Do you drink alcohol? If the answer to this question is positive, consider asking at least the following two questions from the CAGE questionnaire:
   a. Have you ever tried to cut down on your drinking?
   b. Have you ever felt guilty about your drinking?

Patients with a positive response to either question should be referred to an alcohol treatment program.

PATIENT HEALTH QUESTIONNAIRE (PHQ-9)

NAME: _____   DATE:_____

Over the *last 2 weeks*, how often have you been
bothered by any of the following problems?
(use "✓" to indicate your answer)

	Not at all	Several days	More than half the days	Nearly every day
1. Little interest or pleasure in doing things	0	1	2	3
2. Feeling down, depressed, or hopeless	0	1	2	3
3. Trouble falling or staying asleep, or sleeping too much	0	1	2	3
4. Feeling tired or having little energy	0	1	2	3
5. Poor appetite or overeating	0	1	2	3
6. Feeling bad about yourself—or that you are a failure or have let yourself or your family down	0	1	2	3
7. Trouble concentrating on things, such as reading the newspaper or watching television	0	1	2	3
8. Moving or speaking so slowly that other people could have noticed. Or the opposite—being so fidgety or restless that you have been moving around a lot more than usual	0	1	2	3
9. Thoughts that you would be better off dead, or of hurting yourself in some way	0	1	2	3

add columns: _____ + _____ + _____

(Healthcare professional: For interpretation of TOTAL, please refer to accompanying scoring card).   TOTAL: _____

10. If you checked off *any* problems, how
difficult have these problems made it for
you to do your work, take care of things at
home, or get along with other people?

Not difficult at all _____
Somewhat difficult _____
Very difficult _____
Extremely difficult _____

FIGURE 12.1. Patient Health Questionnaire (PHQ)-9. (PHQ9 Copyright © Pfizer Inc. All rights reserved. Reproduced with permission. PRIME-MD ® is a trademark of Pfizer Inc. [www.depression-primarycare.org].)

2. Have you experimented with drugs? If the answer to this question is positive, you should consider referral for treatment of substance abuse.

Screen your patients for bipolar disorder (either bipolar I or bipolar II). Patients with unrecognized bipolar disorder treated with antidepressants are more likely to experience significant adverse side effects, including precipitation of mania.

Bipolar disorder will be associated with previous episodes including the following symptoms:

1. Euphoric mood
2. Hyperactivity
3. Increased libido
4. Decreased need for sleep
5. Racing thoughts
6. Increased sociability
7. Grandiosity

Determine whether the patient is unsafe to self or others. Are any of the following present: suicidal thoughts, homicidal thoughts, assaultive thoughts, inability to care for self or family, or psychotic thinking? If the assessment for suicidal/homicidal thoughts is positive, determine whether the patient has:

1. Access to means for suicide (e.g., a gun in the household)
2. Presence of psychotic symptoms, hallucinations, or anxiety
3. Presence of alcohol or substance abuse
4. Family history of or recent exposure to suicide

Hospitalization should be considered for suicide risk.

Management

Treatment Options: Psychotherapy and Medications

Management decisions in patients with major depression include the use of psychotherapy and/or antidepressant medications.

Psychotherapy

In a review of treatments for depression, the Agency for Healthcare Research and Quality (AHRQ) concluded that cognitive therapy, behavioral therapy, and interpersonal therapy were approximately 50% effective [15].

Antidepressant Medications

1. The most commonly used antidepressant medications are selective serotonin reuptake inhibitors (SSRIs), tricyclic antidepressants (TCAs), heterocyclics, and other agents, such as venlafaxine (Table 12.1).
2. Most medications are associated with a 50% to 60% response rate.
3. The choice of antidepressant is multifactorial.

4. In comparing SSRIs to TCAs, dropout rates are significantly higher for patients taking TCAs due to adverse side effects. In one primary care study that compared an SSRI (Prozac) to a TCA (amitriptyline) it was found that while treatment efficacy was similar, the higher costs of the SSRI were balance by lower costs for outpatient care.

5. The SSRIs are the preferred first-line agents because of their relatively safe profile. There are no compelling data to guide the choice of a specific SSRI. Common side effects include jitteriness, restlessness, agitation, headache, gastrointestinal symptoms, and sleep disturbance.

6. Sleep problems may be alleviated by combining the SSRI with a low dose of trazodone.

7. Sexual dysfunction or weight gain associated with an SSRI may require changing to another agent, such as bupropion.

8. Bupropion has fewer adverse effects on sexual function; however, be cautious when prescribing this medication for patients with anxiety, as it may aggravate these anxiety symptoms.

9. When possible, a reasonable approach to prescribing an antidepressant is to "start low and go slow." This is particularly true for patients who describe high sensitivity to adverse side effects from any medications. Examples of starting doses include paroxetine, 5 to 10 mg; sertraline, 12.5 to 25 mg; fluvoxamine, 25 mg; and fluoxetine, 5 mg.

10. There are no clear predictors of success for any type of therapy.

11. Cautions in prescribing antidepressants include the following:
    a. For patients with underlying bipolar disorder, SSRIs may precipitate mania.
    b. Be cautious about drug–drug interactions.
    c. Advise your patients to avoid discontinuing an SSRI abruptly.
    d. Given the concerns for increased suicidal/homicidal behavior in adolescents, consultation with a psychiatrist is appropriate when considering prescribing an antidepressant for someone in this age group.

12. For patients prescribed an antidepressant, expect an initial response within 2 to 6 weeks; if no response occurs in 6 weeks, consider changing the medication.

13. Nonadherence to medication therapy is a common problem of patients with depression. Only 50% of patients in primary care respond to the first choice of an antidepressant medication. Approximately 20% stop the medication because of adverse side effects, and 30% have no response.

14. Approximately 20% of patients switch medications one or more times, and two-thirds of these will experience an improvement in symptoms.

15. Common actions to take when your patient fails to respond include the following:
    a. Switch to another agent of the same class
    b. Switch to a different class

TABLE 12.1. Antidepressant medications.

Tricyclics and tetracyclics	Initial dose (mg QHS)	Maximum dose (mg QHS)	Common side effects
Amitriptyline/Elavil	25	300	Anticholinergic: dry mouth, drowsiness, cardiac arrhythmia, and weight gain
Imipramine/Tofranil	25	300	Anticholinergic: dry mouth, drowsiness, cardiac arrhythmia, and weight gain
Nortriptyline/Pamelor	25	200	Anticholinergic: dry mouth, drowsiness, cardiac arrhythmia, and weight gain

SSRIs	Initial dose (mg QD)	Maximum dose (mg QD)	Common side effects
Citalopram/Celexa	20	60	Agitation, gastrointestinal distress
Escitalopram/Lexapro	10	20	Agitation, gastrointestinal distress
Fluoxetine/Prozac	20	60	Agitation, gastrointestinal distress
Paroxetine/Paxil	20	60	Agitation, gastrointestinal distress
Sertraline/Zoloft	50	200	Agitation, gastrointestinal distress

Dopamine/norepinephrine reuptake inhibitors	Initial dose (mg)	Maximum dose (mg)	Common side effects
Bupropion/Wellbutrin	75 BID	150 TID	Insomnia, agitation

Serotonin/norepinephrine reuptake inhibitors	Initial dose (mg)	Maximum dose (mg)	Common side effects
Venlafaxine/Effexor	37.5 BID	150/150/75	Agitation, insomnia, gastrointestinal distress
Duloxetine/Cymbalta	20 QD	60 QD	Agitation, insomnia, gastrointestinal distress

Serotonin modulators	Initial dose (mg BID)	Maximum dose (mg BID)	Common side effects
Nefazodone/Serzone	100	300	Drowsiness, dizziness, dry mouth, blurred vision
Trazadone/Desyrel	25	200	Drowsiness, dizziness, dry mouth, blurred vision

Noradrenergic and specific serotonergic modulators	Initial dose (mg QHS)	Maximum dose (mg QHS)	Common side effects
Mirtazapine/Remeron	15	45	Drowsiness, weight gain

    c. Switch to an atypical agent

    d. Combine an SSRI and a TCA

    e. Combine an SSRI and mirtazapine (be cautious about weight gain from mirtazapine)

16. For your patients who are nonresponders, consider the following possibilities:
    a. Nonadherence to the medications
    b. Alcohol or substance abuse
    c. Undiagnosed bipolar disorder; this is especially true for those who experience prominent side effects

17. Regarding duration of treatment:
    a. Antidepressant medication should be taken 6 to 9 months after the first episode of depression; they should be tapered off slowly to minimize side effects over a period of 2 to 4 weeks.
    b. Relapses are common. After a first episode, there is a 40% recurrence rate over the next 2 years; after two episodes, the risk of recurrence is 75% [16].

Depression Disease Management Program

The practice delivery changes likely to be most beneficial are the following:

1. A care manager to assist the primary care physician in patient education, treatment, and treatment monitoring
2. A mental health specialist to provide care management consultation and collaborative care with the primary care physician for more complex cases [17]

Examples of collaborative primary care projects for the treatment of depression include the following:

1. The Robert Wood Johnson Foundation has funded projects related to implementation of chronic care programs in the treatment of depression in primary care settings. The Depression in Primary Care Incentives Demonstration Program is a 5-year national initiative to translate and sustain evidence-based depression care into real-world practice. Materials about the project are available at www.wpic.pitt.edu/dppc/index.htm [18].

2. The MacArthur Foundation has established the Re-Engineering System in Primary Care Treatment of Depression (RESPECT) program [19]. The program includes a website (www.depression-primarycare.org) that has useful clinical tools for patient education and self-management support.

3. The Improving Mood Promoting Access to Collaborative Treatment (IMPACT) program is a collaborative care management program for late-life depression among patients in a primary care setting [20].

   Disease management programs for depression typically use a combination of interventions consisting of patient education programs, provider feedback, provider education programs, multidisciplinary teams of providers, provider reminders, and financial incentives for providers. Practice recommendations from The National Program Office of the Robert Wood Johnson Foundation's Depression in Primary Care Project include the following:

1. Screen your patients for evidence of depression. Systematic screening is recommended to improve detection, treatment, and outcomes of depression in disease management programs. Studies that have assessed the effects of structured screening on the rates of detection of depression have reported 10% to 47% increases in the diagnosis of depression. The two most useful screening questions you can use are:
   a. Are you sad?
   b. Is anything pleasurable?

   Positive answers to one or both should lead to a further inquiry. Positive answers (to the degree of "nearly every day") to both questions are sensitive and specific indicators for major depression [21].

2. Diagnose depression in those who fail the screening test. When screening tests are positive, administer a more specific test to clarify the diagnosis. This includes the use of the PHQ-9 (Figure 12.1), the Beck Depression Inventory, the General Health Questionnaire, or the Zung Self-Assessment Depression Scale.

3. Treat those with an established diagnosis of depression. Use the score on the PHQ-9 to establish who has the diagnosis and who should be treated. Interpretation of the PHQ-9 scores is as follows:
   a. 0–4, no symptoms
   b. 5–9, minor symptoms
   c. 10–14, moderate symptoms
   d. 15–19, moderate to severe symptoms
   e. 20, severe symptoms

   A PHQ-9 score >10 has 90% sensitivity and specificity.

4. Assess the effectiveness of the intervention. You can use the results of the PHQ-9 at the beginning of treatment and within 1, 3, 6, and 12 months. A rough guide for an effective treatment is to expect the score to decrease by 25% to 50% within 6 months of initiating treatment.

5. Co-manage your patients when possible. Use of a care manager and behavioral health specialist can serve as an important adjunct to the structure of the intervention. For example, phone contact by a care manager can be used to assess effectiveness of an intervention and detect problems with medication adherence or adverse side effects.

Strategies to enhance patient education should be part of any disease management program. It is important to support ongoing patient education and self-care responsibilities, which may range from reliably taking medications to participating in cognitive behavioral therapy. Education topics should include the following:

1. The cause, symptoms, and natural history of major depression
2. Treatment options
3. Information on what to expect during the course of treatment
4. How to monitor symptoms and side effects
5. Follow-up protocols
6. Early warning signs of relapse
7. Length of treatment

For patients taking antidepressants, important messages you should give include the following:

1. Side effects from medication often precede benefit and recede over time.
2. Successful treatment often involves dose adjustments and/or a trial of a different medication at some point.
3. It usually takes from 2 to 6 weeks before improvement is seen.
4. Take the medication even after feeling better.
5. Do not stop taking the medication without discussing it with your physician first.

An excellent Web site that contains patient education materials and a self-care action plan is www.depression-primarycare.org/clinicians/toolkits/materials/patient_edu/self_mgmt.

Consider psychiatric consultation for patients:

1. Who fail a reasonable trial of antidepressants
2. Who have severe signs of depression with thought disorder or suicidality
3. Who have a substance abuse problem

Monitoring

Consider applying the monitoring guidelines from the Institute for Clinical Systems Improvement [16]:

1. Assess your patient's progress at least every 1 to 2 weeks for 6 to 8 weeks.
2. To assess how well a system is functioning in the diagnosis, treatment plan, and follow-up, determine from a chart audit:
   a. How well is the diagnosis documented, based on the completion of a PHQ-9 form?

b. How well are ongoing patient contacts documented, based on the frequency of documented contacts?
c. How well are outcomes measured and documented, based on serial PHQ-9 reports?
d. Is the patient responding, based on a decrease in score of 25% to 50% over time? When assessing response to therapy, it is expected that response should be evaluated between 4 to 6 weeks.

When patients do not respond, you should do the following [22]:

1. Re-evaluate the diagnosis, and evaluate for comorbid diagnoses.
2. Determine if the dosage is sufficient.
3. Determine if the duration of treatment is adequate.

HEDIS (Health Plan Employer Data and Information Set) measures for depression include the percentage of primary care patients with three depression visits in the 90 days after initiating antidepressant therapy and the percentage of patients remaining on antidepressants for >6 months [23].

Alternative Therapy

The most commonly used herbal remedies for the treatment of depression are St. John's wort and S-adenosyl methionine (SAM-e). Important observations on the use of St. John's wort include the following:

1. It is more effective than placebo for mild to moderate depression.
2. It should not be used for severe depression.
3. Problems exist with variability of preparations.
4. Long-term data on safety are not available.
5. In combinations with SSRIs, it may lead to the development of serotonin syndrome: agitation, hyperthermia, diaphoresis, tachycardia, and rigidity.
6. Many drugs interact with St. John's wort, including antidepressants, oral contraceptives, and drugs for human immunodeficiency virus.
7. The usual daily dose is 300 mg three times a day.
8. The reported incidence of adverse side effects is less than that of other agents; it has fewer sexual side effects than SSRIs.

Important observations on the use of SAM-e include the following:

1. Randomized controlled trials show SAM-e to be similar in effectiveness to TCAs.
2. Effective oral doses are 400 to 1,000 mg a day.
3. Side effects include decreased appetite, constipation, nausea, dry mouth, diaphoresis, dizziness, and nervousness.

4. Do not combine SAM-e with SSRIs; this may produce the serotonin syndrome.
5. SAM-e is expensive. It can cost $150 per month to take 800 BID; this is typically more than an SSRI costs [23].

Summary

A comprehensive disease management program for depression following the methods of the Chronic Care Model is likely to produce significant improvements in symptoms of depression, physical functioning, health status, satisfaction with treatment, adherence to treatment regimens, and the rate of detection of depression and adequacy of treatment with antidepressants.

References

1. Sullivan M, Simor G, Spertus J, Russo J. Depression related costs in heart failure care. Arch Intern Med 2002;162:1860–1866.
2. Ciechanowski P, Katon W, Russo J. Depression and diabetes: impact of depressive symptoms on adherence, function, and costs. Arch Intern Med 2000;160: 3278–3285.
3. Wells KB, et al. Impact of disseminating quality improvement programs for depression in managed primary care: a randomized controlled trial. JAMA 2000;283:212–220.
4. Katon W, et al. A randomized trial of relapse prevention of depression in primary care. Arch Gen Psychiatry 2001;58:241–247.
5. Simon GE, VonKorff M, Rutter C, Wagner E. Randomised trial of monitoring, feedback, and management of care by telephone to improve treatment of depression in primary care. BMJ 2000;320:550–554.
6. Tutty S, Simon G, Ludman E. Telephone counseling as an adjunct to antidepressant treatment in the primary care system. A pilot study. Eff Clin Pract 2000;3:170–178.
7. Simon GE, et al. Telephone psychotherapy and telephone care management for primary care patients starting antidepressant treatment. A randomized controlled trial. JAMA 2004;292:935–942.
8. Vergouwen AC, Bakker A, Katon WJ, Verheij TJ, Koerselman F. Improving adherence to antidepressants: a systematic review of interventions. J Clin Psychiatry 2003;64:1415–1420.
9. Capoccia KL, et al. Randomized trial of pharmacist interventions to improve depression care and outcomes in primary care. Am J Health Syst Pharm 2004; 61:364–372.
10. Rost K, Pyne JM, Dickinson LM, LoSasso AT. Cost-effectiveness of enhancing primary care depression management on an ongoing basis. Ann Fam Med 2005;3:7–14.
11. http://www.depression-primarycare.org/clinicians/toolkits/materials/patient_ed.

12. Beck AT, Steer RA, Garbin MG. Psychometric properties of the Beck Depression Inventory: twenty-five years of evaluation. Clin Psychol Rev 1988; 8:77–100.
13. Goldberg DP, Blackwell B. Psychiatric illness in general practice. BMJ 1970; 1:439–443.
14. Zung WW, King RE. Identification and treatment of masked depression in a general medical practice. J Clin Psychiatry 1983;44:365–368.
15. Treatment of depression—newer pharmacotherapies. Summary Evidence Report/Technology Assessment, Number 7, March 1999. Agency for Health Care Policy and Research, Rockville, MD. www.ahrq.gov/Clinic/epcsums/deprsumm.htm.
16. Institute for Clinical Systems Improvement (ICSI). Major Depression in Adults for Mental Health Care. Bloomington, MN: Institute for Clinical Systems Improvement (ICSI), 2004.
17. Oxman T, et al. The depression care manager and mental health specialist as collaborators within primary care. Am J Geriatr Psych 2003;11:507–516.
18. www.wpic.pitt.edu/dppc/index.htm.
19. Oxman T, Dietrich A, Schulberg H. The depression care manager and mental health specialist as collaborators within primary care. Am J Geriatr Psych 2003;11:507–516.
20. Unutzer. J, et al. Improving mood-promoting access to collaborative treatment investigators. Collaborative care management of late-life depression in the primary care setting: a randomized controlled trial. JAMA 2002; 288:2836–2845.
21. Kroenke K, Spitzer RL, Williams JB. The Patient Health Questionnaire-2: validity of a two-item depression screener. Med Care 2003;41:1284–1292.
22. Kilbourne AM, Schulbert HC, Post EP, Rollman BL, Belnap BH, Pincus HA. Translating evidence-based depression management services to community-based primary care practices. Milbank Q 2004;82:631–659.
23. Jellin J. Natural Medicines Comprehensive Database. www.naturaldatabase.com.

13
Chronic Pain

Jim Nuovo

Background: Burden as a Chronic Disease

1. Non-cancer–related pain that lasts longer than 3 months is considered chronic pain.
2. According to the National Institutes of Health, chronic pain is the third largest health problem in the world.
3. Approximately 25 million Americans are affected by chronic pain.
4. Chronic pain is one of the most common problems seen in primary care clinics. Pain-related problems account for up to 80% of office visits.
5. Under-recognition and undertreatment of pain can result in significant morbidity; this includes loss of productivity and diminished quality of life.

A high percentage of patients with chronic pain will have comorbid psychiatric diagnoses (e.g., depression, anxiety, and substance abuse disorders). Failure to address the psychosocial issues that accompany chronic pain usually makes treatment programs less effective [1].

Costs

The annual costs associated with chronic pain in the United States exceed $90 billion; these costs are mostly due to medical expenses and loss in job productivity. Annual medical costs are substantially higher for patients with chronic pain and comorbid psychiatric disease [2].

Impact of Disease Management Programs

Chelminski and associates [3] studied the impact of a primary care, multidisciplinary disease management program for opioid-treated patients with chronic non-cancer pain. The study was done as a 3-month uncontrolled clinical trial. They found that their intervention improved their patients' pain, depression, and disability scores.

McCarberg and Wolf [4] studied the impact of cognitive behavioral therapy on patients with chronic pain. Their 8-week randomized trial showed improvement in their patients' perceptions of the severity of pain as well as in their symptoms of depression.

Most studies assessing the impact of a disease management program for chronic pain are focused on the treatment of osteoarthritis. The results of these studies are presented in Chapter 10.

Initial Evaluation

For all patients with chronic pain, the initial evaluation should include the following:

1. A thorough analgesic history, including current and previously used prescription medications, over-the-counter medications, and complementary and alternative remedies.
2. The patient's satisfaction with current pain treatment or health.
3. Whether the pain appears to be neuropathic or non-neuropathic.
   a. Neuropathic pain syndromes are among the most common you are likely to see in your office. Two examples of neuropathic pain syndromes are diabetic neuropathy and postherpetic neuralgia. There are an estimated 3 million people with painful diabetic neuropathy and 1 million people with postherpetic neuralgia. Other examples of chronic neuropathic pain syndromes include degenerative disc disease with peripheral neuropathy, trigeminal neuralgia, phantom limb pain, and complex regional pain syndrome. Common descriptors for neuropathic pain include the following:
      i. Burning
      ii. Sharp
      iii. Aching
      iv. Tingling
      v. Numb
      vi. Skin hypersensitivity
   b. Non-neuropathic pain syndromes are also commonly encountered in the office setting. These include degenerative joint disease, chronic neck and low back pain, fibromyalgia, and tension headaches. Common descriptors for non-neuropathic pain include the following:
      i. Dull or sharp
      ii. Tight
      iii. Knot-like
      iv. Spasms

4. Psychosocial problems that can magnify the pain or make effective treatment more difficult (at minimum, this includes depression, anxiety disorders, sleep disorders, and substance abuse).

Management

Always consider a multidimensional approach for treatment of patients with chronic pain, including:

1. Medications
2. Behavioral interventions such as cognitive behavioral therapy
3. Nondrug modalities such as physical therapy
4. Complementary and alternative therapies
5. Patient education that is condition specific
6. Self-management support (see Chapter 2)

Management that excludes the use of multiple treatment modalities is less likely to be effective in the long run.

Medications

Tricyclic Antidepressants and Antiepileptic Drugs

The two most important medications to consider for patients with neuropathic pain include tricyclic antidepressants (TCAs) and antiepileptic drugs (AEDs). Examples of commonly used TCAs and AEDs are listed in Table 13.1 [5]. Important considerations regarding TCAs include the following:

TABLE 13.1. Commonly prescribed tricyclic antidepressants (TCAs) and antiepileptic drugs (AEDs) for patients with neuropathic pain syndromes.

Category	General mechanism of action	Generic name/brand name
TCAs	Inhibition of norepinephrine reuptake	Desipramine/Norpramin
	Inhibition of norepinephrine and serotonin reuptake	Nortriptyline/Pamelor
		Imipramine/Tofranil
AEDs	Blockade of sodium channel	Amitriptyline/Elavil
		Carbamazepine/Tegretol
		Gabapentin/Neurontin
		Lamotrigine/Lamictal
	Blockade of calcium channel	Gabapentin/Neurontin

1. TCAs are effective in the treatment of neuropathic pain.
2. There is no clear advantage between TCAs and AEDs in the treatment of chronic neuropathic pain. Given the lower cost of TCAs than AEDs, you should consider TCAs as first-line therapy, especially if there is an accompanying sleep disorder.
3. The effectiveness of TCAs is independent of their effects on depression.
4. The full effect may take weeks to occur. It is important to advise your patients of this before they start the medication. Unfortunately, many patients stop taking their TCA well before they have had an adequate trial.
5. The TCAs may also be effective in the treatment of other sources of chronic pain, such as fibromyalgia, low back pain, and headache syndromes.
6. You should prescribe TCAs with caution for the following patients:
   a. The frail elderly. The elderly are more susceptible to the adverse effects of TCAs, such as hypotension.
   b. Patients with suicidal ideation. An intentional overdose with TCAs is often fatal because of seizures and/or dysrhythmias.
7. Other antidepressants have variable efficacy in the treatment of neuropathic pain. Serotonin-specific reuptake inhibitors (SSRIs) used alone are often ineffective in the treatment of chronic pain.

Important considerations regarding AEDs are as follows:

1. The AEDs are effective in the treatment of neuropathic pain.
2. They are classified as first or second generation.
3. There is no clear therapeutic difference between first- and second-generation AEDs in the treatment of neuropathic pain; however, second-generation drugs are generally better tolerated because they cause less sedation.
4. The second-generation AED gabapentin/Neurontin is the most frequently used drug in this class.
5. You should start gabapentin/Neurontin at a low dose and titrate slowly to its maximum dose (if needed). Be cautious about prescribing gabapentin/Neurontin for the elderly and for those with impaired renal function; they are more likely to experience severe sedation.
6. For patients who fail to respond to either a TCA or an AED, you may combine both drugs; however, the risk for adverse side effects, particularly sedation, increases.

Important considerations regarding the use of TCAs and AEDs for non-neuropathic pain include the following:

1. The TCAs are effective for a number of non-neuropathic pain syndromes. These include fibromyalgia, low back pain, and headache syndromes (including migraines) [6,7].

2. The SSRIs and AEDs are generally not effective for non-neuropathic pain.

3. When you are prescribing TCAs or AEDs for neuropathic pain, or TCAs for non-neuropathic pain, the general principle is to start low and go slow. It usually does not require a high dose to achieve therapeutic effect. However, failing to respond to a low dose should prompt careful titration before labeling the medication as ineffective.

Examples of common regimens include the following:

1. Tricyclic antidepressants
   a. Amitriptyline: 10 to 25 mg QHS
   b. Imipramine: 10 to 25 mg QHS
2. Antiepileptic drugs
   a. First-generation: Carbamazepine/Tegretol: 200 mg/day; increase by 200 mg/week; maximum 400 mg TID
   b. Second-generation: Gabapentin/Neurontin: 100 to 300 mg QHS; increase by 100 mg every 3 days; maximum 1,200 mg TID. Dose should be reduced for patients with impaired renal function.

For TCAs and AEDs, the duration of the trial is important to consider before deciding whether the drug is effective. For both, you should consider a trial of at least 6 weeks as being adequate.

Opioids

For patients with chronic nonmalignant pain, your decision to use opioids must be weighed carefully. The World Health Organization (WHO) has published guidelines for the treatment of cancer pain. You can apply the management principles described by the WHO to your patients with chronic nonmalignant pain:

1. Opioids should not be used alone in the treatment of chronic pain.
2. Treatment goals should be established and discussed with the patient.
3. All efforts should be taken to minimize the misuse of opioids, sedative/hypnotics, or other medications for pain.
4. All patients should be encouraged to maximize and maintain optimal physical activity and return to being productive.
5. Help patients increase their self-management skills in coping with pain; this can often result in reducing the severity of pain [8].

In general, when prescribing opioid medications, you should first determine whether the pain can be adequately managed with a short-acting opioid preparation for breakthrough pain, especially if the patient has not yet started taking a TCA and/or an AED. The decision to use longer acting opioids should be based on failing an adequate trial of the short-acting opioids used at appropriate doses.

Longer acting opioids (long-acting morphine, fentanyl patches, methadone, and sustained-released oxycodone) are appropriate under these conditions. Their dosages should be titrated at interval visits. Short-acting, potent opioids (usually oxycodone preparations) may additionally be prescribed for breakthrough pain [9].

The most common pitfalls in prescribing opioid medications include the following:

1. Failure to evaluate the patient/perform an examination
2. Failure to make a diagnosis
3. Failure to document findings in the medical records
4. Failure to establish goals for treatment
5. Failure to monitor refill requests
6. Failure to have a narcotic contract in the record
7. Deviation from a contract
8. Failure to perform a periodic review of diagnosis and treatment
9. Failure to recognize the development of common comorbid psychiatric conditions [10]

Other Drugs

Other drugs commonly prescribed for patients with chronic pain include analgesics such as tramodol and propoxyphene, muscle relaxants, and topical agents such as capsaicin and a lidocaine patch. Although it is reasonable for selected patients to try these medications, overall they are not likely to provide the same results as TCAs and AEDs, particularly to patients with neuropathic pain. You should be especially cautious with patients specifically requesting carisoprodol/Soma as a muscle relaxant. This drug has a particularly high rate of abuse.

Comorbid Conditions

The percentage of your patients with chronic pain who also have depression or anxiety as a comorbid condition is quite high. The percentage is also high for substance abuse. You should be constantly alert for signs of depression, anxiety, and substance abuse disorders. Failing to address these problems will make your treatment program less effective.

Self-Management Support

Holman and Lorig [11] have written extensively on self-management support for patients with chronic disease. The materials in Chapter 2 on self-management also apply to the management of chronic pain. The core self-management skills are:

1. Problem solving
2. Decision making

3. Resource utilization
4. Forming a patient–health provider partnership
5. Taking action
6. Setting goals

Goals that are reasonable to help support your patients with chronic pain are:

1. Prevent or minimize symptoms
2. Reduce pain severity or frequency
3. Improve physical functioning
4. Reduce psychological stress
5. Improve overall quality of life
6. Minimize adverse side effects of treatment [12]

It is not advisable to promise your patient that you will provide complete resolution of their pain. More realistic goals are to reduce the pain severity by 50% and to improve quality of life. An approach to help patients identify goals and support self-management techniques for their chronic pain is available online at http://longbeach.med.va.gov/Our_Services/Patient_Care/cpmpbook/cpmp-4.html. A form to guide the development and implementation of patient-generated goals is provided on this Web site.

There are many other treatment choices for your patients with chronic pain. You should always consider the use of other modalities when appropriate, such as the following:

1. Physical therapy
2. Progressive exercise program
3. Cognitive behavior therapy

Although there have not been a large number of trials on exercise, many of your patients will likely benefit from a progressive program, assuming there are no contraindications to activity. You can guide your patients in a manner similar to that described in Chapters 2, 7, and 9.

The goal of cognitive behavior therapy is to change behaviors, thoughts, and feelings about pain so that there is less pain-related distress. Typically, this includes:

1. Promotion of self-management
2. Relaxation skills
3. Cognitive restructuring
4. Problem-solving skill training

Patient Education

Provide appropriate educational resources for all of your patients with chronic pain. No matter what treatment modalities are used, encourage your patients to learn as much as possible about the management of chronic pain, the importance of self-management, and methods to reduce stress. It is important to adjust your approach to each patient based on what type of information is most appropriate for him or her. Some patients will prefer a class, others a support group, printed materials, or a Web site. For those who are interested in accessing Web-based materials, refer them to the following sites:

1. www.chronicpain.org. The National Chronic Pain Outreach Association, Inc., is a non-profit organization established in 1980. The site includes links to articles and support groups.
2. www.painconnection.org. The National Pain Foundation's Web site focuses on online education.
3. www.nids.nih.gov/disorders/chronic_pain/chronic_pain.htm. The National Institutes of Health maintains this patient information Web site for a variety of health issues related to chronic pain. There are also links to other resources for specific pain syndromes.
4. www.familydoctor.org. The American Academy of Family Physicians' Web site includes patient education materials on a wide variety of topics, including chronic pain.

Before referring patients to any online resource, it is advisable to access the site to see if its approach is consistent with yours.

Referral to a Pain Specialist

Despite initiating a pain management program, there are some patients who require a referral to a specialty clinic. The decision for referral must be based on the unique aspects of each case.

Monitoring

Documenting Pain Severity

Having your patients document the severity of their pain using a standardized pain scale each time they are seen is a reasonable approach in monitoring response to therapy. Although there are many different pain assessment instruments, the visual analogue scale is perhaps the easiest to use (Table 13.2) [13]. The scale is 10 cm long. Patients are asked to point

TABLE 13.2. Visual analogue pain scale.

Ask your patient: "What does your pain feel like?"				
0/none	2/mild	4/moderate	7/very bad	10/unbearable

Source: Data from Von Korff et al. [13].

TABLE 13.3. Subjective units of distress (SUDS) scale.

Ask your patient: "How much does your pain interfere with your abilities to do the things you wish to do each day?"

0/none	2/mild	5/moderate	8/severe	10/unable to carry out usual activities

Source: Data from Wolpe [14].

to the spot that describes the severity of their pain. This is the number that is recorded in the medical record. Some patients have a tendency to report scores above 10. It is important to reorient these patients to the meaning of the scale.

There are also scales used to assess the impact of pain on normal activities. The subjective units of distress scale (SUDS) is a reliable measure of how pain interferes with daily activities (Table 13.3). Again, a 10-point scale is used in which a score of 0 means "no interference" and 10 means that your patient is "unable to carry out usual activities." A self-report of greater than 4 for any particular task usually means that the patient has substantial difficulty with that task and would benefit from an intervention [14].

Other scales to consider include the following:

1. Wong-Baker Faces Pain Rating Scale. This is a series of faces with different expressions of pain. Patients are instructed to point to a face to describe the pain intensity [15].
2. The Pain Disability Index. This is a 26-item self-report on the impact of pain on the ability to perform tasks [16].

Comorbid Conditions

Given the frequency of comorbid conditions, it is important to perform an ongoing assessment for comorbid psychiatric conditions, namely, depression, anxiety, and addictive drug-seeking behavior. Failing to address psychosocial issues often results in derailing the treatment program. It also often results in patients with permanent disabilities. For example, patients with chronic pain who are unemployed for 6 months have a 50% chance of returning to their job; after 1 year, there is only a 10% chance of returning.

When screening for depression, the two most useful questions you can ask are:

1. Are you sad?
2. Is anything pleasurable?

Positive answers to one or both questions should lead to a further inquiry. Positive answers (to the degree of "nearly every day") to both questions are sensitive and specific indicators for major depression [17]. The Patient

Health Questionnaire-9 (see Chapter 12) can be used for patients who "fail" the screening test.

Developing a Pain Contract

Always consider a pain contract as part of an effective pain management program. An example of a pain contract is shown in Table 13.4. Pain contracts should include a termination cause for ongoing care as a consequence for any of the following problems:

1. Forged or altered prescriptions
2. Use of any illicit substances
3. Procuring narcotics from more than one doctor without your knowledge
4. Unwillingness to provide urine samples when requested

TABLE 13.4. Pain medication contract.

Patient's Name:
Medical Record #:
Patient's Phone #:
Primary Care Provider:
My physician and I have agreed that in order to adequately control my pain, I will be taking the following medication(s):
Medication
Strength
Directions
Number of pills given with each prescription
Frequency of refills
Day of month for refills
To ensure uninterrupted service for this/these medications, I acknowledge and agree to the following conditions:
I have told my physician that I want the medication(s) to be filled at _____
Pharmacy, located at _____. Their phone # is:
Once established I will use only this pharmacy; I will not have the prescription transferred to another pharmacy.
I will not have other physicians prescribe the same or similar medications while this agreement is in effect.
I will attend all appointments scheduled for me with my physician.
I will not request the above medication(s) earlier than the agreed date. I will use the medication(s) as prescribed.
I will notify my pharmacy at least 3 working days in advance of the due date.
I am responsible for my medications. Medications that are lost for any reason will not be replaced.
I understand that if I do not meet any of the conditions stated above, my physician may act to discontinue my care at this clinic.
I understand that there are risks associated with the use of narcotic medications, including physical dependence, addiction, and impaired ability to think.

Patient's Name:	Signature:	Date:
Physician's Name:	Signature:	Date:

Compliance with State and Federal Regulatory Boards

In managing our patients with chronic pain, we all need to be aware of federal and state medical board guidelines. The Federation of State Medical Boards (FSMB) has published guidelines for the treatment of chronic pain [9]. The FSMB's policy is based on the principle that "inappropriate treatment of pain, including under-treatment, is a departure from acceptable medical practice." For each patient with chronic pain it is important to document the rationale behind treatment and the results from each examination, and to have a pain contract included in the medical record with a flow sheet to monitor drug use.

Alternative Therapies

There are a large number of complementary and alternative therapies (CAM) for chronic pain. A partial listing of common modalities includes:

1. Acupuncture
2. Biofeedback
3. Chiropractic treatment
4. Meditation
5. Homeopathy
6. Hypnosis
7. Manipulation and massage
8. Visual imagery [18]

Resources for patients seeking CAM can be found on the following Web sites:

1. www.alternative-therapies.com
2. http://medicalacupuncture.org
3. www.aapainmanage.org
4. http://nccam.nih.gov [19]

Summary

Managing chronic pain effectively is an extremely challenging task. Its impact on the quality of life of all patients who are affected by this condition, as well as their families, is substantial. Many patients with chronic pain have comorbid conditions, such as depression, anxiety, sleep disorders, and substance abuse. Failure to recognize and treat these conditions derails effective treatment programs. The management of chronic pain requires a multidimensional approach; no one modality is likely to be effective as the sole treatment. The use of potent narcotics must be weighed carefully, ensuring effective management of pain while avoiding the potential for abuse. Ongoing monitoring of the treatment plan along with the use of a narcotics contract is a means to ensure appropriate care. All patients should be encouraged to learn as much as they can about their condition and the interventions that can improve the quality of their lives. Self-management support should be included in the care of all patients with this condition.

References

1. Workman EA, Hubbard JR, Felker BL. Comorbid psychiatric disorders and predictors of pain management program success in patients with chronic pain. Primary Care Companion J Clin Psychiatry 2002;4:137–140.
2. Greenberg PE, Leong SA, Birnbaum HG, Robinson RL. The economic burden of depression with painful symptoms. J Clin Psychiatry 2003;64: 17–23.
3. Chelminski PR, et al. A primary care, multi-disciplinary disease management program for opioid-treated patients with chronic non-cancer pain and a high burden of psychiatric comorbidity. Available online at www.biomedcentral.com/1472-6963/5/3.
4. McCarberg B, Wolf J. Chronic pain management in a health maintenance organization. Clin J Pain 1999;15:50–57.
5. Ross EL. The evolving role of antiepileptic drugs in treating neuropathic pain. Neurology 2002;55:S42.
6. White KP, Harth M. An analytic review of 24 controlled clinical trials for fibromyalgia syndrome (FMS). Pain 1996;64:211–119.
7. Salerno SM, Browning R, Jackson JL. The effect of antidepressant treatment on chronic back pain: a meta-analysis. Arch Intern Med 2002;162:19–24.
8. Sanders SH, Harden N, Benson SE, Vicente PJ. Clinical practice guidelines for chronic non-malignant pain syndrome in patients II: an evidence-based approach. J Back Musculoskel Rehabil 1999;13:47–58.
9. Position of the Federation of State Medical Boards in Support of adoption of pain management geudelines www.FSMB.org/PDF/1997_grpol_adoption_pain_management.pdf
10. Gallagher R. Opioids in chronic pain management: navigating the clinical and regulatory challenges. J Fam Pract 2004;53:S23.
11. Holman H, Lorig K. Patient self-management: a key to effectiveness and efficiency in care of chronic disease. Public Health Rep 2004;119:239–243.
12. McCarberg B. Contemporary management of chronic pain disorders. J Jam Pract 2004;53:S11–22.
13. Von Korff M, et al. Grading the severity of chronic pain. Pain 1992;50: 133–139.
14. Wolpe J. The Prediction of Behavior Therapy. New York: Pergamon Press, 1973.
15. Wong DL, Hockenberry-Eaton M, Wilson D, et al. Wong's Essentials of Pediatric Nursing, 6th ed. St Louis: Mosby, 2001:1301.
16. Osman A, et al. The pain distress inventory: development and initial psychometric properties. J Clin Psychol 2003;59:767–785.

17. Kroenke K, Spitzer RL, Williams JB. The patient health questionnaire-2: validity of a two-item depression screener. Med Care 003;41:1284–1292.
18. Adams NJ, Plane MB, Fleming MF, Mundt MP, Saunders LA, Stauffacher EA. Opioids and the treatment of chronic pain in a primary care sample. J Pain Symptom Manage 2001;22:791–796.
19. Astin JA, et al. A review of the incorporations of complementary and alternative medicine by mainstream physicians. Arch Intern Med 1998;158: 2303–2310.

Index